GROWTH AND DEVELOPMENT HANDBOOK

Newborn through Adolescent

Barbara L. Mandleco, RN, PhD
Associate Professor
Associate Dean of Research and Scholarship
Brigham Young University
Provo, Utah

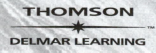

THOMSON
DELMAR LEARNING

Australia   Canada   Mexico   Singapore   Spain   United Kingdom   United States

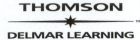

THOMSON

DELMAR LEARNING

Growth and Development Handbook:
Newborn through Adolescence

by Barbara Mandleco

Vice President,
Health Care Business Unit:
William Brottmiller

Editorial Director:
Cathy L. Esperti

Acquisitions Editor:
Matthew Kane

Senior Developmental Editor:
Elisabeth F. Williams

Marketing Director:
Jennifer McAvey

Marketing Coordinator:
Karen Summerlin

Editorial Assistant:
Erin Silk

Production Editor:
James Zayicek

Art and Design Coordinator:
Jay Purcell

For permission to use material from the text or product, contact us by
Tel.   (800) 730-2214
Fax   (800) 730-2215
www.thomsonrights.com

Library of Congress Cataloging-in-Publication Data:

Mandleco, Barbara Hartwig.
   Growth and development handbook : newborn through adolescence / Barbara L. Mandleco.
      p. cm.
   Includes bibliographical references and index.
   ISBN 1-4018-1013-6
      1. Infants—Growth—Handbooks, manuals, etc.
   2. Children—Growth—Handbooks, manuals, etc. 3. Teenagers—Growth—Handbooks, manuals, etc. 4. Child development—Handbooks, manuals, etc. I. Title.

RJ131.M31326 2004
612.6'5—dc21

                                    2003046274

NOTICE TO THE READER

Publisher does not warrant or guarantee any of the products described herein or perform any independent analysis in connection with any of the product information contained herein. Publisher does not assume, and expressly disclaims, any obligation to obtain and include information other than that provided to it by the manufacturer.

The reader is expressly warned to consider and adopt all safety precautions that might be indicated by the activities herein and to avoid all potential hazards. By following the instructions contained herein, the reader willingly assumes all risks in connection with such instructions.

The publisher makes no representation or warranties of any kind, including but not limited to, the warranties of fitness for particular purpose or merchantability, nor are any such representations implied with respect to the material set forth herein, and the publisher takes no responsibility with respect to such material. The publisher shall not be liable for any special, consequential, or exemplary damages resulting, in whole or part, from the readers' use of, or reliance upon, this material.

CONTENTS

APPENDICES:

CONTRIBUTORS

Natalie Annen-Ricks, BSN
Charge Nurse
Neonatal Critical Care Unit
Primary Children's Medical Center
Salt Lake City, Utah
Chapter 3

Mary Heiens Brown, PhD, RN, CPNP
Assistant Professor of Clinical Nursing
University of Texas at Houston
Health Science Center School of Nursing
Houston, Texas
Chapter 1

J. Kelly McCoy, PhD
Assistant Professor
School of Family Life
Brigham Young University
Provo, Utah
Chapter 8

Debra Ann Mills, RN, MS
Assistant Teaching Professor
College of Nursing
Brigham Young University
Provo, Utah
Chapter 5

**Lisa M. Rebeschi, RN, MSN,
Doctoral Student**
Assistant Professor
Southern Connecticut State University
New Haven, Connecticut
Chapter 1

Carolyn C. Reynolds, APRN, MS
Pediatric Clinical Nurse Specialist
Primary Children's Medical Center
Salt Lake City, Utah
Chapter 6

Janice L. Vincent, DSN, RN
Assistant Professor
University of Alabama School of Nursing
Birmingham, Alabama
Chapter 4

Susan O'Connor Von, DNS, RNC
Assistant Professor
Department of Nursing
The College of St. Catherine
St. Paul, Minnesota
Chapter 7

Barbara C. Woodring, RN, EdD
Professor and Associate Dean
University of Alabama School of Nursing
Birmingham, Alabama
Chapter 5

Growth and Development Handbook: Newborn through Adolescent is a book for undergraduate nursing students and practicing nurses that approaches human development from a holistic and family-centered perspective. It provides a learner-oriented approach to understanding and retaining growth and developmental information required to become a safe and caring practitioner while interacting with families and pediatric clients from the newborn period through adolescence.

CONCEPTUAL APPROACH

The idea for this handbook arose from a need to present a succinct summary of human development for the student and practitioner that is easy to use and/or refer to on clinical units. The book can also be used as a supplemental item complementing the students' textbook or as a clinical reference for growth and development content. Practicing nurses will find the text useful as a clinical reference for key information about the development and assessment of their pediatric clients, since normal developmental milestones, health, health promotion, and anticipatory guidance are stressed throughout.

ORGANIZATION OF THE TEXT

Growth and Development Handbook: Newborn through Adolescent offers practical information necessary when providing effective care for the pediatric client; important tips and alerts from seasoned nurses; and

information useful in educating families about home care. The first chapter contains useful information and guides for assessing children. The second chapter reviews theories of human development. Chapters 3 through 8 discuss the major developmental milestones and characteristics of the newborn, infant, toddler, preschooler, school-aged child, and adolescent. Each chapter has summary tables of important developmental indicators, as well as a discussion of the physiological, psychosexual, cognitive, psychosocial, moral, and spiritual development occurring during that particular stage. Health promotion strategies related to nutrition, sleep, rest, activity, dental health, safety, and injury prevention are found throughout these six chapters. In addition, discussions of health screenings and topics related to anticipatory guidance for each age group are also presented.

Appendices

Nine appendices augment *Growth and Development Handbook: Newborn through Adolescent*. They include normal vital signs, growth charts, laboratory values, the Denver II, a family assessment model, the recommended childhood immunization schedule, recommended dietary allowances, sexual maturity ratings, and useful resources.

SPECIAL FEATURES

- *Family Teaching* highlights the significance of keeping family members involved in promoting growth and development of their children.

- *Nursing Tips* help readers apply basic growth and development knowledge to practice by offering useful hints and shortcuts.

- *Nursing Alerts* highlight important information nurses need to be aware of.

- *Eye On* presents cultural, international, and spiritual perspectives related to growth and development.

- *Reflective Thinking* boxes encourage users to examine their own personal views on particular developmental issues and understand the varying viewpoints they may encounter in practice. They also encourage reflection on issues from a personal context, raise awareness of the diversity of opinions, and foster empowerment.

- *Critical Thinking* boxes stimulate thought processes as readers digest chapter content.

CHAPTER 1

Assessment

COMMUNICATING WITH CHILDREN AND FAMILIES

Communication skills are essential in pediatric assessments and interactions with both children and their caregiver(s).

Basic principles to keep in mind are the following:

- Privacy is essential.
- Properly identify yourself, your role, and your purpose.
- Ensure confidentiality, including maintaining safeguards for privacy of computerized patient data.
- Be aware of environmental characteristics such as temperature, noise and light available.
- Begin communication with more general content before getting specific.
- Communicate directly with the child.
- Adolescents may need to communicate without family members present.
- Use open-ended questions appropriately.
- Encourage continued communication with nonverbal gestures such as nodding and eye contact.
- Recognize and be respectful of cultural influences on communication.
- Use interpreters as necessary.
- Silence is an appropriate communication technique.
- Active listening to both nonverbal and verbal cues is an important component.
- Avoid changing focus, falsely reassuring, interrupting, forming prejudged conclusions, and overloading with information.

- Maintain eye-level position with child during communication.
- Transition objects (stuffed animals or toys) may be useful when communicating with children.
- Restate questions as necessary to ensure understanding.
- Writing, drawing, and playing are alternative communication approaches for older children.
- Honesty is important in building a therapeutic nurse/client relationship.

Culturally Sensitive Approaches

Nurses are continually challenged to meet the needs of a multicultural society, and should not only be sensitive to cultural and religious differences, but also should learn about traditions, behaviors, and beliefs of the cultures of families in their domain of influence in order to provide individualized care.

Culture provides children and families with a sort of "blueprint" for living, thinking, behaving, and feeling. It guides the way in which individuals solve their problems and derive meaning from their lives, and is passed from one generation to the other by the family unit.

To provide culturally sensitive care, nurses must evaluate their own feelings, prejudices, and beliefs, and must make a conscious effort to recognize, appreciate, and respect differing views and beliefs of clients. Cultural sensitivity involves an awareness of both cultural similarities and differences.

Guidelines to follow in relation to cultural sensitivity are found in Table 1-1 and Box 1-1.

1

TABLE 1-1 TRADITIONAL COMMUNICATION PATTERNS OF VARIOUS CULTURES

Cultural Group	Communication Styles
Chinese	• Self-expression is repressed. • Silence is valued. • Hesitant to ask questions. • Nonverbal and contextual cues are important. • An individual may smile even if the individual does not understand. • Touching is limited.
Japanese	• Listen empathetically. • Are stoic. • Value politeness, personal restraint, and self-control. • Attitudes, actions, and feelings are more important than words. • Direct eye contact is considered a lack of respect. • Touching is limited.
Vietnamese	• Disrespectful to question authority figures. • Value harmony and modesty of speech and action. • Avoid direct eye contact. • A relaxed concept of time. • Respect titles, family, and generational relationships.
Filipino	• Respect personal dignity, nonverbal communication, and preserving self-esteem. • Avoid direct eye contact, expressions of disagreement, especially with authority figures, and discussion of personal topics. • Small talk is important before serious discussions.
African Americans	• Cautious around and distrustful of the majority. • Value direct eye contact. • Use nonverbal expressions. • Sensitive to incongruence between verbal and nonverbal messages. • Tend to test those in the majority before submitting to their suggestions and care. • May use Ebonics, an English dialect.
Hispanic Americans (Mexican)	• Use direct eye contact. • Use gestures and voice tone changes in speech. • Unassertive if others appear busy or rushed.

continues

TABLE 1-1 *Continued*

Cultural Group	Communication Styles
Hispanic Americans (Mexican) *continued*	• May smile and nod even if do not understand.
	• Perceive touch as reassuring, comforting, and sympathetic.
	• Many are bilingual, but may use nonstandard English.
	• Small talk is important before serious discussion.
	• Appreciate open ended questions and a nondirective approach.
	• It is important for the father to be present when speaking with a male child.
	• Discussions of personal topics are easier if the nurse is of the same gender as the client.
Puerto Ricans	• Value personal and family privacy; questions regarding family are considered presumptuous and disrespectful.
	• A relaxed concept of time.
	• May not use standard English.
	• Many are bilingual.
	• New immigrants and older individuals may speak Spanish.
Cubans	• Most new immigrants are bilingual.
	• Small talk is important before serious discussion.
Native Americans	• Value nonverbal communication.
	• Silence is essential to understanding and respecting another.
	• Direct eye contact is considered insulting.
	• May be reticent in forming opinions of health care providers.
	• Pauses after being questioned are common; they signify thoughtful consideration.
	• Hesitant to discuss personal affairs unless trust has developed and prefer that these discussions occur with a person of the same gender.
	• Sensitive about having their behaviors and words written down.
	• Believe it is wrong to speak for another.
Middle Eastern	• Use silence to show respect.
	• Men and women do not touch each other unless they are in the immediate family or are married.
	• Touching or embracing is common among those of the same gender.
European Americans	• Hugs/embraces are tolerated among intimates and close friends only.

continues

TABLE 1-1 *Continued*

Cultural Group	Communication Styles
European Americans *continued*	• Understanding or agreement is noted by nods. • Use neutral facial expressions in public. • Individuals separate into gender-specific groups at social events, unless the activity is for couples. • Prefer personal space. • Speak warmly and pleasantly and smile to put others at ease. • A firm handshake symbolizes goodwill; a pat on shoulder/back denotes camaraderie.

Adapted from Estes, M. E. Z. (2002). Health assessment & physical examination *(2nd ed). Clifton Park, NY: Thomson Delmar Learning.*

Box 1-1 Surmounting language barriers between health care providers and children/families

A. With an interpreter

1. Determine language(s) and dialect (if relevant) a client is familiar with and speaks at home; the language may not be identical to the one commonly used in their country of origin. Some clients may be multilingual, and a language other than their mother tongue can be used.

2. Avoid using interpreters from groups (countries, regions, religions, tribes) where there may be past or present conflicts.

3. Be sensitive to and make allowances for differences with regard to age, culture, gender, and socioeconomic status between the client and interpreter.

4. Request as verbatim a translation as possible.

5. Be aware that an interpreter not related to the client may request compensation.

B. Without an interpreter

1. Always be polite, formal, patient, and attentive to the client's (or client's family) attempts to communicate.

2. When greeting the client, smile, use the client's complete or last name, indicate your name by saying it while gesturing to oneself, and offer a handshake or nod.

3. Speak in a low and moderate tone.

4. If possible, use words from the client's language.

continues

Box 1-1 *Continued*

5. Use simple words—no idiom, no jargon (medical or otherwise), no slang. Avoid the use of contractions and pronouns, which may be unclear to the client.

6. Give instructions clearly, in simple language (with a minimum of words), and in the correct order.

7. Talk about one topic at a time.

8. Use hand signs freely and act out actions while talking.

9. Check the client's understanding by requesting that he or she describe/illustrate the procedure, pantomime the meaning, or repeat the instructions.

10. Try using Latin phrases or phrases from other languages that have become universal.

11. Write simple sentences in English or another language, since some people understand the written, but not spoken languages, and some accents may be confusing.

12. See if a family member or friend can act as an interpreter for the client. If not, and if the health provider cannot find one, enlist the family in networking to find one.

13. Use phrase books and flash cards.

Adapted from Luckman, J. (1999). Transcultural communication in nursing. Clifton Park, NY: Thomson Delmar Learning.

HISTORY OF CHILD/FAMILY HEALTH

Assessing and taking a history of the child begins in the waiting room, or when obtaining vital signs, observing parent-child interactions, and rating the child's mood and developmental level. All children, regardless of age, should be recognized by their name; whether or not they are directly involved in providing historical information is determined by their developmental level and health status.

An outline for the general health history follows. Headings and questions are traditionally used in the pediatric setting but may be modified or shortened according to situation. The health history traditionally precedes the physical examination.

Chief Complaint

Why is the child being seen today? (The caregiver answer usually is simple: "He has a runny nose.")

Present Illness

Describe the child's signs and symptoms. (Signs and symptoms should be listed in the order mentioned. Specific questions may include: Is the child coughing? What kind? How much? When? How long? How is the child acting otherwise? Has the child been exposed to an illness? What kind of treatment has been used?)

Past History

Birth

Prenatal: How was the mother's health during the pregnancy? Where did she receive prenatal care and for how long? If she had any illnesses or infections, when during the pregnancy did she have them? How were they treated? If she took any medications during her pregnancy, what did she take and when did she start taking them? What is her blood type, the father of the child's blood type, and the child's blood type? Did she receive any X rays during the pregnancy? Was she on any special diet during the pregnancy? If she was hospitalized during the pregnancy, what was the reason? When was she in the hospital and for how long? How many living children does she have? Was she or her doctor worried about this pregnancy? If so, why? How long was this pregnancy?

Natal: How long was labor? Were there any problems? What type of delivery? If anesthesia was used, what kind was it and were there any problems with it? Where was the baby born? What was the weight? What was the baby's condition at birth? Did the baby cry spontaneously? Was the baby blue? Did the baby need oxygen? Who was with the mother during the delivery?

Postnatal: How long did the baby stay in the nursery? Did the baby have any problems in the nursery? If so, what were they? Did the mother and baby come home from the hospital at the same time? Was the baby ever jaundiced or cyanotic? Did the baby have any feeding problems? Did the baby develop any rashes? How much weight did the baby lose?

Allergies

Is the child allergic to any foods? Medications? Insects? Animals? Does the child seem to have any allergies during any particular time of the year? Describe what happens when the child has an allergic reaction. Does the child ever break out into a rash? If so, why?

Accidents

Has the child ever had an accident? If so, where was it (home, school, in car, on bicycle or other sporting equipment)? Describe what happened. How was it treated? Where was the child treated? How did the child react? Have there been any residual problems?

Illnesses

Has the child had any infections? When? Where? How was it treated? How was it followed up? Has the child had any childhood diseases? If so, what diseases did the child have (measles, mumps, roseola, chickenpox, whooping cough)? Has the child ever had any X rays?

Surgeries

Has the child ever had any surgery? If so, when? For what condition? What was the outcome?

Hospitalizations

If the child has ever spent any time in the hospital, what was the reason? Where was the hospital? Has the condition resolved? Are there any residual problems?

Immunizations

Has the child had any immunizations? Which ones has the child had? Did the child have any reactions to the immunizations? If so, what was the reaction? Has the child received any boosters? If so, which ones? Has the child ever been tested for tuberculosis? If so, how? When? What was the result?

Family History

Family Members

What is the mother's age and health status? What is the father's age and health status? What are the ages and genders of this child's siblings? What is the health status of each?

Family Diseases

Within the immediate family (grandparents, first aunts/uncles, parents, siblings) are any of the following conditions present?

Eyes, ears, nose, throat: Nosebleeds, sinus problems, glaucoma, cataracts, myopia, or strabismus? Any other problems not listed?

Cardiorespiratory: Is there any asthma? Hay fever? Tuberculosis? Hypertension? Heart murmurs? Heart attacks? Strokes? Anemia? Rheumatic fever? Leukemia? Pneumonia? Emphysema? Any other problem not listed?

Gastrointestinal/Genitourinary: Does anyone have any ulcers? Colitis? Kidney infections? Bladder infections? Any other problem with the gastrointestinal or genitourinary system not listed?

Musculoskeletal: Does anyone in the family have any of the following: dislocated hips, club foot, muscular dystrophy, arthritis? Any other problems with bones, joints, or muscles not listed?

Neurological: Does anyone have seizures? Mental retardation? Mental problems? Epilepsy? Any other problems not listed?

Special senses: Is anyone blind or deaf?

Chronic: Does anyone have diabetes? Cancer/tumors? Thyroid problems? Congenital anomalies?

General: Are there any medical problems in the family that are important to know about?

Social History

Where does the family live? In a house? Apartment? Room? How large is the place where they live? Is there a yard? Is it fenced? Does anyone live with the family (grandparents, aunts, etc.)? Does the father and/or mother work? Full or part time? What are their occupations? If no one works, how are they supported? Is there any outside help? Does the child go to day care? Preschool? School? What are the relationships of the family like (happy, sad, chaotic, depressed, violent)?

Review of Systems

Skin

Does the child have any rashes? Birth marks? Discolorations?

Eyes, Ears, Nose, Throat

Does this child have any persistent nosebleeds? Frequent sore throats or colds (more than 4 a year)? Pneumonia? Trouble breathing? Epistaxis? Nasal discharge? Frequent earaches? Difficulty hearing? Pain? Ear discharge? Myringotomy? Do the child's eyes ever cross? Do they tear excessively? Have there been any eye injuries? Discharges? Puffiness? Redness? Has the child ever worn glasses? Any difficulty swallowing? Dental defects? Swollen glands? Masses? Stiffness in the neck? Neck asymmetry?

Cardiorespiratory

Does the child have any trouble breathing? Running? Finishing a 3 to 4 oz bottle without tiring (if an infant)? Cough? Hoarseness? Wheezing? Does the child turn blue? Have there been any heart defects? Heart murmurs? "Heart trouble"? Pain over the heart or in the chest?

Gastrointestinal

Does the child have any problems with diarrhea? Constipation? Bleeding around the rectum? Bloody stools? Pain? Vomiting? What has the appetite been like? Abdominal pain or distension? Jaundice?

Genitourinary

Does the child have a straight, strong urinary stream or does the urine just dribble out? How often does the child urinate? Is there any pain? Is there any discharge? How much does the child void during the day? Does she (an older girl) menstruate? If so, what was the age of onset? How often does she menstruate? Are there any problems?

Neurological

Has the child ever had a seizure? A fainting spell? Tremors? Twitches? Blackouts? Dizzy spells? Frequent headaches? Any incoordination? Numbness?

Musculoskeletal

Has the child ever broken any bones? Had any sprains? Complained of pain in the joints, swelling, or redness around the joints? Difficulty moving extremities or in walking?

Special Senses

Does the child see well? Hear well? Does the child seem clumsy? Can the child see the blackboard from where he or she sits in the classroom? Does the child fall or walk into doors?

Chronic Conditions

Does the child have any long term disease? If so, describe the child's disease.

General

Does the child have any other problems you would like to talk about?

Habits

Nutrition

How would you describe the child's appetite (good, fair, varied)? Is the child breast fed or bottle fed? If the child is receiving formula, what kind is it? How much and how often does the child eat in a 24 hour period? How is the formula prepared? What kinds of food (meat, fruits, vegetables, cereals, milk, eggs, juices, sweets, snacks) and how often does the child eat? What are the portion sizes? Does the child take vitamins? If so, what kind? How often? How much? Does the child feed himself or herself? Does the child use a cup? Utensils? Would you describe the child as messy? Does the child eat with the family? What is the emotional climate (relaxed, rushed, tense) of the family meals? What are the child's favorite foods? What foods does the child dislike?

Elimination

Describe the child's bowel and bladder patterns (frequency, consistency, color, discomfort). Is the child toilet trained? If not, is it planned in the future? When? If the child is toilet trained, describe any problems. If the child is toilet trained, does the child have any accidents? If so, when do they occur? How frequently do they occur?

Rest and Sleep

Where does the child sleep? What time does the child go to bed at night? What time does the child wake up in the morning? Does the child wake up during the night? If so, how often? Describe what the child does. Describe how the parent responds. Does the child have any nightmares? Night terrors? Does the child nap during the day? If so, when? How long does the child nap? How many hours does the child sleep in a 24 hour period? Does the child seem to need more sleep than he or she is getting?

Play and Activity

What types of play or games is the child involved in during the day? How often? If an older child: Does the child participate in sports, team activities, and/or regular exercise? Ask child and parent to describe the child's friendships.

Safety and Accident Prevention

Questions to use related to child proofing the home are found in Box 1-2 .

Development

How does the child's development compare with siblings and peers? When did the child first roll over? Sit? Stand? Walk? Talk? What grade is the child in at school? Does the child like school? What does the child like to do in school? Does the child have any playmates?

Personality

How would you describe the child's personality (quiet, outgoing, independent, dependent)? How does the child cope with stress (withdraw, aggressive, etc.)? Describe the child's temper. Describe how the child handles anger, fear, jealousy. How does the child relax? How does the child separate from parents? How does the child react to new situations? How does the child react to discipline? How does the child relate to baby sitters or others?

Family Relations

How do members of the family get along? How are disagreements handled within the family? What activities do the family participate in together? How often? What methods are used in the family for discipline? Are there any siblings?

Box 1-2   Questions about childproofing the environment

1. Would you tell me how you have childproofed your home?
2. Do you have gates on the top and bottom of the stairs?
3. Are the slats on the crib less than $2^3/_8$ inches apart?
4. Have you taken the crib mobile down and taken out the bumper pads (applies to infants who are trying to pull up)?
5. Is all sleepwear flame retardant?
6. Is the hot water thermostat turned down to 120° Fahrenheit?
7. Have you installed potty locks to keep the toilet lid down?
8. Do you keep curtain and blind strings out of reach?
9. Have you placed all sharp items such as razors and knives out of reach of the child?
10. Do you monitor your child in the bathtub?
11. Do you always drain the water in the tub after getting out?
12. Have you placed cushioned covering on the tub's water faucet and drain lever?
13. Do you use a nonskid bath mat in the tub?
14. Are there outlet covers on every outlet in the house?
15. When you are cooking, do you keep the pot or pan handles turned in?
16. Have you taken tablecloths off all tables?
17. Do you keep the phone cord out of reach?
18. Is the slack taken up on all electrical appliance and lamp cords?
19. If you have a raised hearth, have you covered it with bumpers, pads, or towels?
20. Are all of your plants out of reach?
21. Are slip protectors under all rugs?
22. If you have a pool in the yard, is it fenced in, or is there a protective cover on top?
23. Do you empty pails that contain liquid after using them?
24. Are medications, cosmetics, pesticides, gasoline, cleaning solutions, paint thinner, and all other poisonous materials out of the child's reach?
25. Do you have your local poison control telephone number next to each phone?
26. Do you have syrup of ipecac in the house? Do you know why it is used and its expiration date?
27. Do you have smoke detectors close to or in the child's bedroom, and on each floor of the house?
28. Do you have a fire extinguisher on each floor?
29. Have you devised and practiced an escape route plan in case of fire?
30. Are you CPR trained?
31. What would you do in case of an emergency?
32. Where do you place your child's car seat—in the front or back seat, facing front or rear? Do you place your child in the car where an air bag is supplied?
33. Does your child use protective gear such as a helmet or knee and elbow pads if participating in an activity in which injuries may occur?
34. Do you keep plastic dry cleaner overwraps, latex balloons (unattended by a caregiver), plastic trash bags, and grocery bags out of the child's reach?

PHYSICAL ASSESSMENT

General Guidelines

The physical assessment of a pediatric client must be performed as opportunities present. Therefore, be prepared with all equipment, including stethoscope, tape measure, penlight, and tongue blade, when entering a client's room. The assessment should begin immediately. The client's skin color, position, and gait (if the child is observed walking) should be noted, as well as the caregiver's response and caregiver-child interaction. If an infant is sleeping, it is a good time to listen to his or her heart sounds. Rapport can be established with the caregiver and child by talking first with the caregiver and then with the child.

The nurse can use play therapy as necessary to accomplish the assessment. Listening to the caregiver's or a stuffed toy's heart and lungs can show children, especially toddlers, that it does not hurt. The nurse can then attempt to obtain resting heart rate, heart sounds, respirations, and breath sounds. The child also can assist with the assessment if possible. Since preschoolers and older children like to listen to their own heart sounds, this is an opportunity to teach about the body, and how to keep it healthy, and to validate the child's normalcy.

Invasive procedures and painful areas or procedures should be saved until the end of the assessment. What constitutes invasive varies with age groups. For example, examining ears, mouth, and nose is invasive to toddlers. Genitourinary system and abdominal procedures are invasive to school-aged children and adolescents. If the child refuses to cooperate, the nurse must use a firm approach and perform the examination as quickly as possible. Regardless of the order in which the assessment is performed, it must be charted in a logical head-to-toe format.

General Appearance

Note the overall appearance of the child. For example, is the child small, obese, well nourished, awake, alert, cooperative, developmentally appropriate for age, lethargic, or distressed? What is the client's state of consciousness?

Skin

Inspect and palpate the skin for color. (Remember that room color, gown color, and lighting affect observation. Evaluate for jaundice in natural lighting of a window; cyanosis blanches momentarily, bruises do not.) Also note pigmentation, temperature, texture, moisture, and turgor.

Note and describe all lesions for the following:

Location—exactly where on body
Pattern—clustered, confluent, evanescent, linear
Size—measured in centimeters
Color—red, pink, brown, white, hyperpigmented, or hypopigmented
Elevation—raised (papular), flat (macular), fluid filled (vesicular)
Blanching—do they pale when pressure is applied?

Hair

Note color, texture, distribution, quality, and loss. Look in hair behind the ears for nits.

Nails

Note color, cyanosis, shape, and condition of nails. Clubbing is determined by checking nail angle. The normal angle is 160 degrees. An angle of 180 degrees or larger is seen in clubbing caused by hypoxia.

Head

Inspect and palpate, feeling for bogginess, sutures, and fontanels. In children under two years of age, measure anterior fontanel in two dimensions; usually is 4 to 5 cm by 3 to 4 cm, but should be at least 1 cm by 1 cm. Normally, the fontanels should feel flat. In states of dehydration, fontanels may be sunken. In states of increased intracranial pressure, fontanels may be bulging. Measure frontal occipital circumference (FOC) until the child is 36 months old or if its size is important to the child's condition after 2 years of age. Always plot FOC and note size, shape, and symmetry of the head.

Palpate the scalp for tenderness and lesions.

Neck

Inspect for swelling, webbing, nuchal fold, and vein distension. Palpate for swelling, carotid pulse, trachea, and thyroid.

Ears

Inspect for shape, color, symmetry, helix formation, and position. The top of the ear should go through an imaginary line from the inner canthus to the outer canthus of the eye to the occiput. Palpate for firmness and pain and observe for and describe any discharge from the ear canal. Assess for gross hearing. Infants less than 4 months of age startle to sound. Older infants turn to localize the sound of jingling keys and other objects. Use the whisper test with verbal and cooperative children.

Eyes

Inspect for position, alignment, lid closure, inner canthal distance (average = 2.5 cm), epicanthal folds, and slant of fissure. Note dark circles under the eyes (usually present in children with allergies).

> Brows—note separateness, nits
> Lashes—note if they curve into eye
> Lids—note color, swelling, lesions, discharge
> Conjunctiva
> > Palpebral (should be pink)—note redness, pallor
> > Sclera and bulbar—note injection, redness, color (should be white; yellow in jaundice, blue in osteogenesis imperfecta)
> Pupils—note shape, size, and briskness of reaction to light by constricting directly and consensually and accommodation for near and far vision
> Iris—note color, roundness, any clefts or defects
> Extraocular movements (EOMs)
> > Six cardinal fields of gaze—Hold chin and have child's eyes follow your finger, moving in the shape of an H. Note asymmetric eye movement or nystagmus; a few beats of nystagmus in the far lateral gaze are normal.
> > Corneal light reflex—Hold light 15 inches from bridge of nose and shine on bridge. It should reflect in the same place in each eye in normally aligned eyes.
> > Cover–uncover test—Check for movement when one eye is covered and the other is gazing at a distant object. Remove cover and note movement of covered eye. Repeat using a near object.
> Gross vision—Newborns blink and hyperextend their necks to light. Infants who can see fix on and follow objects. Grossly assess older children's vision by having them describe what they see on the wall or out the window.

Face

Note color, symmetrical movement, expression, skin folds, and swelling.

Nose

Inspect for color of skin, any nasal crease, nasal mucosa, any discharge and its color, and patency. Flaring of nares may be a sign of respiratory distress. Assess turbinates by shining a light into the nares while pushing up gently on the tip of the nose (red and swollen indicates possible upper respiratory infection; pale and boggy indicates possible allergic rhinitis). Palpate sinuses for tenderness. Frontal sinuses are not developed completely until approximately 8 years of age.

Mouth

Inspect all areas. Note number and condition of teeth. Observe tonsils for swelling (grade 1+ indicates mild swelling; grade 4+ indicates touching, or "kissing," tonsils), color (should be same color as buccal mucosa), and discharge. Examine the hard and soft palate for color, patency, and lesions. The uvula should rise symmetrically; a bifid uvula could indicate a submucosal cleft. Note tongue shape, size, color, movement, and inspect for any lesions (most common lesions are white and are thrush). Note breath odor.

Thorax and Lungs

Inspect for symmetry, movement, color, retractions, breast development, and type and effort of breathing. Breathing is predominately abdominal until age 7 years. Note nasal flaring and use of accessory muscles. Retractions usually start subcostal and substernal, then progress to suprasternal and supraclavicular, and lastly intercostal, indicating severe distress. Palpate for tactile fremitus (increased in congestion and consolidation). Percuss for resonance (sound becomes dull with fluid or masses). Auscultate side to side for symmetry of sound. Infants breathe deeper when they cry; toddlers and preschoolers can breathe deeper when they blow bubbles or try to "blow out the light" of your pen light. Assess all fields. Listen to the back to assess the lower lobes in children younger than 8 years of age. Auscultate in the axillae to best hear crackles in children with suspected pneumonia. Normal sounds are vesicular or bronchovesicular. Infants' breath sounds are louder and more bronchial because they have thin chest walls.

Describe adventitious sounds as follows:

Rhonchi—a continuous, low-pitched sound with a snoring quality

Crackles—intermittent, brief, repetitive sounds caused by small collapsed airways popping open

Fine crackles—soft, high-pitched and brief

Coarse crackles—louder, lower-pitched and slightly longer than fine crackles

Wheezes—musical, more continuous sounds produced by rapid movement of air through narrowed passages. Usual progression of wheezing starts with expiratory wheezes only, then inspiratory wheezes with decreased expiratory wheezes, then inspiratory wheezes only (airways are collapsing on expiration), and finally, no sounds because there is little air movement.

Stridor—inspiratory wheeze heard louder in neck than in chest, usually right over trachea

Infants with upper airway congestion can have sounds transmitted to lungs because they are obligate nose breathers. Listen to their lungs when they are crying and breathing through their mouths to decrease the amount of transmitted noise and better assess their breath sounds.

Cardiovascular System

Inspect for point of maximum impulse (PMI), cyanosis, mottling, edema, respiratory distress, clubbing, activity intolerance, and tiring with feeds. Palpate PMI and brachial, radial, femoral, and pedal pulses.

Auscultate the following areas with bell and diaphragm of the stethoscope:

Aortic area:
Right second intercostal space (ICS) at right sternal border (SB)

Pulmonic area:
Left second ICS at left SB

Erb's point:
Left third ICS at left SB

Tricuspid:
Left fifth ICS at left SB

Mitral:
Left fifth ICS at left midclavicular line

S_1 correlates with the carotid pulse and is best heard at the apex of the heart. S_2 is best heard in the aortic and pulmonic areas (base of heart). Quality of sound should be crisp and clear. Heart rate should be normal for age and condition and synchronous with the radial pulse. Rhythm should be regular or may slow and speed up with respirations in young infants. Auscultate with the child in two positions if possible. Auscultate for muffled or additional sounds and note where they are best heard.

Murmurs should be assessed for the following:

Location—where heard best on the chest wall

Timing in cardiac cycle—continuous, systolic, or diastolic

Grade—I/VI to VI/VI
  I/VI—very faint, have to really tune in
  II/VI—quiet, but can hear soon after
    placing stethoscope
  III/VI—moderately loud
  IV/VI—loud
  V/VI—very loud, may be heard with
    stethoscope partially off chest
  VI/VI—can hear without stethoscope

Pitch—high (best heard with the
  diaphragm), medium, or low (best
  heard with the bell)

Quality—harsh, blowing, machinery-like,
  musical

Radiation—does it radiate, and if so
  where (listen to back, axillae, and
  above clavicles)

Abdomen

Inspect for pulsation, contour, symmetry, peristaltic waves, masses, and normal skin color. Auscultate before palpating so normal bowel sounds are not disturbed. Listen in all four quadrants for a full minute. Normal sounds should be heard every 10 to 30 seconds (4 to 5 sounds per minute). Less than 4 per minute indicates decreased bowel sounds. Listen for a full 5 minutes before concluding that they are absent.

Percuss for dullness over the client's liver and full bladder. The rest of the abdomen should percuss tympani. Palpate using light pressure first. Have the child bend the knees up while lying on his or her back to relax the abdomen. Use the child's hands under your hands if the child is very ticklish or tense. With deep palpation, support the child from the back, then palpate. Start in lower quadrants and move upward to detect an enlarged liver or spleen. Note areas of tenderness, pain, or any masses.

Anus

Inspect the skin and perineum for excoriation, bruising, discoloration, or tears.

Genitourinary System

Female genitalia—Note redness,
  excoriation, discharge and odor.

Male genitalia—Note if circumcised or uncircumcised. (If uncircumcised, see if foreskin is retractable.) Note position of meatus. Close off the canals and feel for the testes or any masses in the scrotal sac. If you feel a mass other than the testes, transilluminate for fluid.

Lymphatic System

Nodes should be firm, small (1 cm or less), freely moveable, and nontender. Palpate preauricular, postauricular, anterior and posterior cervical chains, supraclavicular and subclavicular, axillary, and inguinal lymph nodes with pads of fingers.

Musculoskeletal System

Incorporate assessment into the examination. Observe walking, sitting, turning, and range of motion in all joints. Observe spinal curvature and mobility. Exaggerated lumbar curve is normal in toddlers. Note sacral dimples or tufts of hair at the base of the spinal column. Note symmetry and movement of the extremities.

Test muscle strength. Strength is graded on a 0 to 5 scale. Normal muscle strength is grade 5.

  0—no contraction noted
  1—barely a trace of contraction
  2—active movement without gravity
  3—active movement against gravity
  4—active movement against gravity and
    resistance
  5—active movement against full
    resistance without tiring

Note size, color, temperature, and mobility of joints. Examine palmar creases. Note extra digits and deformities.

Note stance and gait. Bowed legs (genu varum) are normal in toddlers until approximately age 2 years. Knock-knees (genu valgum) are normal from 2 until approximately 6 to 10 years. Note foot deformities. Stroke the side of the foot to see if it returns to a neutral position. Check for dislocatable hips using Barlow's test and Ortolani's maneuver in infants. Also look for uneven skin folds.

Neurological System

Observe grossly for speech and ability to follow directions in an older child. In an infant, observe activity and tone. In ambulatory patients, observe gait and balance.

Check deep tendon reflexes. These are graded from 0 to 41.

4+—very brisk, hyperactive
3+—brisker than average
2+—normal
1+—decreased
0—absent

Use a percussion hammer or the side of the stethoscope diaphragm to elicit the following responses:

DEEP TENDON REFLEX	PROCEDURE	RESPONSE
Biceps	Hit antecubital space	Forearm flexes
Triceps	Bend arm at elbow, hit triceps tendon above elbow	Forearm extends
Patellar	Strike patellar tendon	Lower leg extends
Achilles	Hold foot lightly, hit Achilles tendon	Foot flexes downward
Cranial nerves	Most are integrated into routine examination and are not specifically tested.	

INFANT REFLEXES

Reflex	Age	Assessment
Babinski	Birth to 2 yr	Stroke bottom of foot; toes fan
Galant	Birth to 4–8 wk	Stroke infant's side; hips swing to that side
Moro	Birth to 3–4 mo	Arms extend, fingers fan (if asymmetrical, brachial plexus injury should be suspected); if Moro persists beyond 6 mo, brain damage should be suspected
Palmar grasp	Birth to 4 mo	Put your finger in infant's palm from ulnar side; infant closes fingers around your finger
Rooting	Birth to 4 mo (up to 12 mo during sleep)	Stroke infant's cheek and corner of mouth; infant's head turns in that direction
Sucking	Birth to 4 mo (7 mo during sleep)	Infant has reflexive sucking to stimuli

Neurovascular System

Assess closely in children with intravenous (IV) lines in extremities, and those in casts, restraints, and in traction. Note color and size of extremity and compare with unaffected extremity. Check pulses bilaterally for equality of strength. Check capillary refill time by pinching a toe or finger and noting the time it takes for the color to return. They should have brisk, immediate blood return. Both congestive heart failure and dehydration can increase capillary refill time. Assess for any alterations in sensation or increased pain.

Refer to Appendix A for normal vital signs of children.

Growth Measurements

One of the most important areas in assessing children is the measurement of physical growth. The pediatric nurse should measure weight, height/length, head circumference, skinfold thickness, and arm circumference. Measurements are plotted on growth charts to determine percentiles to compare an individual child's measurements with that of the general population.

The National Center for Health Statistics (NCHS) has developed growth charts according to age. One growth chart is to be used for children from birth to 36 months of age. In this age group, the weight by age, recumbent length by age, weight for length, and head circumference by age are plotted. Another growth chart is to be used for children ages 2 to 18 years. In this age group, weight by age and stature by age are plotted. See Appendix B.

The NCHS uses the 5th and 95th percentiles as the parameters for determining if children fall outside of the normal limits for growth. Those below the 5th percentile are considered underweight and/or small in stature and those above the 95th percentile are considered overweight and/or large in stature. Children whose measurements fall outside normal limits should be followed more closely, especially when genetic factors are not involved.

Recumbent length should be measured when using the birth to 36-month growth chart. Lay the child supine on a papered surface, and mark where the top of the child's head and the bottom of the child's heel touch the paper. The distance between the marks, measured with a tape measure, is the recumbent length.

Height is measured when using the 2 to 18 year growth chart, and taken when the child is standing upright. To measure height most accurately, remove the child's shoes, and make sure the child's head is in the midline and facing straight ahead. There should be no flexion of the knees, slumping of the shoulders, or raising of the heels during the measurement. The most accurate measurements are taken with a wall-mounted stadiometer.

Use a balanced scale to measure weight. Children should be weighed nude when using the birth to 36-month growth chart. If a child is wearing something heavy, such as a cast or an IV board, document that with the weight. Always remember safety issues.

Head circumference is measured from birth to 36 months of age. The measurement should be taken at the greatest circumference, which is slightly above the eyebrows and ear pinna and around the occipital prominence at the back of the skull. A paper tape measure should be used to give the most accurate data.

Chest circumference is measured primarily for comparison with head circumference. Chest circumference is measured at the nipple line midway between inspiration and expiration.

Measuring skinfold thickness is sometimes used to assess body fat. Calipers are used in one or more of the following sites: triceps, subscapula, abdomen, upper thigh, and suprailiac. An average of at least two measurements from each site is used.

The measurement of arm circumference is an indirect assessment used to evaluate nutrition. The arm circumference is measured with a paper tape measure, which is placed vertically along the posterior upper arm until the same measurement appears at the acromial process and olecranon process.

NUTRITIONAL ASSESSMENT

Nutritional status affects the general health of a child and has a direct influence on a child's growth, development, cognition, and learning. A nutritional assessment is an essential component of a complete health history, and should include information about dietary intake, and a clinical assessment of nutritional and biochemical status.

The following topics should be evaluated:

- Usual mealtimes
- Which family member is responsible for meal preparation and shopping
- How much money is allotted for groceries each week
- How most foods are prepared (e.g., baked, fried, broiled, microwaved)
- How often the family eats out (frequency of fast food restaurants)

- Favorite foods, snacks
- Cultural practices/ethnic foods
- Food/beverage dislikes
- Description of child's usual appetite
- Feeding habits
- Breastfeeding
- Past medical history including any emotional difficulties
- Medication history
- Supplemental vitamins, herbs, iron, fluoride
- Food allergies
- Special diets
- Recent weight gain/loss
- Types of routine exercise

Additional information to obtain for young infants includes the following:

- Birth history (e.g., birth weight, history of prematurity, small for gestational age)
- Past medical history, especially in terms of gastrointestinal disturbances
- Feeding difficulties such as excessive fussiness, colic, regurgitation, difficulty swallowing/sucking

Dietary Intake

A thorough diet history should also be obtained. Food intake can be recorded by using a food diary and/or a food frequency record.

Record the following types of information in a food diary:

- Times of meals and snacks
- Description of food items including the actual food, amount, and method of preparation
- With whom the child ate
- Related factors such as associated activity, place, persons, feelings, hunger

Record the following types of information in a food frequency record:

- Food group (breads/cereals/pasta, milk/cheese/yogurt, vegetables, fruits/juice, protein foods, fats/oils/sweets)
- Numbers of servings per day or week in each of the food groups
- Serving size

Clinical Assessment

Another component of the nutritional assessment is the clinical examination of the child. This provides information regarding signs of adequate nutrition or deficiencies. Assessment of the skin, hair, mouth, teeth, eyes, neck, chest, abdomen, cardiovascular system, neurological system, and musculoskeletal system can be useful in determining possible nutritional deficits or excesses (see Table 1-2). Anthropomorphic measurements of height, weight, head circumference, skinfold thickness, and arm circumference are essential components.

Biochemical Analysis

Blood chemistry levels of hematocrit and hemoglobin (indication of anemias), albumin (protein malnutrition), blood urea nitrogen (negative nitrogen balance), creatinine (high protein intake), lead (water consumption containing lead), glucose (dehydration, acidosis), and cholesterol (dietary-fat intake) should be analyzed. Normal values for these tests are located in Appendix C.

CALCULATING DAILY CALORIC REQUIREMENTS	
Body Weight (kg)	Caloric Expenditure/Day
Up to 10	100 kcal/kg
11–20	1,000 kcal + 50 kcal/kg for each kg above 10 kg
More than 20	1,500 kcal + 20 kcal/kg for each kg above 20 kg

These formulas are not appropriate for neonates less than 2 weeks old or for children with conditions associated with abnormal losses. Children with disease, prior surgery, fever, or pain may require additional calories above maintenance. Children who are comatose or immobile may require fewer calories.

TABLE 1-2 PHYSICAL SIGNS ASSOCIATED WITH NUTRITIONAL DEFICITS

Body Part	Normal Appearance	Physical Signs	Nutritional Deficit/Excess
Skin	Uniform color, smooth, firm	Depigmentation, scaling, dry appearance, edema, pallor	Vitamin A, protein, riboflavin, vitamin B_{12}, excess sodium
Hair	Shiny, strong, not easily plucked	Dull, dry, thin, alopecia depigmentation	Protein, calories, vitamin C
Mouth	Lips smooth, pink, not chapped; tongue rough texture, no lesions; teeth white, no cavities; gums firm, pink; mucous membranes moist, pink, smooth	Lips reddened, swollen, cracked; tongue—glossitis; teeth brown, pitted, with caries; gums spongy, bleeding, swollen; mucous membranes with ulcers	Riboflavin, vitamin C, niacin, fluoride; excess carbohydrates, excess vitamin A
Eyes	Clear, bright, moist membranes	Pale conjunctiva, night blindness, corneal drying	Vitamin A, riboflavin
Neck	Thyroid not visible	Thyroid enlarged, grossly visible	Iodine
Chest	Chest is almost circular; lateral diameter increases in proportion to anteroposterior diameter in children	Depressed rib cage, protrusion of sternum	Vitamin D
Abdomen	Abdomen is slightly protruded; older children have flat abdomen	Abdominal distension, poor musculature	Protein, calories
Cardiovascular system	Heart rate and blood pressure within normal limits	Tachycardia, palpitations, arrhythmias, increased blood pressure	Potassium, magnesium; excess sodium
Neurological system	Alert, emotionally stable, intact reflexes	Irritable, listless, lethargic, diminished or absent deep tendon reflexes	Thiamin, niacin, vitamin C, vitamin E
Musculo-skeletal system	Firm muscles, bilaterally equal strength, normal spinal curves, symmetric and straight extremities, full range of motion	Weak, wasting appearance, kyphosis/lordosis/scoliosis, bowing of extremities	Protein, calories, vitamin D, calcium, vitamin A

DEVELOPMENTAL ASSESSMENT

Evaluation of developmental functioning is an essential component of any pediatric assessment. Purposes of the developmental assessment are to: (1) validate a child is developing normally, (2) detect problems, (3) identify caregiver/child concerns, and (4) provide an opportunity for anticipatory guidance/teaching relative to expected and age appropriate behaviors. The developmental assessment may be completed either before or after the physical examination.

Several assessment measures are listed in Table 1-3. These measures evaluate a variety of aspects, including fine and gross motor skills, social and language skills, behavior, temperament, cognition, memory, and the child's home environment. Screening procedures using these measures quickly and reliably identify children whose development is below normal and may also be used to monitor developmental progress. Most measures can be administered in a variety of settings with a minimal amount of preparation. Although all measures listed are valid and reliable, some may not be standardized on children of lower socioeconomic status or of different ethnic groups. Caution should always be taken to guarantee administration is accurate; directions and explanations to caregivers and children need to be clear and concise. Following administration, ask caregivers if the child's performance was typical, since retesting/rescreening may be necessary if the behavior was atypical. All results should be communicated to caregivers carefully so misunderstandings and misinterpretations are kept to a minimum. Before administering any measure, it is essential to read and follow instructions carefully.

FAMILY ASSESSMENT

Family assessment involves collecting data about family structure, and relationships and interactions among individual members. Data are systematically collected using predetermined guidelines or questions, and then classified and analyzed according to their meaning.

Two commonly used instruments for developing a family database are the genogram and the ecomap.

A genogram is a format for drawing a family tree that records information about family members and their relationships over a period of time, usually three generations. It also records the health history of all members (morbidity, mortality, and onset of illnesses), thus revealing information about genetic and familial diseases. Figure 1-1 is an example of a genogram/family tree.

An ecomap is a visual representation of a family in relation to the community. It demonstrates the nature and quality of family relationships and what kinds of resources or energies are going in and out of the family. Figure 1-2 shows a family ecomap. This schematic is useful in identifying the strengths of family networks and resources they have available during stressful times or crises.

An in-depth family assessment requires a significant amount of time, and every family does not need a comprehensive assessment. However, when a family is at risk for dysfunction, such an assessment may be required. Referral to other health care professionals and community organizations is appropriate in these situations. Information can be obtained through interviewing and questioning, observing interactions between members, and utilizing a family assessment instrument.

Several family assessment instruments are available. Many have been developed by family theorists, mostly nonnurses, and are used by the health care team to obtain information about family systems. However, nurses have created some instruments, two of which are the Calgary Family Assessment Model (Wright & Leahey, 1994) and the Friedman Family Assessment Model (Friedman, 2002).

The Calgary Family Assessment Model

The Calgary Family Assessment Model (CFAM) combines nursing and family therapy concepts and is based on systems, cybernetics, communication, and change

TABLE 1-3 DEVELOPMENTAL ASSESSMENT MEASURES FOR INFANTS AND CHILDREN

Test Name	Ages	Features Evaluated
Carey-Revised Infant Temperament	4 – 8 months	Temperament, patterns of feeding, sleeping, elimination, responses to different situations
Denver Articulation Screening Exam	2.5 – 6 years	Intelligibility; articulation of 30 sound elements
Denver II (Found in Appendix D)	Birth – 6 years	Personal-social, fine motor-adaptive, language, gross motor
Developmental Profile II	Birth – 9 years	Physical, self-help, social, academic, communication skills
Early Language	Birth – 3 years	Auditory expressive and receptive, visual components of speech
Goodnough-Harris Drawing Test	5 – 17 years	Child's drawing of a person: analyzed for body parts, clothing, proportion, perspective
HOME (Home Observation for Measurement of the Environment)	Birth – 6 years	Organization, play materials, parental control, stimulation, punishment or restriction
McCarthy Scales of Children's Abilities	2.5 – 8.5 years	Intellectual and motor development, memory, quantitative perceptual performance, general cognition

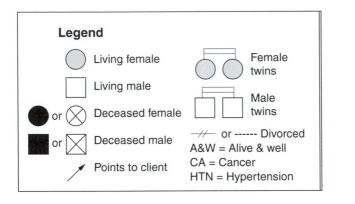

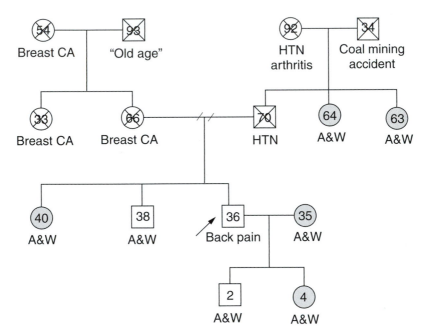

Denies family hx of heart dz, CVA, TB, DM, kidney dz, blood disorders, migraine H/A, gout, thyroid dz, asthma, allergic disorders, obesity, drug addiction, AIDS, violence, mental illness.

Figure 1-1 Family Genogram

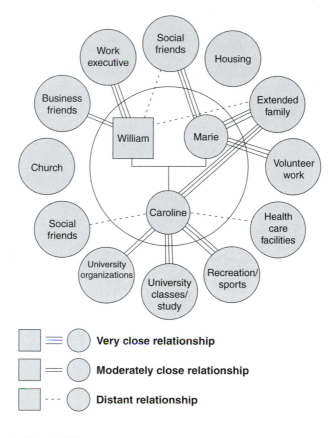

Figure 1-2 Family Ecomap

theories. As illustrated in Figure 1-3, the model consists of three major categories: structural, developmental, and functional. The assessment questions are organized into these groupings. The first major category is the family structure, which has internal, external, and contextual components. Structure includes the composition of the family, the connection among family members, and the family's context. Family development, the second major category, includes assessment of family stages, tasks, and attachments. The third area for assessment is family functioning, which includes instrumental and expressive subcategories. Instrumental aspects of family functioning are activities of daily living such as sleeping, eating, meal preparation, etc. Expressive areas include emotional functioning, communication patterns, problem-solving methods, beliefs, and alliances. The CFAM is broad in perspective, though it focuses on internal relations within the family rather than on the family's relationship with the community. Although assessment of every element is not always necessary, following this guide ensures that data about the family are not presented as isolated facts.

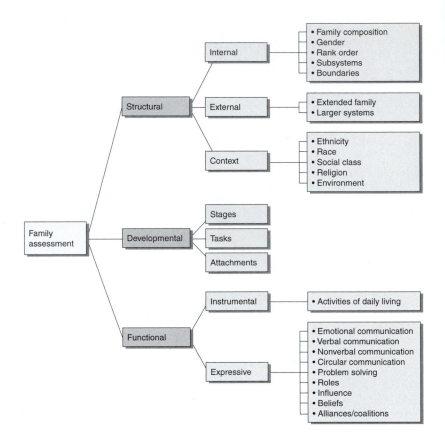

Figure 1-3 The Calgary Family Assessment Model. From *Nurses and Families: A guide to family assessment and intervention,* by L. M. Wright and M. Leahy. (1994). Philadelphia: F. A. Davis. Used with permission.

Friedman Family Assessment Model

The Friedman Family Assessment Model is based on the structural-functional theory, as well as on developmental and systems theory. This model views the family as just one of the basic units of the wider society, along with such institutions as those involving religion, education, and health. Its main focus is the family's structure and functions, and the family's relationships with other social systems. The Friedman Family Assessment Model consists of six broad categories of interview questions:

1. Identifying data (family last name, composition, ethnic background, religious identification, social class status)

2. Developmental stage and history of the family

3. Environmental data (characteristics of the home, neighborhood and larger community, geographic mobility, family's social support system)

4. Family structure (role structure, family values, communication patterns, and power structure)

5. Family functions (affective, socialization, reproductive, economic, health care)

6. Family coping (current stressors, coping strategies used, dysfunctional adaptive strategies used, problem areas in which family has achieved mastery)

Each category contains numerous subcategories. This assessment exists in a short and a long form. The short form is in Appendix E. This assessment is broad and general, and is especially useful for viewing families in the context of their community.

REFERENCES

Friedman, Bowden, & Jones. (2002). *Family nursing: Research, theory, & practice* (5th ed.). Upper Saddle River, NJ: Pearson Education, Inc.

Wright, L., & Leahy, M. (1994). *Nurses and families: A guide to family assessment and intervention.* Philadelphia: F.A. Davis.

SUGGESTED READINGS

Behrman, R., & Kliegman, R. (2002). *Nelson's essentials of pediatrics* (4th ed.). Philadelphia, PA: W.B. Saunders.

Berkowitz, C. (2000). *Pediatrics: A primary care approach* (2nd ed.). Philadelphia, PA: W.B. Saunders

Estes, M. E. Z. (2002). *Health assessment & physical examination* (2nd ed.). Clifton Park, NY: Thomson Delmar Learning.

Johnson, K., Oski, F. (Eds.). (1997). *Oski's essential pediatrics.* Philadephia, PA: Lippincott-Raven.

Murray, R., & Zentner, J. (2001). *Health promotion strategies through the lifespan* (7th ed.). Upper Saddle River, NJ: Prentice Hall.

Potts, N. & Mandleco, B. (Eds). (2002). *Caring for children and their families.* Clifton Park, NY: Thomson Delmar Learning.

Rebeschi, L., & Brown, M. (2002). *The pediatric nurses' survival guide* (2nd ed.). Clifton Park, NY: Thomson Delmar Learning.

CHAPTER 2

Theoretical Approaches to the Growth and Development of Children

Understanding human development is an essential part of the nursing process. Knowledge of normal behavior for specific age groups allows for individualizing assessments and care plans. Emphasis on promoting and maintaining health, anticipatory guidance related to human development, and assisting children and families achieve optimal development are all important aspects of pediatric nursing. Knowledge of several principles, issues, and theories helps us understand holistic optimal development and care. Various principles and issues that are interwoven within the major developmental theories follow. Each theory is summarized, and ideas on how the nurse can apply the theories to practice are presented.

to the physiological, psychosocial, and cognitive changes occurring over one's life span due to growth, maturation, and learning, and assumes that orderly and specific situations lead to new activities and behavior patterns.

The five stages and age ranges of human development relating specifically to pediatric nursing are found in Table 2-1.

PRINCIPLES OF GROWTH AND DEVELOPMENT

Eight principles provide a framework for studying human development. These principles are summarized in Table 2-2.

GROWTH, MATURATION, AND DEVELOPMENT

Growth refers to a physiologic increase in size through cell multiplication or differentiation. This is most obviously seen in weight and height changes occurring during the first year of life. Maturation refers to changes that are due to genetic inheritance rather than life experiences, illness, or injury, and that allow children to function at increasingly higher and more sophisticated levels as they get older. Development refers

Reflective Thinking

Principles of Development

Do you agree that development is orderly, sequential, directional, unique, and interrelated? Do you think development becomes increasingly differentiated, integrated, and complex as children get older? Are children competent? Do new skills predominate? Why? Provide examples other than those suggested in the text.

TABLE 2-1 STAGES, AGE RANGES, AND CHARACTERISTICS OF HUMAN DEVELOPMENT RELATED TO PEDIATRIC NURSING

Stage	Age	Characteristics
Infant	Birth to 1 year	Period of rapid growth and change; attachments to family members and other caregivers are formed; trust develops.
Toddler	1 to 3 years	Motor ability, coordination, sensory skills developing; basic feelings, emotions, a sense of self, and being independent become important.
Preschooler	3 to 6 years	Continued physiological, psychological, and cognitive growth; better able to care for selves, interested in playing with other children; beginning to develop a concept of who they are.
School age	6 to 12 years	Interested in achievement; ability to read, write, and complete academic work advances; understanding of the world broadens.
Adolescent	12 to 19 years, or later	Transition period between childhood and adulthood; physiological maturation occurs, formal operational thought begins; preparation for becoming an adult takes place.

TABLE 2-2 PRINCIPLES OF GROWTH AND DEVELOPMENT

Principle	Explanation
Development is orderly and sequential.	Maturation follows a predictable, universal timetable.
	Developmental changes occur rapidly during the first year of life and slow during middle and late childhood.
	Example: Children crawl before walking and walk before running.
Development is directional. Cephalocaudal Proximodistal	**Cephalocaudal:** from head downward (areas closest to the brain/head develop first followed by the trunk then the legs and feet).
	Example: Head control is followed by sitting then crawling and walking.

continues

TABLE 2-2 *Continued*	
Principle	**Explanation**
continued	**Proximodistal:** from the inside out (controlled movements closest to the body's center [trunk, arms] develop before controlled movements distant to the body [fingers]). *Example*: The grasp changes from using the entire hand (palmar grasp) to just using the fingers (pincer grasp).
Development is unique.	Every child has a unique timetable for physiological, psychosocial, cognitive, and moral development. *Example*: Some children can name four colors by the time they are 3 years old whereas other cannot name four colors until they are 4½ years old.
Development is related.	Physiological, psychosocial, cognitive, and moral aspects of development affect and are affected by one another. *Example*: Central nervous system maturity is necessary for cognitive development; children cannot be independent in toileting if they are not aware of the urge to void and cannot independently remove their clothing.
Development becomes increasingly differentiated.	Responses become more specific and skillful as the child gets older. *Example*: Infants react to pain with their entire body by crying and withdrawing, whereas a child is able to localize the pain, identify its source, and withdraw only the extremity experiencing the pain.
Development becomes increasingly integrated and complex.	As new skills are gained, more complex tasks are learned. *Example*: Infant's cooing is followed by babbling before these sounds are refined into understandable speech of a child.
Children are competent.	They possess qualities and abilities ensuring their survival and promoting their development. *Example*: Children make their needs known to caregivers in increasingly sophisticated ways so others know if they are cold, hungry, or in pain.
New skills predominate.	Children have a strong drive to practice and perfect new abilities especially when they are young and not capable of coping with several new skills simultaneously. *Example*: When children are learning to walk, talk, or feed themselves with utensils, their attention and effort is focused on developing that one skill; they do not usually learn to walk, talk, and feed themselves at the same time.

Family Teaching

Principles of Development

- Teach caregivers that development, although orderly and sequential, may vary in individual children, so some preschoolers may have advanced language skills and others may not.

- Remind caregivers of the importance of connections that exist among physiological, psychosocial, and cognitive development. For instance, children need to know what it feels like to have a wet diaper and to be able to tell the caregiver that they are wet before they can be success-fully toilet trained.

ISSUES OF HUMAN DEVELOPMENT

Theories of growth and development are often considered from the perspective of seven issues. These issues help explain how development occurs and what humans are like. They also answer questions related to the importance of biology or the environment on development, whether children are inherently good, bad, or actively involved in their own development, if development occurs gradually or abruptly, if children are

Reflective Thinking

Experiences and the Child

What do you think the impact of providing young children with experiences formerly reserved for older children (academic preschool, computer technology) has on developing specific skills, habits, or relationships? What impact does political and social change have on a child's development in countries experiencing loss of traditional cultural values?

more similar than different from one another, or if one's personality or way of interacting with others remains stable throughout life. The issues are presented in Table 2-3.

THEORIES OF HUMAN DEVELOPMENT

The following theoretical views present ways of examining human development during childhood and adolescence. Although each theory may describe only one aspect of development, holistic pediatric care assumes that all are important and need consideration when providing nursing interventions. Each theory focuses on particular areas of human development and has underlying assumptions, principles, strengths, and weaknesses that can help guide practice. Figure 2-1 provides a visualization of all theories discussed. Even though the figure is portrayed as a circle, consider it a sphere, with each part of the sphere a three-dimensional necessary part of the whole.

Psychoanalytic Perspective

These theories describe and define motivations and inner workings of the human mind during development, and answer questions related to the origin and development of personality and the outward expression of the inner self. Stages of development, unconscious motivation for behavior, and conflicts within the personality are emphasized (Sigelman, 1999). The psychoanalytic perspective is divided into the psychosexual (Freud), psychosocial (Erikson), and interpersonal (Sullivan) theories of development.

Freud and Psychosexual Development

The psychosexual theory emphasizes the importance of unconscious motivation and early childhood experiences in influencing

TABLE 2-3 ISSUES OF HUMAN DEVELOPMENT

Issue	Question asked	Beliefs	Comment
Nature versus Nurture	What influence does biology (nature) and the environment (nurture) have on an individual?	**Nature**: development is predetermined by genetic factors and not altered by the environment (eye color, body type).	Both are important; contribution of each depends on aspect of development studied.
		Nurture: development can take different pathways depending on the experiences an individual has over the life course.	Concern is how do both factors interact to produce developmental differences and changes, rather than the importance of one over the other.
Continuity versus Discontinuity	What is the nature of developmental change?	**Continuity**: change is orderly and built upon earlier experiences; development is gradual; early and late development are connected.	Both are true, as when children grow older they become taller, run faster, and learn more about the world around them (continuity) and also, as they grow older, they change from a nonverbal infant to a preschooler who uses language (discontinuity).
		Discontinuity: development is a series of discrete steps/stages that elevate the child to a more advanced/higher level of functioning as he/she gets older; early and late development are not connected.	
Passivity versus Activity	Are children passively shaped by the external environment or internally driven and active participants in their development?	**Passive**: child rearing beliefs, practices, and behaviors cause children to be either shy or assertive; children can learn by watching and listening to others.	Both behaviors may operate in a child depending on the situation he/she is in.
		Active: children purposefully, creatively, and actively seek experiences to control, direct, and shape their development; children can modify caregiver, peer, and teacher behavior.	

continues

TABLE 2-3 *Continued*

Issue	Question asked	Beliefs	Comment
Critical versus Sensitive Period	How important are different time periods in development? Are some phases more important than others in developing particular abilities, knowledge, or skills?	**Critical Period**: a limited time span when a child is biologically prepared to acquire certain behaviors. **Sensitive Period**: a time span that is optimal for certain capacities to emerge when the individual is especially receptive to environmental influences.	The first 3 years of life are important for language, social, and emotional development. If there is little or no opportunity for experiences in these areas during this time, difficulties may arise in these areas later in life. However, some behaviors can be modified during early development if children have positive experiences that counteract these early deficiencies.
Universality versus Context Specificity	Does culture influence development? Are there some aspects of development that apply to all children in all cultures?	**Universality**: humans follow similar developmental pathways regardless of their culture. **Context Specificity**: children are different because of their cultural values, beliefs, and experiences.	Language is acquired and used at 11–14 months of age and cognitive changes occurring during 5–7 years of age prepare children for schooling or higher learning. However, some societies encourage early walking whereas other cultures carry or swaddle infants, thereby reducing the chance of walking until older.

continues

TABLE 2-3 *Continued*

Issue	Question asked	Beliefs	Comment
Assumptions of Human Nature	Are children inherently good, evil, or neither?	**Innate Purity**: children are inherently good and born without an intuitive sense of what is right and wrong.	Emphasis on positive or negative aspects of a child's character reflect an individual's orientation and assumptions about human nature. If one believes children are inherently caring and helpful or on the other hand selfish, child rearing practices would vary. Permissive parents may believe children should be allowed to develop without interference whereas authoritarian parents may take an approach that would combat and control their child's selfish and aggressive impulses.
		Original Sin: children are inherently evil and selfish egotists who must be controlled by society.	
		Tabula Rasa: children enter the world as a blank slate without inborn tendencies and are molded by life experiences.	
Behavioral Consistency	Do a child's basic behavioral traits change according to the setting?	**Consistency**: individual personality characteristics and predispositions cause children to behave similarly no matter the setting.	Children's behavior sometimes does change according to the situation and who/what is present (friend in need, angry caregiver, teacher), but for many children, their core personality really does not change.
		Inconsistency: children's behavior changes from one setting to another.	

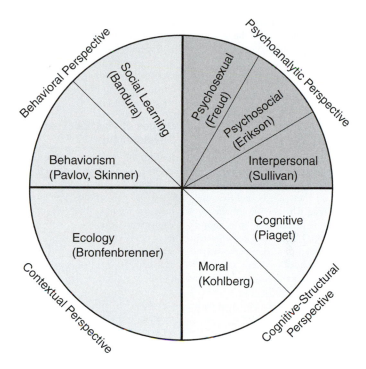

Figure 2-1 The Eclectic Nature of Human Development

behavior and describes concepts related to personality and stages of development (Freud, 1933).

Central to Freudian theory is the notion that two basic biological instincts (life and death) motivate behavior, must be satisfied, and compete for supremacy (Freud, 1933). The life instinct is responsible for such activities as eating and breathing, and behavior that expresses self preservation, love, and constructive conduct. The death instinct is a destructive force expressed by self centered and cruel behavior, hate, aggression, and destructive conduct. These instincts have three components: id, ego, and superego (Freud, 1933).

During infancy, all psychic energy resides in the id, the inborn element of personality that is driven by selfish urges. The id obeys the "pleasure principle," and is oriented toward maximizing pleasure and immediately satisfying needs. The id is manifest as the irrational, selfish, impulsive part of personality (Freud, 1933).

The ego operates according to the "reality principle," allows individuals to be successful, and includes memory, cognition, intelligence, problem solving, compromising, separating reality from fantasy, and incorporating experiences and learning into future behavior. Ego development continues during childhood and throughout the life span (Freud, 1933).

The third component of personality is the superego or conscience, which emerges when the child internalizes caregiver or societal values, roles, and morals. Superego development becomes apparent in the preschool and school-aged years when the child learns socially acceptable behavior. The superego strives for perfection rather than for pleasure or reality. After the superego emerges, children have a conscience that tells them the difference between right and wrong. The superego also serves as a disciplinarian by creating feelings of remorse and guilt for transgressing rules, and self praise and pride for adhering to rules (Freud, 1933).

Conflict among the id, ego, and superego is inevitable. Mature, healthy personalities, however, are in a dynamic balance, with the id communicating its basic needs, the ego restraining the id until realistic ways are found to satisfy these needs, and the superego determining whether or not the ego's problem-solving strategies are morally acceptable. Freud believed defense mechanisms, such as regression, displacement, projection, and sublimation were created to repress painful experiences or threatening thoughts coming from the id's unsatisfied needs, and which were not managed by the ego or superego (Freud, 1933).

To Freud, the most important life instinct was the sex instinct, which changed its character and focus according to biological maturation. As the sex instinct's psychic energy (libido) shifts from one part of the body to another, the child passes through five stages

of development: oral, anal, phallic, latency, and genital (Table 2-4). Each stage is related to a specific body part (erogenous zone) that brings primary pleasure to the child during that stage. According to Freud, adult personality is profoundly impacted by how each stage is managed.

Stages of Psychosexual Development

During the oral stage (birth to 1 year), the infant is preoccupied with activities associated with the mouth such as sucking, biting, chewing, and satisfying hunger. Freud believed infants received satisfaction and enjoyment from these oral behaviors and later development was affected by how well oral needs were met as well as how closely attached the infant was to the mother who usually met these needs (Freud, 1933).

During the anal stage (1–3 years), sphincter muscles are maturing and children develop the ability to eliminate and retain fecal material. Sexual urges are gratified primarily by learning to voluntarily defecate. Freud suggested that methods caregivers use to toilet train children during this period may have long lasting effects on personality (Freud, 1933).

TABLE 2-4 STAGES OF FREUD'S PSYCHOSEXUAL DEVELOPMENT

Stage	Age	Characteristics
Oral	Birth to 1 year	Receives satisfaction from oral needs being met; attachment to mother important because she usually meets infant's needs
Anal	1 to 3 years	Learning to control body functions, especially toileting
Phallic	3 to 6 years	Fascinated with gender differences, childbirth; Oedipus/Electra complex
Latency	6 to 11 years	Sexual drives submerged; appropriate gender roles adopted; learning about society
Genital	12 years and older	Sexual desires directed toward opposite gender; learns how to form loving relationships and manage sexual urges in societally appropriate ways

During the phallic stage (3–6 years), the child's psychic energy is redirected to the genitals. Children are curious about childbirth, fascinated with anatomic differences, and find pleasure in their own genitals. The phallus (penis) assumes a critical role in the development of both boys and girls. Girls wish they had a penis (penis envy) and occasionally believe they once had one that was removed by a jealous, hostile mother. Boys fear losing their penis due to an attack or injury by others (castration anxiety). During these years, children also develop a strong incestuous desire for the caregiver of the opposite gender. The Oedipal complex (attachment of a boy to his mother) and Electra complex (attachment of a girl to her father) produce anxiety that must be resolved and controlled. Resolution and control allows children to identify with the caregiver of the same gender and fosters male and female identity (Freud, 1933).

During the latency stage (6–11 years), sexual drives are submerged, appropriate gender roles are adopted, and the Oedipal/Electra conflicts are resolved. Since by now the superego has developed sufficiently to keep the id under control, children in this period rapidly learn about society and themselves while developing useful skills. They increasingly identify with the same-gender caregiver and become intensely involved with their same-gender peers. Energies are directed toward school, play, and increasing their problem-solving abilities (Freud, 1933).

Freud's last period, the genital stage, begins at puberty (about age 12) and lasts throughout adulthood. Sexual desires reemerge due to physiological changes, fluctuating hormone levels, and changing social relationships. Before mature adult adjustment is possible however, turmoil and adaptation are necessary. The adolescent vacillates between dependence/independence from parents, learns how to form loving relationships, and manages sexual urges in societally appropriate ways. These psychic conflicts are necessary for fully functioning and mature adult personality development (Freud, 1933).

Reflective Thinking

Psychosexual Development

Which points of Freud's theory of psychosexual development do you agree or disagree with? Provide examples. How relevant and current is Freud's theory today? Explain your thinking.

Application

Freud helps us understand others by acknowledging that all behavior is meaningful and may hide inner needs or conflicts. It is especially important to teach this information, as well as normal behavior for the various stages, to parents. Since during infancy comfort and pleasure are obtained through the mouth, when hungry, infants should be promptly fed (if not NPO). Providing plastic or rubber rings or other toys suitable for teething infants is also appropriate.

Toddlers are gratified by controlling body excretions. Therefore, it is wise to provide a child-sized potty chair and avoid starting toilet training during periods of illness or stress. In addition, toddlers should be reprimanded carefully if toilet training is difficult or if the child has accidents. Finally, parents need to be flexible and patient in toilet training and begin when the toddler indicates readiness.

Preschool children are concerned about sexuality and initially identify with the parent of the opposite gender. Parents should be taught that curiosity about gender differences and masturbation is normal. School-aged children and adolescents should be encouraged to have contact with friends, and their questions answered honestly. Privacy for both school age and adolescent clients should be ensured during physical examinations or when they are changing clothes or showering in gym class.

Erikson and Psychosocial Development

Erik Erikson (1902–1994) acknowledged the contribution of biologic factors to development, but felt that the environment, culture, and society were also important. His psychosocial (epigenetic) theory of development stresses the complexity of inter-relationships existing between emotional and physical variables during one's lifetime (Erikson, 1963). Erikson agreed with many of Freud's ideas regarding basic instincts and the three components of personality (id, ego, superego). In addition, he believed development was stage-like, and conflict resolution was necessary at each stage in order for the individual to successfully advance to the next stage. Erikson's first five stages of development and the approximate ages of each stage correspond closely with those outlined by Freud an other theorists (Table 2-5). Erikson differs from Freud, however, in that he believes children actively adapt to and explore their environment instead of being controlled and molded by caregivers and society; and that children are rational creatures whose actions, feelings, and thoughts are controlled primarily by the ego.

For Erikson, lifespan development consisted of eight sequential stages. Five of these stages describe infants through adolescents (Table 2-6). Each stage is dominated by major developmental conflicts or crises related to societal demands and expectations that must be addressed or resolved before the individual can progress to the next stage. The resolution of each conflict or crisis might be positive (favorable and growth enhancing), or negative (unfavorable, frustrating, and making later development difficult). Erikson believed that major conflicts occurring during each stage are rarely completely resolved. Instead, they are of primary or dominant importance during a particular stage and then become less important or dominant as other conflicts arise in later stages. In addition, he suggested that conflict is rarely completely resolved positively. Rather, the positive resolution predominates over the negative resolution. Failure to successfully master a crisis or developmental task does not destine the child to failure since delayed mastery is possible. It is true, however, that difficulty at one stage may affect progress through later stages (Erickson, 1963).

Stages of Psychosocial Development

Erikson's first stage, trust versus mistrust, occurs during infancy (1 month to 1½ years) when the basic task is to establish trust rather than mistrust in relation to oneself and others. Infants whose needs for comfort, food, and warmth are effectively and consistently met by a nurturing caregiver learn that the world is not only predictable, but safe, reliable, and trustwothy. If caregivers are unpredictable, inconsistent, inadequate, or convey a sense of confusion or chaos, the child learns to view the environment with mistrust or wariness, and may demonstrate restlessness, crying, whining, sleep disturbances, vomiting, or diarrhea (Erikson, 1963).

During the toddler years (1½ to 3 years), autonomy versus shame and doubt occurs. Autonomy develops as children discover their new abilities while improving language and motor skills and learning competencies related to bathing, eating, toileting, and dressing. Shame occurs if assertiveness and independence are considered unacceptable or ineffective by caregivers. Doubt occurs if children learn to mistrust not only themselves, but also others in the immediate environment. Children demonstrating dependency and constantly needing approval for their actions have not resolved this conflict (Erikson, 1963).

The third developmental stage (3–6 years) is initiative versus guilt. Initiative refers to a person's independently beginning an activity rather than merely responding to or imitating others. It occurs when a child tries out new ways of combining activities, invents creative ways to use skills and abilities, imagines what other people or things are like, and takes responsibility for one's own actions. Guilt occurs when caregivers frequently reprimand behaviors reflecting initiative. Children experiencing guilt may become passive, reluctant, or refuse to participate in activities (Erikson, 1963).

The major developmental task of the school age years (6–11 years) is industry versus inferiority. Industry involves mastery of social, physical, and intellectual skills, and

TABLE 2-5	COMPARISON OF STAGE THEORIES OF HUMAN DEVELOPMENT				
Age Period	**Freud**	**Erikson**	**Sullivan**	**Piaget**	**Kohlberg**
Infancy (Birth to 1 year)	Oral (Birth to 1 year)	Trust/Mistrust (Birth to 1½ years)	Infant (Birth to 1½ years)	Sensorimotor (Birth to 2 years)	Preconventional (Birth to 7 years)
Toddler (1 to 3 years)	Anal (1 to 3 years)	Trust/Mistrust (continued)	Infant (continued)	Sensorimotor (continued)	Preconventional (continued)
		Autonomy/ Shame-Doubt (1½ to 3 years)	Early Childhood (1½ to 6 years)	Preoperational (2 to 7 years)	
Preschool (3 to 6 years)	Phallic (3 to 6 years)	Initiative/Guilt (3 to 6 years)	Early Childhood (continued)	Preoperational (continued)	Preconventional (continued)
School age (6 to 12 years)	Latency (6 to 12 years)	Industry/Inferiority (6 to 12 years)	Late Childhood (6 to 9 years)	Concrete Operations (7 to 11 years)	Conventional (7 to 12 years)
			Preadolescence (9 to 12 years)		
Adolescence (12 to 19 years)	Genital (12 years and older)	Identity/Role Confusion (12 to 18 years)	Early Adolescence (12 to 15 years)	Formal Operations (12 years and older)	Postconventional (12 years and older)
			Late Adolescence (15 to 19 years)		

TABLE 2-6	STAGES OF ERIKSON'S PSYCHOSOCIAL THEORY OF DEVELOPMENT	
Stage	**Age**	**Characteristics**
Trust versus Mistrust	1 month to 1½ years	Learns world is good and can be trusted as basic needs are met
Autonomy versus Shame and Doubt	1½ to 3 years	Learns independent behaviors regarding toileting, bathing, feeding, dressing; exerts self; exercises choices
Initiative versus Guilt	3 to 6 years	Goal directed, competitive, exploratory behavior; imaginative play
Industry versus Inferiority	6 to 11 years	Learns self worth as gains mastery of psychosocial, physiological, and cognitive skills; becomes society/peer focused
Identity versus Role Confusion	12 to 18 years	Develops sense of who I am; gains independence from parents; peers important

orientation toward and competition with peers. Attention and energy are devoted to learning academic skills and social roles, as the child becomes less family focused and more society and peer focused. Inferiority develops when school-aged children are ridiculed by peers, don't measure up to adult or their own expectations, or lack certain skills so they are not always the best, first, fastest, or smartest (Erikson, 1963).

Adolescence (12 to 18 years) is characterized by identity versus role confusion. Identity involves achieving a sense of who one is intellectually, cognitively, behaviorally, and emotionally. Erikson believed identity is attained as the young person's view of who one is becomes consistent with others' views, and requires resolution of subconflicts, including finding one's own political, social, economic, and religious ideology, adopting an appropriate gender identity, making an occupational or vocational choice, and adopting behaviors consistent with one's own self concept. Identity formation affects commitments and decisions made later in life.

Role confusion occurs when the adolescent is unable to acquire a sense of direction, self, or place within the world (Erikson, 1963).

Erikson identified three other stages beyond identity versus role confusion that occur during adulthood. They are intimacy versus isolation, generativity versus stagnation, and integrity versus despair. In each of these stages, as with the earlier stages, conflict needs to be resolved before the next stage is reached.

Application

Erikson's theory provides a means of assessing and gaining insight into developmental crises children and adolescents face, and allows us to use this knowledge to teach caregivers behaviors they can expect to see. It also helps us realize the importance of societal influences on health and behavior, and that psychosocial development is a lifelong process.

Erikson's theory is easy to apply to practice. Health care provides a variety of situations and opportunities where a child's

👁 Eye On:

Psychosocial Development

The culture and beliefs that people grow up with will affect how they trust and express autonomy, initiative, industry, and identity. Reflect how you navigated these stages, then compare your findings to someone else's who comes from a different cultural background.

Critical Thinking

Using Psychosocial Development in Practice

How would you identify children having difficulty developing trust, autonomy, initiative, industry, or identity? What suggestions would you give parents to help them help their children positively resolve each developmental crisis?

progression through stages can be facilitated, and caregivers taught how to encourage positive resolution of each developmental crisis. Since meeting basic needs (feeding, bathing, changing) in a timely and appropriate fashion during infancy results in the development of trust, it is critical that feeding and hygiene needs be met promptly.

For toddlers, familiar daily routines help foster independence and self control. Allowing opportunities for the child to independently dress, feed, and do self-hygiene care is important.

Preschoolers like to initiate activities and remain curious and interested in the world around them. Opportunities to explore, ask questions, and create should be provided. Accepting children's choices and negative expression of feelings, answering their questions, and allowing them to play with unfamiliar equipment so their curiosity is satisfied and their knowledge about experiences broadened is important.

For school-aged children, involvement and success in a variety of activities provide a sense of self-worth and value. School work, hobbies or activities, opportunities to interact with their peers, and adjustments to new limitations should all be part of the school-aged child's experience.

Adolescents are searching for who they will become independent from their parents. Adolescents should be as autonomous as possible, and encouraged to take responsibility for their own actions. Parental involvement and guidance in the life of adolescents is important.

Family Teaching

Erikson's Theory

- Teach parents to meet infants' basic needs in a timely and appropriate manner.

- Allow opportunities for toddlers to be independent.

- Provide preschoolers with a variety of experiences where they can explore, ask questions, and create.

- Encourage school-aged children to interact with peers.

- Support adolescents' choices, be available to listen, and offer guidance.

Sullivan and Interpersonal Development

Harry Stack Sullivan (1892–1949) focused on interpersonal relations as important motivators and the source of psychological health. His interpersonal theory posits that self concept is the key to personality development. He acknowledged the importance of the environment (especially the home), and also emphasized the role of social approval and disapproval in forming a child's self concept. Sullivan believed personality development was largely the result of childhood experiences, interpersonal encounters, and the mother–child relationship. How well physiological needs were met in an interpersonal situation affected not only one's sense of satisfaction and security, but also prevented anxiety (Sullivan, 1953).

Stages of Interpersonal Development

Sullivan describes seven stages of interpersonal development (Sullivan, 1953); six relate specifically to infants through adolescents (Table 2-7). Sullivan believed each stage prepared the personalty for the next stage and failure to successfully achieve stage activities limited personality development and opportunities for a successful life. Refer to Table 2-5 for a comparison of Sullivan's first six stages with Freud's and Erikson's stages.

The first stage (infant) encompasses birth to when the child is able to use words that convey the same meaning to the child as they do to others (18 months). The primary task revolves around learning to rely on others, especially the primary caregiver, to gratify physiological needs and achieve satisfaction. When basic needs are met, infants are in a state of well being. If these needs are not met, a fear-like state occurs, manifested by excessive crying or difficulties eating or sleeping. Infants are sensitive to others' attitudes and emotions while these needs are being met. Sullivan felt one's self image emerged according to how the infant interpreted the mother (primary caregiver)–infant relationship when these needs were met. "Good me" feelings occur when acceptance is sensed; "bad me" feelings occur when the infant experiences anxiety while interacting with caregivers. Excessive anxiety may cause children to believe they are bad, leading to feelings of inferiority or depression. "Good me" and "bad me" fuse around 18 months of age; but the dominant "me" can change with situational or maturational crises (Sullivan, 1953).

During the early childhood stage (18 months to 6 years), children are able to communicate better with others, thereby facilitating interpersonal relationships. As children learn to recognize signs indicating

TABLE 2-7   STAGES OF SULLIVAN'S INTERPERSONAL THEORY OF DEVELOPMENT

Stage	Age	Characteristics
Infant	Birth to 18 months	Learns to rely on others, especially mother; "good me/bad me" emerges
Early Childhood	18 months to 6 years	Learns to clarify communication; recognizes approval/disapproval; delays gratification
Late Childhood	6 to 9 years	Increasing intellectual abilities; learns to control behavior and own place in the world
Preadolescence	9 to 12 years	Vulnerable to teasing; "chum" important
Early Adolescence	12 to 15 years	Mastering independence; develops relationships with persons of opposite gender
Late Adolescence	15 to 19 years	Masters expression of sexual impulses; forms responsible and satisfying relationships with others

approval/disapproval of their behavior, they learn about controlling personal desires, delaying gratification, and accepting interference from others. Excess parental disapproval during this time may cause children to view themselves and the world as negative and/or hostile.

The third stage, late childhood (6–9 years), is characterized by increasing intellectual ability and developing internal control over behavior. Children learn to pay attention to others' wishes, form satisfying relations with peers of both genders, and sometimes oppose rules. They also learn to accept subordination from authority figures (parents, teachers, other adults) and develop a sense of their own status and role in society (Sullivan, 1953).

During preadolescence (9–12 years), children participate in an expanding world that provides confrontation with rules and knowledge about themselves. They realize their status within the peer group is based on performance, are vulnerable to teasing, and become interested in relating closely to a peer of the same gender, which Sullivan calls the "chum." Preadolescents who do not have a chum may experience difficulty with relationships later (Sullivan, 1953).

During early adolescence (12–15 years), independence is mastered and satisfying relations with members of the opposite gender are established as attempts are made to integrate sexual urges with other aspects of personal relationships. Early adolescents may demonstrate a variety of behaviors including rebellion, dependence, cooperation, and collaboration as they become independent.

The sixth stage is termed late adolescence (15–19 years). Sullivan believes initial feelings of love for the opposite gender emerge here, as the individual learns to master expression of sexual impulses, form responsible and satisfying relationships, and use communication skills in interactions.

Application

Sullivan emphasizes the significance of interpersonal relations with others on personality development, and meeting the child's basic needs in a timely and appropriate fashion. This does not mean, however, that caregivers protect children from all discomforts or meet needs before they are expressed. The key is to relieve unpleasant feelings associated with basic needs so feelings of security and attachment result in a "good me" rather than a "bad me." Sullivan also has helped us realize the important place chums have in a school-aged child's life, and how this experience is critical for developing interpersonal relationships later in life.

Nurses need to teach caregivers about Sullivan's theory so they may help their child develop a healthy personality, and realize the importance that they, the caregivers, have in a child's life.

Family Teaching

Sullivan

- Teach caregivers that their interactions with children should be positive, nurturing, and consistent.

- Remind caregivers that children need special friends during the school age years to share experiences, secrets, and dreams.

Reflective Thinking

Contributions of the Psychoanalytic Perspective

Consider the contributions the psychoanalytic perspective makes to the study of human development. Do you think that caregivers influence young children as much as Freud, Erikson, and Sullivan suggest? Why or why not? How would you explain children who grow up in dysfunctional environments but who overcome adversity and become well-adjusted and psychologically healthy adults?

Behavioral Perspective

The behavioral perspective posits that human actions and interactions come from learned responses to environmental stimuli. Behavioral theorists look for ways to alter or control the environment to change, modify, or teach desired behaviors. The past or unconscious motives are not related to behavior and learning does not depend on maturation. These theorists believe children randomly respond to the environment consistent with developmental capabilities, and rewards and/or punishment influence behavior. Behavior resulting in punishment, pain, disappointment, or frustration often is discontinued, whereas behavior that is rewarded or viewed positively is retained and repeated in similar situations. The behavioral perspective is divided into behaviorism (operant conditioning) and social learning (Crain, 2000; Sigelman, 1999).

Skinner and Operant Conditioning

Operant conditioning, a term originated by B. F. Skinner (1904–1990), involves behavioral changes due to either negative (punishment) or positive (reinforcers) consequences rather than just the occurrence of a stimuli. If behavior is rewarded, the likelihood of it reoccurring increases; if behavior is punished, chances are it will not reoccur. Positive reinforcement includes friendly smiles, praise, or special treats/privileges; punishment includes criticism, a frown, or withdrawal of privileges. Skinner discovered that behavioral change became more permanent when consequences were provided intermittently rather than continuously, and believed development involved constantly acquiring new behaviors or habits due to reinforcing or punishing stimuli. He emphasized why behaviors occur rather than simply describing the behavior seen (Skinner, 1953).

Bandura and Social Learning

According to social learning, children learn by imitating and observing others (a model), as well as by conditioning. Social learning theorists also believe behavior is influenced by the environment and learned through various experiences. However, they do not believe behavioral change is a mindless response to stimuli. Rather, they suggest personality, past experiences, relationships with the model, the situation itself, and cognition impact behavioral change (Bandura, 1977).

Bandura believes modeled behavior can be weakened or strengthened depending on whether it is punished or rewarded. Bandura suggests observational learning (learning that results from merely watching others), where children acquire a variety of new behaviors when "models" are merely pursuing their own interests and not attempting to teach, reward, or punish, is another important method of learning behaviors. For example, research has shown children who watch television violence frequently are more aggressive than those children who do not watch very much television violence (Murray & Zentner, 2001). Finally, Bandura found children tend to model behavior of children and adults of their same gender more often than not, and males model behavior of others more often than females do (Crain, 2000; Sigelman, 1999).

Application

Positive behaviors should be reinforced by encouragement, praise, and other rewards, and behaviors needing to be altered or removed from a child's repertoire can be extinguished by either ignoring or punishing.

Family Teaching

Behavioral Perspective

- Reprimanding children for their unacceptable behavior should be consistent and appropriate.

- Children will model behavior they see in their parents even if parents talk to children about not modeling that same behavior.

Some academic and preschool programs and parents use behavior modification and time-out activities to modify and change undesirable behavior in children. Conditioning can also help develop new or extinguish undesirable behavior by providing specific guidelines, determining available reinforcers, identifying responses acceptable for reinforcement, and planning how reinforcers will be scheduled so behavior is repeated.

Critical Thinking

Children and the Media

How would the behavioral perspective explain the effect the media (television, movies, videos, newspapers, the Internet) has on children and adolescents relative to violence, drug use, and promiscuity? What might you do to help caregivers concerned about this issue?

Reflective Thinking

Behavioral Perspective

How would you use social learning and conditioning to change a child's behavior and attitudes toward responsibility and accountability?

Cognitive-Structural Perspective

Cognitive-structural theorists are concerned with how children learn to reason, use language, and think, rather than what they learn. These theorists believe cognitive development is the result of the interaction between central nervous system maturation and active involvement with the environment. They also believe children constantly adapt to their world by integrating new knowledge with existing knowledge. The most significant cognitive-structural theorists are Jean Piaget and Lawrence Kohlberg.

Piaget and Cognitive Development

Jean Piaget (1896–1980) began studying children's intellectual development during the 1920s. He was fascinated by the process and steps children took as they discovered, reinvented, understood, and acquired knowledge of the world around them. He felt that from the moment of birth, children not only acted upon and transformed their environment, but also were shaped by the consequences of their actions. This constant interplay was responsible for intellectual growth.

Piaget believed intellectual growth followed an orderly progression based on the child's maturational level, experiences with physical objects, interactions with caregivers, other adults and peers, and an internal self-regulating mechanism that responded to environmental stimuli. He used several terms (schema, assimilation, accommodation, equilibrium) to describe cognitive development (Piaget, 1963).

To Piaget, interactions with the environment caused people to organize patterns of thought (schema), which they used to interpret or make sense of their experiences. For example, young children who believe the sun is alive because it moves are operating on the schema that moving things are alive. As children develop, they may regard other moving objects they see (wind up toy, animals) as alive as well, thereby demonstrating assimilation, or interpreting new information in terms of existing information. As they get older, children continually encounter animate and inanimate objects, and learn all objects are not alive. For example, trees do not move from one area of the yard to another even though they are alive. This more adequate understanding of differences between nonliving and living objects reflects accommodation, or revising, readjusting, or realigning existing schema to accept this new information. Assimilation and accommodation result in equilibrium, or harmonious relationships between thought processes and the environment (Piaget, 1963; Wadsworth, 1989).

Stages of Cognitive Development

According to Piaget, cognitive development occurs gradually, sequentially, and without regression. He postulated that development moves from simple to complex, begins with concrete situations and objects, and proceeds to abstraction. Piaget suggested cognitive development passes through four stages and several phases within some of these stages. Stages represented increased integration and organization, and although sequential, children could pass through them at different rates. Table 2-8 presents Piaget's stages of cognitive development. Refer back to Table 2-5 to compare Piaget's stages with Freud, Erikson, and Sullivan.

During the sensorimotor stage (birth to age 2), cognitive functioning is begun and sensory and motor capabilities are used to gain a basic understanding of the world. Infants learn goal-directed behavior, alternate ways of achieving a goal, the connection between cause and effect, and that they can make things happen. Infants also acquire a primitive sense of who they are and their relation to others, and realize objects con-

TABLE 2-8   STAGES OF PIAGET'S THEORY OF COGNITIVE DEVELOPMENT

Stage	Age	Characteristics
Sensorimotor	**Birth to 2 years**	
Reflexive	Birth to 1 month	Predictable, innate survival reflexes
Primary Circular Reactions	1 to 4 months	Responds purposefully to stimuli; initiates, repeats satisfying behaviors
Secondary Circular Reactions	4 to 8 months	Learns from intentional behavior; motor skills/vision coordinated; recognizes familiar objects
Coordination of Secondary Schemes	8 to 12 months	Develops object permanence; anticipates others' actions; differentiates familiar/unfamiliar
Tertiary Circular Reactions	12 to 18 months	Interested in novelty, repetition; understands causality; solicits help from others
Mental Combinations	18 to 24 months	Simple problem solving; imitates
Preoperational	**2 to 7 years**	
Preconceptual	2 to 4 years	Egocentric thought; mental imagery; increasing language
Intuitive	4 to 7 years	Sophisticated language; decreasing egocentric thought; reality-based play
Concrete operations	**7 to 11 years**	Understands relationships, classification, conservation, seriation, reversibility; logical reasoning limited; less egocentric thought
Formal operations	**11 years and older**	Capable of systematic, abstract thought

tinue to exist even after they are out of sight (object permanence). For example, 6-month-old infants will continue to look for a rattle that has been dropped on the floor even though they cannot see it.

The sensorimotor stage is divided into six phases. The reflexive phase (birth to 1 month) is characterized by innate survival reflexes (sucking, grasping) becoming more efficient and generalized. During the primary circular reaction phase (1–4 months), the infant performs more complex, repetitive behaviors that may be responses to chance events centering on the infant's own body (following objects that disappear, expecting disappeared objects to reappear). They initiate and repeat satisfying behavior, and learn how their body feels. During this phase infants commonly look and reach for objects. From 4 to 8 months, (secondary circular reaction phase), the infant learns from intentional behavior (shaking rattle to hear sound), usually explores the world from a sitting position, and begins to show some understanding of objects (recognizes familiar objects, searches for objects when they disappear). Motor skills and vision become further coordinated and interest in the environment increases. The coordination of secondary schemes phase (8–12 months) occurs when the infant understands concepts of space and object permanence, learns to direct actions toward an intended goal (searches for hidden objects; drops, throws, examines objects), and anticipates actions of others (caregiver comes with crying). They can differentiate objects (caregiver and stranger; familiar toy and unfamiliar toy), and begin developing habits. The tertiary circular reactions phase (12–18 months) is characterized by interest in novelty and repetition (continually hitting toy hammer on variety of surfaces or objects), awareness that objects which are out of sight continue to exist, understanding of causality (if I throw my toy out of the crib, I cannot reach it), and ability to solicit help (obtain an unreachable toy). Between 12 and 18 months, solutions to problems will be discovered, objects will be increasingly explored to learn how they work, and new behaviors developed. During the mental combinations phase (18–24 months), young children are able to think before acting and use memory for simple trial and error problem solving. They can name and locate familiar objects, predict effects when observing causes, imitate behavior, and demonstrate symbolic and ritualistic play (Piaget, 1963).

During the preoperational stage (2–7 years), children use language and have a growing understanding of the past, present, and future. However, they have not yet developed the concept of irreversibility. That is, if one of two clay balls that are the same size is flattened in front of the child, the child will not believe the two clay balls still contain the same amount of clay. Children do not fully grasp the relationship between objects and events, and do not understand the process of transition (if A is less than B, and B is less than C, then A is less than C). Their thought is egocentric (unable to take another's perspective); they are easily fooled, respond to events and objects according to how they appear, are not able to understand the fundamental relationships among and between phenomena, and intermingle fantasy with reality. By the end of the stage they begin to realize others do not always perceive the world as they do (Piaget, 1963).

Piaget divides the preoperational stage into two phases, the preconceptual and intuitive phases. The preconceptual phase (2-4 years) is characterized by increasing use of language, egocentric thought, symbolic play, and mental imagery. During the intuitive phase (4–7 years), the child demonstrates more sophisticated language development, decreasing egocentrism, incessant questioning, and more reality-based play. Children during this phase cannot focus on more than one aspect of a situation at the same time, are easily deluded by appearances, believe every question has a simple and direct answer, can concentrate either on the parts or the whole of an object but cannot relate to both at the same time, and cannot reverse actions, situations or physical properties of objects (i.e., wide and tall containers do not contain the same amount of water even if the child is shown that the containers have the same volume). They also believe inanimate objects have human feelings and are capable of human actions, assume everything has been created either by humans or a supernatural force, use symbolic play (pieces of wood become boats, trucks, cars, animals), and act out events experienced in their everyday life (Piaget 1963).

Children acquire and use mental activities in the concrete operations stage (7–11 years) and begin understanding the basic properties of and relationships between objects and events. Their capability for logical reasoning is limited to their experiences. However, they are able to classify objects into several categories (size, shape, color), and understand the principle of conservation (things are the same even though shape or arrangement changes). They can also understand seriation according to a principle (arrange buttons according to size). Children in this stage tend to solve practical problems through trial and error, understand reversibility (a lump of clay contains the same volume when it is shaped into a ball or rolled into a rope), focus on several dimensions at the same time (color, size, shape), develop intricate rules, see others' viewpoints, and understand others' intentions (Piaget 1963).

The formal operations stage (12 years and older) is characterized by systematic and abstract thought. Because they may enjoy thinking about hypothetical issues, children and adolescents in this stage may become idealistic. Their developing deductive reasoning abilities allows them to consider alternate solutions before choosing the correct answer. Their developing inductive reasoning ability allow them to organize and construct theories about their ideas. Children and adolescents in this stage move from what is real to what is possible, and can project themselves into and plan for the future. Finally, they have a better understanding of mathematics and scientific principles (proportion, variables) and are able to establish personal values and rules (Piaget, 1963).

Application

During the sensorimotor stage infants use sight and motor skills to learn about the environment and become familiar with their abilities. Manipulative toys, mobiles, and bright pictures or photographs are helpful since young children in this stage receive comfort from these objects. The environment should be safe, and opportunities provided for exploring and manipulating objects. During the preoperational stage children become more verbal but are limited in thought processes. Therefore, careful explanations of experiences in language the child will understand are important. Children also need to be reassured that they are not responsible for illnesses in themselves or others.

School-aged children are in the concrete operations stage. This means they are capable of mature thought, but need to manipulate or see objects to understand how they are related, change, or interact. Details are important when providing explanations, but care should be taken so the child understands the discussion.

Adolescents are capable of abstract thought (formal operations). Therefore, providing complete and clearly understood information, both verbally and in writing, is important. However, since all adolescents may not have developed mature abstract

Family Teaching

Cognitive Development

- Remind caregivers their children may learn at different rates and in different ways. Even though adolescents are capable of formal operational thought, some still may use concrete operations.

- Encourage caregivers and family members to use simple language when talking with young children and help them understand that directions may need to be repeated several times, or paired with a demonstration. Encourage family members to be patient with children's questions as that is the way they learn about the world.

Reflective Thinking

Cognitive Development

Think about experiences in your own life that provide examples of Piaget's concepts of assimilation and accommodation. Describe them. Provide examples of formal and concrete operational thought. Do you use concrete operational thought more or less than formal operational thought? Explain your position.

thought, information may need to be presented at a more concrete or individualized level.

Kohlberg and Moral Development

Lawrence Kohlberg (1927–1987) formulated a theory of moral development that described changes in thinking about moral judgments and reflected societal norms and values. In developing his theory, he asked children and adults to resolve a series of moral dilemmas, thereby challenging them to choose between obeying a rule, law, or authority figure and taking action to serve a human need that conflicts with these rules, laws, or authority figures. For example, should a mother who cannot afford an expensive drug that would save the life of her child steal the drug from a pharmacy? Kohlberg was interested in the underlying rationale for the moral decisions rather than the decision itself (Kohlberg, 1963).

He also believed moral development was influenced by internal and external factors. Internal factors included empathy, intelligence, impulse control, and the ability to judge behavior. External factors included rewards, punishment, family structure, and parent/peer contacts (Lewis & Volkmar, 1990). Finally, he suggests moral growth progressed through universal and invariant sequences of three broad levels, each containing several stages (Kohlberg, 1963). Table 2-9 presents Kohlberg's stages of moral

development. Refer back to Table 2-5 for a comparison of Kohlberg's stages with Freud, Erikson, Sullivan, and Piaget.

Stages of Moral Development

The first level (preconventional morality), characterized by an egocentric focus, is divided into three stages. During stage 0 (premoral stage; birth to 2 years), impulses rule behavior. Infants and young children are unable to differentiate right from wrong. What is good is pleasant or exciting; what is bad is painful or feared. Stage 1 (2–3 years) is the punishment and obedience orientation stage. During this stage, behaviors, decisions, and conformity to rules are based on fear of punishment rather than respect for authority ("I do it because you tell me to and I don't want to be punished"). A child's "goodness" and "badness" are defined by consequences; the more severe the punishment, the more "bad" the act. During stage 2, called the instrumental realistic orientation stage (4–7 years), rules are obeyed to gain rewards or satisfy personal objectives. Sometimes the child does something to please others, but other times, children will make decisions and behave out of self satisfaction and self concern; something is done to get something in return ("I do it because it makes me feel good"). There is no feeling of gratitude, loyalty, or justice (Kohlberg, 1963).

The second level (conventional morality) is seen in the school years. Here, the child is concerned with maintaining and valuing the rules and expectations of the family, group, or society. Conformity and loyalty are reflected in good behavior and societal approval. Stage 3 is interpersonal concordance orientation, or the "good boy," "good girl" orientation (7–10 years). Here, behavior and decisions are evaluated on the basis of one's intent ("he means well") and concerns about others' reactions ("I'll do it because you expect it and will give me something"). Behavior may also be evaluated on the basis of how the other person feels ("I know what it's like to be cold, so I'll give you my sweater"). Stage 4 (10–12 years), authority and social order maintaining orientation, is characterized by believing laws should be

TABLE 2-9   STAGES OF KOHLBERG'S THEORY OF MORAL DEVELOPMENT

Stage	Age	Characteristics
Preconventional Level	**Birth to 7 years**	
Premoral Stage	Birth to 2 years	Cannot differentiate right from wrong
Punishment and Obedience Orientation Stage	2 to 3 years	Conforming behavior based on fear of punishment
Instrumental Realistic Orientation Stage	4 to 7 years	Conforming behavior based on rewards
Conventional Level	**7 to 12 years**	
Interpersonal Concordance Orientation Stage	7 to 10 years	Behavior evaluated on intent and other's reactions
Authority and Social Order Maintaining Orientation Stage	10 to 12 years	Obeys out of respect for laws, authority
Postconventional Level	**12 years and older**	
Social Contract/Legalistic Orientation Stage	12 years through adolescence	Believes laws should further human values and express majority views
Universal Ethical Principles Orientation Stage	Adolescence through adulthood	Right/wrong defined on universal, comprehensive, and consistent, yet personal ethical principles

obeyed because they are law and take precedence over any personal wishes, good intentions, or group beliefs. People conform to societal expectations because they want to preserve the social order, rather than because they are afraid of being punished (Kohlberg, 1963).

The third level is postconventional morality (12 years and older), with a universal focus where right, wrong, and moral values are defined autonomously and in terms of broad principles of justice that may conflict with authority figures or written laws. Stage 5 (social contract legalistic orientation) reflects awareness that just laws should be followed because they further human values and express the majority will. On the other hand, laws compromising human rights or dignity are unjust and

should be challenged. Social rules are not the only reason for behavior and decisions; there are higher moral principles (equality, justice, due process) which also need consideration. Stage 6 (universal ethical principle orientation) is attained by few. Right and wrong are defined on universal, comprehensive, and consistent, yet personal ethical principles. These ethical principles are abstract moral guidelines that include respect for individual rights and transcend any law or social contract. People at this stage are able to see the perspective of anyone affected by a moral decision and can make a decision considered fair for everyone. They believe there is a higher order than the social order, and accept pain, death, and injustice as an integral part of existence (Kohlberg, 1963).

Family Teaching

Moral Development

- Explain to caregivers and other family members how moral development changes during childhood and why children of certain ages respond the way they do.

- Teach caregivers appropriate ways to help children learn ethical behavior.

- Provide examples of appropriate disciplinary practices caregivers can use for children of various ages based on their level of moral development.

Reflective Thinking

Moral Standards

Think about a moral dilemma that has affected you. Why do some people have higher moral standards than others? Apply your answer to Kohlberg's theory. How can you assist children and adolescents to develop high moral standards?

Application

Although Kohlberg offered age guidelines for his stages, they are approximate and many people do not reach the highest stage (Crain, 2000; Sigelman, 1999). Therefore, adults need to understand the stage a particular child is in relative to moral development. Parents need to be educated about normal behavior at each stage so behavioral expectations are appropriate and discipline is fair. For example, young children may stop hitting each other because of fear of being punished rather than because it is morally wrong, and show no remorse for their behavior. Parents also need to know that only when young children show interest in another's well being will they truly understand why it is wrong to hit others. In addition, children may participate in an activity for the wrong reason (to please others, to avoid punishment), and not fully understand the decisions they are making. Therefore it is important to give clear and specific reasons for requests and be patient if there are questions or more information is needed. When moral dilemmas arise (should I do it if it is against my parent's wishes?), clarifying, explaining, and validating concerns may help contribute to moral development.

Spiritual Development

There is minimal research on spiritual development, and what has been published is criticized. However, Fowler (1974) has identified seven stages of faith development; five can be associated with the child's psychosocial, cognitive, and moral development. Table 2-10 describes the five stages most appropriate for children and adolescents.

Contextual Perspective

The contextual perspective adopts a broader focus by viewing human development as a lifelong process affected by other individuals or groups of individuals, and the historical, cultural, political, and economic context one lives in. Ecological theory is an example of the contextual perspective.

Ecological theory stresses the importance of understanding how relationships between the individual and a variety of environmental systems affect human development. The theory proposes that changes in the environment produce changes in the individual, and changes in the individual produce changes in the environment. These interchanges occur simultaneously and continuously. Children are seen as active participants in creating their environments, and though biology is important, the main emphasis is on environmental systems. Development is viewed as continuous; experiences throughout the life span are important. However, situational influences have more impact on develop-

TABLE 2-10 FOWLER'S STAGES OF FAITH

Stage	Description
0: Undifferentiated	During infancy when there is no concept of right or wrong, no convictions to guide behavior, and no beliefs. Establishing trust with the primary caregiver serves as the basis for developing faith.
1: Intuitive-projective	During the toddler years, religious gestures and behaviors of others are imitated without comprehending the significance or meaning of the activities. During the preschool years however, the values and beliefs of parents are assimilated, and parental attitudes toward religious beliefs and moral codes are conveyed to children. Children tend to follow parental beliefs because they are part of their daily life rather than from an understanding of their basic concepts.
2: Mythical-literal	Most school-aged children are interested in religion and accept the existence of a deity. Requests to an omnipotent being are expected to be answered, and important. Faith can be articulated, but sometimes is questioned.
3: Synthetic-convention	Adolescents become increasingly aware of spiritual disappointments and recognize that prayers are not always answered. Some begin to question established parental religious standards and drop or modify some religious practices.
4: Individuating-reflexive	Adolescents become more skeptical and start comparing religious standards of their parents with others as they determine which to adopt and incorporate into their own set of religious values. Religious standards are compared with scientific viewpoints. Many are uncertain about religious ideas and will not gain insight until late adolescence or early adulthood.

ment than individual characteristics, and there are culture-bound principles explaining differences between individuals raised in different cultures (Asian, Italian, Swedish) and at different historical time periods (1920s, 1950s, 1980s).

Bronfenbrenner and Ecological Theory

Urie Bronfenbrenner (b. 1917) offers an organizational framework for examining the environmental influences on human development (Bronfenbrenner, 1979). For him,

the child's world is like a set of nested Russian dolls, with three systems (microsystem, exosystem, macrosystem) ranging from the most immediate setting or context (family, peer group), to the more remote setting or context (the government). The developing individual, embedded within the center of these systems, has a unique heritage (physical appearance, maturation rate, emotionality, innate intelligence, physical health, gender), which is different from any other person. As individuals mature, they impact and are impacted by these changing systems and relationships differently.

Reflective Thinking

Family Experiences

Is personality shaped by family experiences? If so, why are children from the same family often so different from one another?

The broadest context or system affecting development is the macrosystem. This system is large, enduring, and contains cultural and subcultural ideologies and beliefs. Although macrosystem effects may not be obviously apparent in the life of any one individual, the macrosystem profoundly affects development (Bronfenbrenner, 1979). For example, children living in poverty or an inner city ghetto (the macrosystem) are exposed to beliefs and values that are different than those of children living in an affluent suburb.

The exosystem, or middle system, indirectly affects development. It includes social settings the individual never directly experiences even though these experiences provide an important influence (Bronfenbrenner, 1979). Examples of the exosystem are caregiver work settings, social networks, or educational level; one's neighborhood (including environmental noise or pollution); and community decision-making bodies. For example, when a caregiver travels a great deal or works different shifts, the child's family life may change. Children can be affected by whether or not a caregiver's work is satisfying or stressful, or if the caregiver has supportive social relationships. If a planning and zoning commission decides to build a highway through a neighborhood playground, the child's recreational life may change.

The microsystem is the child's immediate environment and includes daily interactions with others (family, peers, teachers, neighbors, religious leaders) or community resources (school, church) (Bronfenbrenner, 1979). The importance of the microsystem changes across development; during infancy, the family and home are of primary importance, whereas in middle childhood and adolescence, the peer group and school become more important.

The mesosystem is the interrelationship among two or more microsystems. For example, the interrelationship among the home, school, and peer group make up a child's mesosystem. For an adult, the mesosystem typically consists of family, employment situations, and friends. If the mesosystem has positive interrelationships, development will progress normally and optimally. If the mesosystem has negative interrelationships, development may not progress normally or optimally.

Application

In the ecological theory, the child is viewed holistically, as a member of a unique family, neighborhood, and cultural belief system

Critical Thinking

Developmental Theories

How do the issues discussed in the early part of the chapter relate to the theories described in the later part of the chapter? That is, how does Freud or Erikson or Bandura or Piaget view the child—active or passive; innately pure or of original sin? How would Bronfenbrenner view the impact culture has on a child?

Reflective Thinking

Theory of Human Development

If you could develop a theory of human development, what would you propose? Upon which theoretical orientation do you lean most heavily in constructing your theory? What personal experiences have you had that might influence the developmental theory you would construct?

that all impact development. Ecological theory also suggests the important influence parents have on their children. It reminds us that home and cultural environments are not the same, and why those home resources and facilities must be assessed before discharge or prescribing home treatment/procedures.

Finally, ecological theory helps us understand that human development can proceed along several different pathways depending on the interplay of internal/external forces within the individual. All children in the same family really may come from different families, since a first child's experiences with parents may be different than a second or third child's experiences in the same family. Bronfenbrenner also reminds us that the influence children have on parents and other family members is as important as the effect family members and parents have on children. It also teaches us to realize that stress or illness in one family member will affect the entire family system.

Therefore, nurses implementing Bronfenbrenner's perspective will need to understand children in their environmental context, teach this information to parents, and allow for family differences. Other nursing considerations include educating parents and other family members (especially siblings), and appropriately conveying understanding and support of parents struggling with setting priorities relative to family and work commitments.

There is no single principle, issue, or theory capable of holistically explaining human development. Therefore, it is important that nurses be aware of the contribution each makes to understanding development, and apply each in context. For example, behaviorists and social learning theorists help us understand how various stimuli, reinforcers, and models influence behavior. Psychoanalytic theory helps us understand the unconscious mind, reasons for abnormal behaviors, and the importance of the past in influencing present behavior. Erikson helps us realize the best solution to a stage crisis is not always positive; exposure to the negative conflict is sometimes inevitable and helpful. The cognitive theories, oriented toward explaining how we acquire and process information and become knowledgeable about the world, help us learn not only what to expect cognitively from children of all ages, but also help us understand how to challenge and stimulate learning at any age. Ecological theories remind us of the importance of the family, culture, and society in development. It is essential that nurses develop an eclectic approach to human development, borrowing and using whatever is appropriate with individual children and their families as they practice holistic care.

REFERENCES

Bandura, A. (1977). *Social learning theory.* Englewood Cliffs, NJ: Prentice-Hall.

Bronfenbrenner, U. (1979). *The ecology of human development.* Cambridge, MA: Harvard University Press.

Crain, W. (2000). *Theories of development: Concepts and applications,* (4th ed.). Upper Saddle River, NJ: Prentice Hall.

Erikson, E. (1963). *Childhood and society* (2nd ed.). New York: Norton.

Fowler, J. (1974). Toward a developmental perspective on faith. *Religious Education, 69,* 207-219.

Freud, S. (1933). *New introductory lectures in psychoanalysis.* New York: Norton.

Kohlberg, L. (1963). The development of children's orientation toward a moral order: I Sequence in the development of moral thought. *Vita Humana, 6,* 11–33.

Lewis, M., & Volkmar, F. (1990). *Clinical aspects of child and adolescent development* (3rd ed.). Philadelphia: Lea and Febiger.

Murray, R., & Zentner, J. (2001). *Health assessment and promotion strategies through the lifespan* (7th ed.). Upper Saddle River, NJ: Prentice Hall.

Piaget, J. (1963). *The origins of intelligence in children.* New York: Norton.

Sigelman, C. (1999). *Life-span human development* (3rd ed.). Pacific Grove, CA: Brooks/Cole.

Skinner, B. F. (1953). *Science and human behavior.* New York: Macmillan.

Sullivan, H.S. (1953). *The Interpersonal Theory of Psychiatry.* New York: Norton.

Lewis, M., & Volkmar, F. (1990). *Clinical aspects of child and adolescent development* (3rd ed.). Philadelphia: Lea and Febiger.

Wadsworth, B. (1989). *Piaget's theory of cognitive and affective development* (4th ed.). New York: Longman.

SUGGESTED READINGS

Angoff, W. (1988). The nature-nurture debate, aptitudes, and group differences. *American Psychologist, 43*, 713–720.

Behrman, R., & Kliegman, R. (2002). *Nelson's essentials of Pediatrics* (4th ed.). Philadelphia, PA: W. B. Saunders.

Bronfenbrenner, U. (1986). Ecology of the family as a context for human development: Research perspectives. *Developmental Psychology, 22*, 723–742.

Brooks-Gunn, J., Duncan, G., & Aber, L. (Eds.). (1997). *Neighborhood poverty: Context and consequences for children.* New York: Russell Sage Foundation.

Child Development and Developmental Psychology. These journals are two leading research journals in the field of child development and discuss the research interests of developmentalists over the years.

Colby, A., & Kohlberg, L. (1987). *The measurement of moral judgement. Vol 1: Theoretical foundations and research validation.* Cambridge, U.K.: Cambridge University Press.

Collins, W., Macoby, E., Steinberg, L., Hetherington, E., & Bornstein, M. (2000). Contemporary research on parenting: The case for nature and nurture. *American Psychologist, 55*(2), 212–232.

Cooper, M. (1989). Gilligan's different voice: A perspective for nursing. *Journal of Professional Nursing, 5*(1), 10–16.

Crews, F. (1996). The verdict on Freud [*Review of Freud evaluated: The completed arc*]. *Psychological Science, 7*, 63–68.

Emde, R. N. (1992). Individual meaning and increasing complexity: Contributions of Sigmund Freud and Rene Spitz to developmental psychology. *Developmental Psychology, 28*, 347–359.

Gilligan, C. (1977). In a different voice: Women's conceptions of self and of morality. *Harvard Educational Review, 47*(4), 481–517.

Harris, J. (1998). *The nurture assumption: Why children turn out the way they do.* New York: Free Press.

Kohlberg, L. (Ed). (1973). *Collected papers on moral development and moral education.* Cambridge, MA: Moral Educational Research Foundation.

Mullahy, P. (1970). *Psychoanalysis and interpersonal psychiatry: The contributions of Harry Stack Sullivan.* New York: Science House.

Murray, R., & Zentner, J. (2001). *Health promotion strategies through the lifespan* (7th ed.). Upper Saddle River, NJ: Prentice Hall.

Potts, N. & Mandleco, B. (Eds). (2002). *Caring for children and their families.* Clifton Park, NY: Delmar.

Walker, L. (1989). A longitudinal study of moral reasoning. *Child Development, 60*(1), 157–166.

Whitener, L., Cox, K., & Maglich, S. (1998). Use of theory to guide nurses in the design of health messages for children. *Advances in Nursing Science, 20*(3), 21–35.

CHAPTER 3

Growth and Development of the Newborn

The neonatal or newborn period is defined as the first 28 days of life. This chapter will present the normal physiological, psychosocial, and cognitive development that occurs during the newborn period. Nursing care of the normal newborn will also be presented.

PHYSIOLOGICAL DEVELOPMENT

General Appearance

The newborn's head, which is one-quarter of the total body size, may appear out of proportion to the body and be misshapen due to the labor and delivery process (molding; Figure 3-1). A caput succedaneum may be present as well, especially after a long labor. A caput is the swelling of the soft tissues of the scalp. The swelling may extend across the suture lines, is evident within 24 hours after birth, and usually resolves within a few days. The collection of blood between the skull bone and the periosteum as a result of the rupture of blood vessels secondary to head trauma from the birth process may result in a cephalhematoma. A cephalhematoma develops 24–48 hours after birth, does not cross the suture lines (Figure 3-2) and may take 2–3 weeks to resolve.

Eyelids may be puffy and eye color indistinguishable. In addition, the newborn has a large, round abdomen with an umbilical area that may protrude for several weeks until the cord stump falls off.

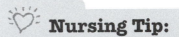

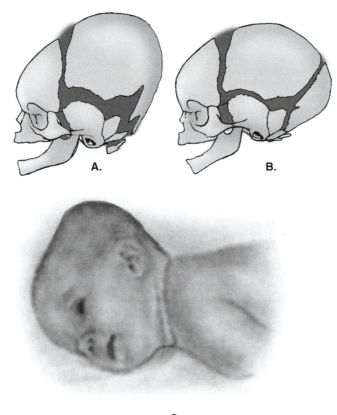

Figure 3-1 Molding. (A) Movement of Cranial Bones During Labor. (B) Cranial bones return to their proper placement in 2 to 3 days. (C) Infant Exhibiting Molding.

The extremities may appear short in comparison to the body, but hands should be able to touch the upper thighs when extended. The legs may appear to be bowed and the newborn typically remains in a position with the extremities flexed. The skin is delicate, often mottled, or acrocyanosis, the bluish discoloration of the hands and feet caused by the instability of the peripheral circulation, system may be presemt.

The soft spots, or fontanels, occur at skull bone junctions or suture lines, and allow the head to adapt to the pelvis shape during delivery and for brain growth over the coming year (Figure 3-3). The posterior fontanel typically closes by 3 months of age, while the anterior fontanel closes around 8–18 months of age.

Neurological System

The initial neurological examination should include observation of the newborn's position and response to handling and stimulation, as well as a determination of gestational

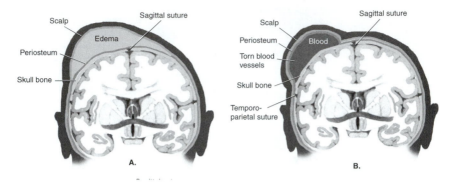

Figure 3-2 (A) Caput Succedaneum and (B) Cephalhematoma

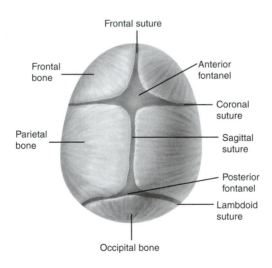

Figure 3-3 Placement of Sutures and Fontanels

age. The use of the Ballard score assists in determining the gestational age of the newborn. For accuracy and validity the examination should be completed within the first 12 hours of life (Ballard, Khoury, Wedig, Wang, Eilers-Walsman, & Lipp, 1991); (refer to Figure 3-4 for the Ballard Assessment Scale of Gestational Age). After the determination of gestational age, the newborn can be classified as (1) large for gestational age (LGA), (2) appropriate for gestational age (AGA), or (3) small for gestational age (SGA). Newborns who are above the 90th percentile are classified as LGA. The AGA newborn is one who lies between the 10th and 90th percentile. The SGA newborn will fall below the 10th percentile. Gestational age assessment

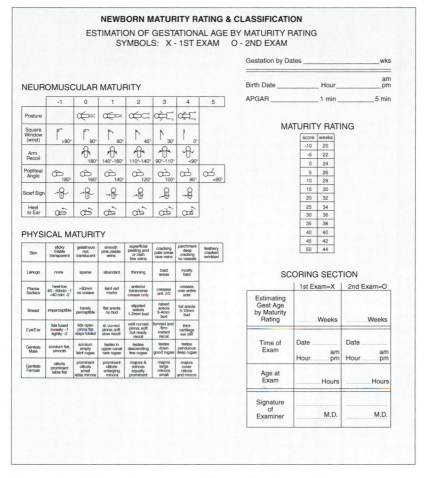

Figure 3-4 Ballard Assessment Scale. Courtesy of Mead Johnson Nutritionals.

assists in determining appropriate care, since immaturity may not be related to size, and influences neurological development and functioning.

Most of time the newborn is in a sleep state with short periods of wakefulness between those sleep states. As the newborn advances to the infant stage, the periods of wakefulness will increase, allowing for more interactions with caregivers. The newborn is able to respond to the environment and stimulation by changing expression (smiling, grimacing, crying), but caregivers may need assistance in deciphering what these signals mean for their baby.

Primitive, innate behaviors seen in the newborn are known as reflexes. Deep tendon reflexes can be elicited in the newborn but have limited value. The reflexes serve a variety of purposes, and can be categorized into localized or generalized, and then further separated into those that are of a primitive or survival nature. Refer to Table 3-1 for newborn reflexes.

TABLE 3-1	NEONATAL REFLEXES			
Reflex	Stimuli	Response	Disappears	Pathology If Abnormal
Localized Reflexes				
Eyes				
Blinking or corneal reflex*	Sudden appearance of a bright light or approach of an object toward cornea	Infant blinks	Persists throughout life	Neurological damage
Doll's eye	Head moved slowly to right or left	Eyes lag behind and do not immediately adjust to new position of head	As ability to fixate develops	Neurological damage
Pupillary*	Bright light shines toward pupil	Pupil constricts	Persists throughout life	Neurological damage
Nose				
Sneeze*	Irritation or obstruction in nasal passages	Sneezing	Persists throughout life	Neurological damage
Mouth and throat				
Cough	Irritation of laryngeal or tracheobronchial tree mucous membranes	Coughing	Persists throughout life	Neurological damage
Extrusion	Depressing or touching the tongue	Tongue is forced outward	4 Months	

* Survival reflex

continues

TABLE 3-1 *Continued*

Reflex	Stimuli	Response	Disappears	Pathology If Abnormal
Gag*	Food, suction, or passing a tube stimulating the posterior pharynx	Gagging	Persists throughout life	Neurological damage
Rooting°	Stroke or touch cheek	Head turns toward stimuli	Approximately 4 months	Central neurological system disease (frontal lobe lesion)
Sucking*	Object touching lips or placed in mouth	Sucking	7 Months	Prematurity; CNS depression in full-term breastfed newborn whose mother has ingested barbiturates
Yawn	Decreased oxygen	Baby yawns	Persists throughout life	

* Survival reflex

continues

TABLE 3-1 *Continued*

Reflex	Stimuli	Response	Disappears	Pathology If Abnormal
Extremities				
Babinski[†]	Lateral aspect of the sole is stroked from heel upward and across ball of foot	Hypertension of the toes	1 Year	Cerebral palsy
Grasp[†]	Palms of hands or soles of feet are touched near base of digits	Flexion of hands and toes	8 Months	
Palmar Grasp[†]	Stimulate the palm	Object is grasped	4 Months	Frontal lobe lesions

[†]Primitive reflex

continues

TABLE 3-1 *Continued*				
Reflex	**Stimuli**	**Response**	**Disappears**	**Pathology If Abnormal**
Plantar grasp [†]	Place the thumb at the base of the newborn's toes	Toes will curl downward	8 Months	Cerebral palsy; obstructive CNS lesion (abscess, tumor)
Mass Reflexes				
Crawl	Infant placed on abdomen	Makes crawling movements with arms and legs	6 Weeks	Neurological damage
Dance or step [†]	Newborn is held upright, one foot is allowed to touch a flat surface	Alternate stepping movements	4 Months	Cerebral palsy

[†] Primitive reflex

continues

TABLE 3-1 *Continued*				
Reflex	**Stimuli**	**Response**	**Disappears**	**Pathology If Abnormal**
Moro†	Sudden changes in position or jarring	Arms extend, head moves back, fingers spread apart with thumb and forefinger forming a "c" followed by arms being brought back to center with hands clenched, spine and lower extremities extended	3–4 Months	Neurological damage
Placing	Held upright; dorsal surface of the feet touch the edge of the table	Flexion of the knees and hips and movement of the legs up the table surface	4 Months	Breech paralysis; cerebral cortex abnormalities

† primitive reflex

continues

TABLE 3-1 *Continued*

Reflex	Stimuli	Response	Disappears	Pathology If Abnormal
Tonic neck	Head turned to one side when supine	Arm and leg extend on the side head is turned toward; arm and leg flexed on opposite side	3–4 Months	Neurological damage
Trunk incurvation (Galant)	Firmly stroke the back in a downward motion for about 5 cm (2 in.), when in prone position	Body curves to the side of the stimulus. Important to check both sides.	2–3 Months	Spinal cord lesion

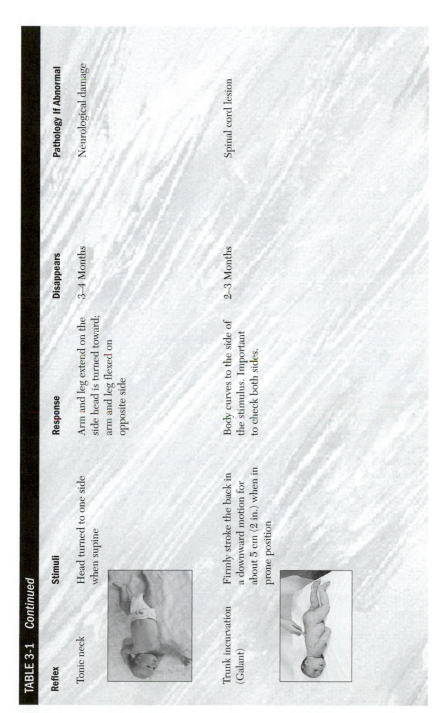

Cardiorespiratory System

Lung compliance in the newborn is affected by anatomy. Mediastinal structures, in conjunction with a relatively large heart, reduce the space available for lung expansion. The newborn's large abdomen also will affect lung space by increasing upward pressure on the diaphragm. The structures of the thorax, including weak intercostal muscles, horizontally positioned ribs, and high diaphragm restrict lung expansion space. Finally, airway resistance is affected by the length, radius, and number of airways. Since the newborn has smaller airways and is an obligatory nose breather, any obstruction causes respiratory distress.

The respiratory rate is usually 30–60 breaths per minute. The respirations are primarily abdominal and shallow, with irregular depth and rhythm. Short periods of apnea may be seen. The newborn's state of consciousness will also affect the respiratory pattern. When the newborn is in a deep sleep, the respiratory pattern is quite regular. Irregular breathing is more noticeable when the newborn is in a light sleep or active state.

The heart rate will initially accelerate up to 180 beats per minute following the first breath. This increase is for a brief period and after 4 hours of life, stroke volume and heart rate decrease and approximate normal ranges (Walther, Benders, & Leighton, 1993). The heart rate will range from 100 beats per minute while asleep to 150 beats per minute while awake. The blood pressure is affected by the changes in blood volume that occur during transition, birth weight, and activity state.

Gastrointestinal System

Gastrointestinal system motility gradually matures during the first few years of life, and is significantly slower in the newborn period than in the adult period. Stomach capacity is approximately 60 mL and will increase during infancy. The emptying time of the stomach is 2½–3 hours, and increases to 3–6 hours during infancy.

The liver remains functionally immature until approximately 1 year of age (Vanderhoof, Zach, & Adrian, 1994). Because the liver has reduced bile salt secretion and the pancreas works less efficiently in the newborn, fat is not absorbed well.

After delivery, excess hemoglobin is destroyed by the reticuloendothial system and not replaced. When the erythrocytes are broken down, the end products of metabolism are formed, and hemoglobin becomes a protein, consisting of globin and heme. Unconjugated (indirect) bilirubin is formed in the liver and spleen from these byproducts, and then binds to albumin in the plasma (Maisels, 1994). Since newborn albumin has limited binding capacity, a significant amount of unconjugated bilirubin accumulates and plasma concentrations may become elevated.

The liver also contains specialized cells that will remove unconjugated bilirubin from the bloodstream and convert it to conjugated (direct) bilirubin. Since conjugated bilirubin is water soluble, it can then be excreted through the stool as bile (Maisels, 1994). However, the newborn's immature liver is not always able to adequately alter and remove the excess bilirubin, and as it accumulates, visible jaundice (the yellowish discoloration of the skin and eyes caused by excess bilirubin) occurs.

Physiologic or normal jaundice shows a gradual rise in bilirubin of 8 mg/dL at 3–5 days after birth, and falls to normal levels the second week of life. Abnormal jaundice is seen with an extreme elevation in bilirubin within the first 24 hours of life. If the unconjugated level is >12 mg/dL when the baby is formula-fed, >14 mg/dL if the baby is breast-fed, or if the jaundice is persistent past 2 weeks of age further evaluation is warranted. Causes of pathologic jaundice may include fetal–maternal blood group incompatibility, nonspecific hemolytic anemias, sepsis, polycythemia, or infants of diabetic mothers.

Phototherapy, or the use of special high-intensity fluorescent lights, is generally an effective method of reducing serum bilirubin

⚡ Nursing Alert:

Eye and Skin Care During Phototherapy

The eyes of the newborn need to be protected while under phototherapy. The patches should be removed periodically, and the eyes and skin under the patches observed for irritation and breakdown. The skin should be examined for pressure areas and evidence of breakdown. The newborn should be repositioned every 2 hours. The newborn may experience loose stools and increased urine output, which may lead to dehydration and excoriation of the skin in the perianal area.

levels and preventing kernicterus. The phototherapy light oxidizes the unconjugated bilirubin in the skin, which then becomes soluble in water and is excreted in the stool and urine. The newborn's eyes should be shielded with special patches to prevent possible retinal damage when undergoing phototherapy, and the genital area covered with a surgical mask to provide protection to the gonads, since maximum exposure is accomplished when the newborn is unclothed.

Genitourinary System

The kidneys are responsible for the regulation of fluid and electrolyte balance, arterial blood pressure, and the removal of some toxins. The fetus does not begin urine production with glomerular filtration until 9–12 weeks' gestation, with renal development continuing until 36 weeks' gestation. The term newborn's kidneys have a full complement of nephrons and even though the glomeruli are small, the surface area for filtration, in respect to body weight, is higher than the adult's. The newborn's renal tubules are short, narrow, and less able to concentrate urine due to the inability to reabsorb water, sodium, glucose, and other solutes back into the blood; the ability to concentrate

urine completely will not be achieved until 3 months of age.

Urine output depends on the glomerular filtration rate and tubular reabsorption of water. Normal urinary output for a newborn is 1–3 mL/kg/hour (Brion, Satlin, & Edelmann, 1994). This is equivalent to approximately 2–6 voidings per day. The urine output is typically low during the first day of life and increases as daily intake increases. Renal function should be evaluated in a newborn that does not void in the first 24 hours of life. Normal newborn urine values are identified in Table 3-2.

Male genitals are evaluated for the presence of testes and the appearance of the rugae on the scrotal sac. Prior to 36 weeks' gestation, the scrotum is small with few rugae (folds), the testes have not descended to the scrotum, and remain in the inguinal canal. The term newborn, however, will demonstrate a pendulous scrotum covered with rugae, with testes palpable in the lower portion of the scrotal sac. If the scrotum is distended, the use of a transilluminator may reveal a hydrocele or a collection of fluid between the parietal and visceral layers of the tunica vaginalis, the outermost covering of the testes. No treatment is usually necessary unless the hydrocele persists beyond the first year of life. Caregivers may need reassurance that this is normal and will soon disappear.

Some male infants undergo circumcision, the surgical removal of the foreskin. When performed on the newborn this is considered an elective procedure, and the decision to have the newborn male circumcised is

TABLE 3-2	NORMAL VALUES FOR NEWBORN URINE
Color	Pale yellow
Glucose	Negative
pH	4.5–8
Protein	<5–10 mg/dL
RBC	Negative
Specific gravity	1.001–1.020
WBC	Negative

Family Teaching

Circumcision Care

The immediate care of the circumcised newborn is dependent on the procedure performed. *If the Plastibell was utilized,* it is left on the penis. Instruct the caregiver to gently lift the ring and squeeze warm water from a cotton ball on to the tip when changing the diaper. The ring will fall off in 7–10 days when the circumcision has healed—do *not* pull it off. *If the ring was not used,* there may be gauze on the penis. This may or may not be replaced depending on the person who performed the circumcision. Diapers should be changed often so urine and stool do not irritate the site. A thin layer of petroleum jelly may be applied to prevent the diaper from adhering to the circumcision site. Yellow exudate may be seen on the second day after the circumcision. This is granulation tissue and is normal and should not be removed.

Nursing Tip:

Care of the uncircumcised newborn

The caregiver should be instructed to wash the outside of the penis to decrease the chance of odor and infection. **Smegma,** a collection of cells that shed from the outer layer of skin, gathers under the foreskin. Odor and infection may develop if the smegma is not removed. In the uncircumcised male the foreskin remains intact. The foreskin may not be retractable until the child is around 3 years of age. The caregiver must be cognizant of this so that they do not attempt to retract the foreskin and cause damage.

Eye On:

Circumcision

Male Jewish newborns may be circumcised on the 8th day of life at a religious ceremony. The circumcision is performed by a mohel, a person trained on performing circumcisions. Anesthesia is not used. The infant is often given a bit of wine as part of the ceremony. Parents should be taught circumcision care prior to leaving the hospital even though the circumcision is done in the home

left up to the parents. Factors that may affect their decision include cleanliness, tradition, possible prevention of cancer, and personal preference. As with any surgery there are risks (hemorrhage, infection, injury to the penis, urethra, and scrotum, deformity, scarring).

The appearance of female genitalia depends on subcutaneous fat deposition and gestational age. The newborn less than 36 weeks' gestation has a prominent clitoris. The labia majora is small and widely separated. The term newborn will have the clitoris and labia minora covered by the labia majora. Vernix caseosa may be present between the labia, and sometimes the hymenal tag may protrude from the floor of the vagina.

Musculoskeletal System

The term newborn exhibits hypertonic flexion of all extremities. Flexion development occurs in the lower extremities first; therefore, during examination, the legs should be assessed first. To assess flexation, place the newborn on a flat surface with the legs in flexion while manipulating the hip joint and placing a hand on the newborn's knees. After flexing the legs, extend them onto the flat surface and release. The full-term newborn's legs should recoil and quickly return to a flexed position. When examining the elbows, flex them by holding them for 5 seconds and then extend them. The term newborn's elbows form an angle of less than 90° and rapidly recoil back to a flexed position. Because a healthy but fatigued newborn may elicit a slower response, this test should be delayed for the first hour after birth.

Muscles in the extremities are not well defined, and muscle tone is not fully developed. Therefore, the newborn cannot support the full weight of the head, and head lag is seen if the newborn is pulled from a supine to a sitting position (Figure 3-5). However, in the prone position, the newborn is able to slightly raise the head. The hands should reach to the upper thighs when the upper extremities are extended. The legs should be equal length with symmetrical gluteal skin folds.

Intrauterine positioning of the newborn's feet may result in a talipes deformity or clubfoot. Usually, no treatment is needed if the foot can easily be manipulated to midline. When the foot cannot be aligned readily, an orthopedic consult should be considered. The spine, examined with the newborn in a prone position, should be straight and flat.

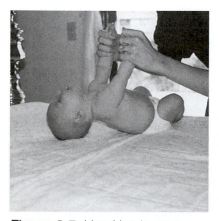

Figure 3-5 Head lag is seen when the newborn is supine and the body lifted.

The base of the spine should be closely observed for any deformities such as spina bifida (a congenital defect in the walls of the spinal cord caused by a lack of union between the laminae of the vertebrae). The newborn will gain approximately 5–7 ounces per week, and head circumference and length will increase 1 inch per month.

Integumentary System

The skin is delicate and often mottled, or acrocyanosis may be present. The skin should be observed for other characteristics such as color and color change that may occur during activity, racial features, rashes, milia, birthmarks, and petechiae. Milia are small white papules on the nose, face, forehead, and upper torso caused by the plugging of the sebaceous gland. Petechiae are small, pinpoint, nonraised, perfectly round, purplish red spots, which are a result of an intradermal or submucosal hemorrhage. Petechiae may be a normal finding if located in the area of the presenting part. If found elsewhere, an investigation of possible causes, such as sepsis, should be pursued. A mongolian spot is an irregularly dark pigmented area on the posterior lumbar region that has no clinical significance but may be noted in African American, Asian, and Native American newborns. Desquamation, or peeling of the skin, may also be present. The degree of peeling depends on the maturity of the newborn with preterm newborns experiencing less and postterm newborns experiencing more. Telangiectatic nevi are capillary hemangiomas commonly called "stork bites," which are sometimes found on the nape of the neck and the bridge of the nose. These will disappear with time. Nevus flammeus, or port wine stain, is a hemangioma or vascular tumor that will not disappear with time. Some newborns may experience a transient newborn rash that is characterized by a red macular base with a white vesicular center, referred to as erythema toxicum.

Table 3-3 provides a summary of the normal and acceptable variations found when performing a newborn assessment.

TABLE 3-3   SUMMARY OF NEWBORN PHYSICAL ASSESSMENT

Area Assessed	Normal Findings	Acceptable Variances
Head	Anterior fontanel diamond-shaped, soft/flat Posterior fontanel triangle-shaped Head circumference 33–35 cm (13–14 in)	Molding Caput succedaneum Cephalhematoma Puncture mark from internal scalp electrode Head circumference 32.5–37.5 cm (12.5–14.5 in)
Face/Eyes	Symmetrical facial features/movement Eyes symmetrical in shape, placement and movement	Eyelid edema Subconjunctival hemorrhage
Thorax	Symmetrical movement Circumference equal to or less than head circumference Nipples symmetrical Breath sounds clear and equal bilaterally Heart with regular rate and rhythm S2 split	Breast engorgement (male and female) Supernumerary nipples Noticeable ribs on deep inspiration *Functional* heart murmur
Abdomen	Soft, nondistended Umbilical cord with two arteries and one vein Bowel sounds present	Irregular bowel sounds Reducible umbilical hernia

continues

TABLE 3-3	*Continued*	
Area Assessed	**Normal Findings**	**Acceptable Variances**
Genitalia	**Male**	
	• Meatal opening in center of glans	Hydrocele (accumulation of fluid in the scrotal sac)
	• Strong, arching urinary stream	Testes at external inguinal ring
	• Penile erection when voiding or with stimulation	
	• Scrotum with rugae and pink or dark brown in color (depends on ethnic background)	
	• Both testes descended	
	Female	
	• White or pink vaginal discharge	Vaginal/hymenal tag
	• Edematous clitoris and labia majora	Fusion of labia minora
	• Increased pigmentation	
Anus/rectum	Patent anus	Meconium within 48 hours
	Meconium passage by 24 hours	
Extremities	Flexed position	Extended knees if breech
	Symmetrical and equal movement	
	Full range of motion	
	Hands reach upper thighs when upper extremities are extended	
Spine	Straight	
	Moves head from side to side when prone	
	Can lift head when prone	

PSYCHOSOCIAL DEVELOPMENT

Erik Erikson has divided the human life span into eight stages. The first stage, which includes the newborn, is trust versus mistrust. Here, the newborn relies on others to fulfill needs and develops basic trust when the caregivers meet these needs. Through a supportive, nurturing, and loving environment, the newborn will form an attachment to the caregiver and develop positive relationships (refer to Chapter 1 for more information).

However, the development of attachment between the newborn and caregiver requires more than just being fed and having biological needs met. Attachment depends on emotional responses as well. For example, reports from various orphanages and foundling homes from the early 1900s showed that infants who lacked interaction were retarded in physical growth, language, and intellectual development (Kalat, 1993). These infants were also socially inept and unresponsive to their environment. Twenty minutes of extra handling per day has been reported to result in earlier exploring and grasping behavior by the infant (Murray & Zenter, 2001).

response. High-frequency signals are more likely to produce a response, but it may be a distress response whereas lower intensity signals inhibit distress.

In addition, the newborn is sensitive to touch and handling. If a newborn is quiet, a rapid, intrusive touch will elicit an alert state. When the newborn is upset and crying, a slow soft touch will be calming. If some form of central nervous system irritation exists, there is increasing irritability with stimuli (especially tactile stimulation), and further evaluation is required.

The newborn's response to various stimuli affects the caregiver–infant bond. Since nonverbal communication between caregiver and infant are the initial stages of attachment, caregivers should provide the newborn with stimuli that evoke a response, thus enhancing attachment. Caregivers should also be taught to look for cues that the infant may be overstimulated or becoming habituated.

Habituation, the ability to decrease responses to disturbing stimuli, is a defensive state that the newborn may enter in response to noxious stimuli. Habituation protects the newborn from overstimulation and frees energy to meet physiologic demands. A newborn who cannot habituate will continue to react vigorously to repeated stimuli.

COGNITIVE DEVELOPMENT

T. Berry Brazelton (1994) has shown that the newborn has the ability to interact with the environment and signal needs and gratitude when those needs are met. The newborn as young as 12 days of age is able to imitate facial and manual gestures of adults and prefers sharply contrasting colors (black, white, red), large squares, medium-bright objects, and ovoid objects with eyes and a mouth.

The newborn also has the ability to respond to auditory stimuli by turning the head and "looking" with the eyes to find the source. The frequency and intensity of the auditory stimulus, however, affect the

HEALTH SCREENING

Required screening for newborns differs from state to state. The most common requirements involve phenylkentonuria and congenital hypothyroidism; galactosemia; and sickle cell disease (Galvis, 2000). Check with your institution regarding screenings mandated in your state.

The AAP suggests that all newborns go through a hearing screen to identify possible hearing loss. The AAP and the Joint Committee on Infant Hearing (1995) suggest the goal of universal detection of hearing loss before 3 months of age and appropriate intervention at no more than 6 months of age (AAP, 1999).

HEALTH PROMOTION

Shortly after birth, all newborns receive ophthalmic drops or ointment. Even though the incidence of mothers infected with gonorrhea at the time of delivery is less than 3%, the importance of preventing blindness makes this procedure mandatory for all newborns (Murray & Zentner, 2001).

Hemorrhagic disease of the newborn due to vitamin K deficiency may be prevented by administering phytonadione within 1 hour of birth. The dosage is usually 1 mg intramuscularly for the full-term newborn or 0.5 mg for preterm infants (Pillitteri, 2003). Prior to discharge from the hospital, the newborn should have a screening blood test to rule out the presence of phenylketonuria (PKU) and hypothyroidism.

Immunizations

Immunizations to promote disease resistance and prevention are also essential for all newborns and infants. Caregivers should be informed of the importance of obtaining recommended immunizations and should receive a written schedule of when immunizations are due (see Appendix F for immunization schedule). Recommendations for routine well baby check-ups vary among practitioners. Some primary care providers will see the breastfed newborns at 1 week of age to check their weight; others will have all newborns return to the office at 2 weeks of age. Finally, caregivers should receive a recommended schedule for follow-up care.

Nutrition

The American Academy of Pediatrics (AAP) recommends breastfeeding for the first 6–12 months of life (AAP, 1997). Breast milk has many advantages over formula such as (1) requiring no mixing; (2) being the correct temperature; (3) requiring no sterilization; (4) being easily digested; (5) its fats are well absorbed; (6) having antibodies and immunoglobulins to many types of microorganisms, which are passed from mother to

---

Family Teaching

Colostrum

Explain to the mother that breast milk does not come in until the 2nd or 4th day. Until then, the newborn gets nutrients from colostrum, a product the breast produces prior to milk.

Critical Thinking

I Don't Think I Can Do It

Christine, the first-time mother of a 4-hour-old infant says she wants to breastfeed her baby. However, she does not think that she can do it because her milk has not "come in" yet, and her mother and sisters were not able to breastfeed their infants. What would you tell her?

---

baby; and (7) being cost effective. Many women, however, choose not to breastfeed for a variety of reasons. The mother who chooses not to breastfeed should not be made to feel guilty because of her decision. If breastfeeding is not selected, commercial formulas are available that attempt to mimic human milk. However, most commercial formulas have a slightly higher renal load and higher protein intake that may alter the blood urea nitrogen level and serum or urine level of amino acids (Murray & Zentner, 2001). Cow's milk should not be used to feed infants until recommended by the primary care provider since the composition of cow's milk is designed for a rapidly growing animal and differs significantly from human milk or commercial formula. Cow's milk contains more protein, fat, sugar, calcium, sodium, potassium, magnesium, sulfur, and phosphorous than human milk or commercial formulas. The caregivers should be instructed on these differences and the importance of maintaining the newborn and infant on breast milk or commercial formula.

Family Teaching

Breastfeeding

1. Breasts may be firm but feel softer after nursing.
2. Nurse at least 10–15 minutes on each side.
3. To prevent nipple tenderness, hold infant correctly: cradle hold, football hold, or side-lying down.
4. Make sure the newborn's lips are behind the nipple, encircling the areola.
5. Release the suction before the newborn is removed from the breast by placing a finger in the side of the mouth and between the jaws.
6. After nursing, express a little breast milk, massage into the nipples and areola, and allow to air dry.
7. Avoid using soap, alcohol, or creams on breasts or nipples. Express droplet of breast milk and allow to air dry, especially for cracks and reddened areas on nipples. Clean with water during showering or bathing.
8. Baby's urine should be light yellow with soft yellow stools.
9. Burp baby between breasts and at the end of feeding.

Bottle Feeding

1. Formula should be iron-fortified.
2. All the newborn's nutritional needs are met by formula. Cereal, juice, or other baby foods are not necessary.
3. Formula comes in three forms: ready to feed, concentrated liquid, and powdered.
4. Be sure formula is diluted correctly if in concentrated or powder form. Never add more or less water to the formula than is recommended by the manufacturer because this can be very dangerous for the newborn.
5. Once opened or mixed, a can of formula or prepared bottle should be refrigerated and used within 48 hours.
6. If the newborn drinks part of a bottle, it can be left at room temperature, but it must be used within 1 hour.
7. Avoid adding fresh formula to a partially used bottle or reuse a bottle that has been out for longer than 1 hour.
8. Avoid heating bottles in a microwave. This leads to uneven heating and can cause severe burns to the newborn's mouth and throat.
9. Most babies are satisfied in about 20 minutes. Feedings should not last longer than 30 minutes.
10. Burp after half of the feeding and again at the end of the feeding.
11. Never prop the bottle or leave the newborn unattended.
12. Avoid allowing the newborn to drink from a bottle for long periods, especially when sleeping. This practice can cause "nursing bottle syndrome" or the development of dental caries and has also been linked to an increased incidence of otitis media.

Soy protein may be substituted for milk protein when newborns have lactose intolerance. Symptoms include abdominal pain, diarrhea, distension, and flatus after ingesting milk products. Special formulas have also been developed to meet the needs of babies with PKU, fat malabsorption problems, or those requiring increased calories (e.g., preterm infants). The choice of formula is often decided by the pediatrician and hospital staff unless the caregivers request a specific formula.

The method of feeding is important, but the procedure for feeding may also have a significant impact on the newborn. Feeding time is crucial to the development of the caregiver–newborn attachment, since it is a time for the newborn and caregiver to interact and learn about each other. If the newborn remains in the crib or in an infant seat with the bottle propped, the attachment process can be delayed. If the newborn is held and cuddled during feeding, both caregiver and newborn experience a feeling of closeness as well as close eye contact.

In past years, newborns were placed on a specific feeding schedule. However, current practice is on-demand feeds which involves feeding the newborn when hungry instead of according to a prearranged time schedule. Because formula is digested more slowly, formula-fed newborns will go longer between feedings and usually establish a pattern of feeding every 3–4 hours, whereas a breastfed newborn may nurse every 1½–3 hours. For the first few feedings, the newborn may only consume ½–1 ounce, and progresses to 6–8 feedings of 2–3 ounces per feeding after the first week of life. By 1 month of age, the newborn is eating 5–6 feedings per day and taking 3–4 ounces per feeding.

Elimination

The first stool of the newborn, meconium, is black and tarry, and usually is passed within the first 24 to 48 hours after birth. By the third day of life, the transitional stool is passed. It is green brown to yellow in color. If the newborn is breastfed, the stool then becomes yellow to golden yellow in color,

looks pastey, like bird seeds, and has a sour milk odor. If the newborn is formula fed, the stool is pale to light yellow in color, firmer than the stool of the breast-fed newborn, and has a strong odor.

Newborns should also void within the first 24 hours of life. After that, most newborns have 6 to 8 wet diapers per day and pass stools at least once a day. (Breastfed newborns may have more frequent stools.)

Hygiene

When changing the diaper of a female, instruct caregivers to wipe from front to back so feces do not contaminate the vaginal area. Keeping the diaper clean and dry is the best prevention against diaper rash, and the AAP recommends using plain water and absorbent cotton or fresh washcloth. There is no need to use commercial wipes. However, if they are used, the wipes should be designed for babies not adults since adult wipes contain alcohol that can dry babies' skin.

The causes of diaper rash include:

- Too much moisture next to skin
- Chafing or rubbing
- Prolonged skin contact with urine, feces, or both
- Use of antibiotics (yeast infection)
- Allergic reaction to diaper material

Symptoms of diaper rash can be mild to severe and include red skin; painful open sores; and rash around abdomen, genital area, or inside the skin folds of thighs and buttocks. Treatment includes changing diaper often, using clear water to clean diaper area, and applying a thick layer of protective ointment or cream (zinc oxide or petrolatum). Caregivers should contact a health care practioner if the rash doesn't go away within 48–72 hours or gets worse, including open sores and blisters (AAP, 2000).

Rest and Sleep

Term newborns have two sleep states: deep and light. During deep sleep, the eyes are firmly closed and still, no rapid eye movements occur, and little or no motor activity is present, except for occasional startles. During light sleep, rapid eye movements occur during a 10-second interval, and activity ranges from stretching to minor twitches. The newborn will sleep between 16 and 19 hours a day, with sleep cycles averaging 45–50 minutes. The term newborn begins and ends in light sleep (Brazelton, 1994).

Circadian rhythm, the cyclic variations in bodily functions that occur in a 24-hour period, is controlled by the central nervous system. Often the newborn's "clock" will not coincide with the family's and can result in conflict and disruption. This discrepancy may lead the family to perceive the newborn as "difficult." However, through alterations in care giving and patience, the infant's schedule can become synchronous with the family's rhythms.

In 1992, the AAP recommended the supine or side-lying position for sleep for infants (2002). However, newborns with craniofacial abnormalities and gastroesophageal reflux should be positioned prone. In recent studies from various countries, the side or back sleeping position has shown a large and sustained decrease in the incidence of sudden infant death syndrome (SIDS). The type of bedding the newborn is placed on has also been implicated in SIDS with a higher incidence occurring on soft bedding such as pillows, comforters, blankets, or sheepskin (Willinger, Hoffman, & Hartford, 1994).

Activity and Play

Newborns attend to sounds, sights, tastes, and smells as well as different kinesthetic and tactile sensations. They can also discriminate among squares, rectangles, circles, and crosses, and prefer black, white, and red instead of bright colors. Newborns like to look at faces rather than objects, and can tell the difference between different facial expressions. They can distinguish between their mother's voice and that of others, and are probably able to discriminate among sounds of different pitch, intensity, and duration. Neonates can also detect the direction from which sounds come and turn their head toward the sound they hear. If a continuous sound is presented, they become bored.

Within a few days of birth, they also recognize recurrent situations and respond to changes in their routines. Although newborns are usually quiet, they are alert and interested in their environment, are sensitive to touch, and learn to calm themselves when comforted by gentle motion, touch, sucking, and swaddling. Therefore, newborns need gentle touching, holding, and eye contact. In fact, nurturing contact from consistent caregivers facilitates emotional attachment as well as physical development. Rocking, singing, talking, comforting, cuddling, playful interactions, and giving love during everyday activities (bathing, dressing, diapering) help development. It is also important to allow newborns many opportunities to watch family members and look at human faces, especially the eyes, as well as a variety of changing scenes and colors. Providing a mirror and mobiles that move and have a sound will help facilitate interest in the environment. Since too much stimulation is not

Family Teaching

Sleeping

1. Explain the American Academy of Pediatrics recommendation for "back to sleep":
   a. Do not position newborn prone.
   b. Position newborn supine or side-lying.
2. Provide information on the type of bedding to avoid:
   a. Soft bedding
   b. Pillows
   c. Comforters
   d. Sheepskin
   e. Water beds
3. Explain that overswaddling or increased room temperature, in combination with the prone position, may increase the likelihood of SIDS threefold.

helpful, newborns need periodic breaks and times when they can rest (Murray & Zentner, 2001.

Safety and Injury Prevention

Newborns can wiggle into a variety of unsafe positions. Therefore, the only place to leave a newborn unattended is in the crib with the side rails up. Therefore one hand should always be kept on the newborn when on top of any object, since he/she can quickly roll off. Other safety concerns for the newborn are drowning, suffocation, burns, or motor vehicle accidents.

Bathing can be a fun time for the caregiver and newborn, but the newborn should never be left unattended. Therefore, caregivers should be taught to not answer the phone or door bell when bathing the newborn, unless the newborn is bundled up and taken with the caregiver.

Motor vehicle accidents can plague every age group, and all children need to be properly restrained. Recent information has shown the front passenger seat is dangerous; so the neonate should be secured in a car seat in the rear, facing backward. Caregivers should know how their car seat is installed and how it works prior to use. If the family is involved in an accident, the car seat needs to be removed from service, even if there is no visible damage. Placing the crib away from heat sources, using warm-air vaporizers cautiously, covering unused electrical outlets, and not holding the newborn

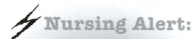

Nursing Alert:

Pacifiers for Newborns

When a pacifier is used, it should be of solid, one-piece construction. It should not be tied to a string or rope and placed around the newborn's neck as this poses a strangulation hazard.

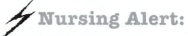

Nursing Alert:

Water Temperature for Bathing

Water heaters should be set no higher than 120°F. Exposure to hot water for even a brief time may result in second or third degree burns. At a water temperature of 155°F, a burn can occur in 1 second. At a temperature of 120°F, a burn occurs in 5 minutes. After filling the bath tub, turn the hot water off first and then the cold. The water temperature should always be checked before the newborn is placed in the tub.

while drinking hot liquids will also help prevent injury or accidents.

Since the incidence of recurrent otitis media and respiratory infections has been linked to secondhand smoke, smoking around the newborn should be avoided. If family members need to smoke, they should go outside, and avoid smoking in the car if a newborn or older infant is present.

ANTICIPATORY GUIDANCE

Thermoregulation

The newborn is capable of maintaining body temperature but not as effectively as a more mature person. Therefore, the newborn is more vulnerable to underheating and overheating because of a relatively large body surface area, poor thermal insulation, limited shivering response, and increased metabolic rate.

Heat exchange occurs through convection, conduction, radiation, evaporation, and over a heat gradient, or from a higher to lower temperature. The transfer of heat between a solid surface and air or liquid is convection. This type of heat exchange would occur between the newborn and

Family Teaching

Keeping the Newborn Warm

1. Explain how the newborn loses heat:
   a. Convection
   b. Conduction
   c. Radiation
   d. Evaporation
2. Provide information on how to reduce heat exchange:
   a. Reduce the area exposed during a bath.
   b. Limit exposure to drafts created by doors, ventilation systems, and traffic flow around the newborn's bed.
   c. Warm solid surfaces between the newborn by placing a blanket on the scale or counter.
   d. Place the newborn's crib on an inside wall in the room, away from the window.
   e. Block sunlight on the newborn in the car to prevent overheating.

Reflective Thinking

Overdressing

You enter a room to find the thermostat set at 80°F. The newborn is dressed in a t-shirt, sleeper, socks, and bundled in a quilt. How do you approach the mom to explain how overdressing and overbundling can affect the newborn's temperature? What if the mom states she's doing this because of her cultural background?

liquid during a bath or when exposed to drafts. Conduction of heat occurs between two solid objects that come in contact with each other. For example, when the infant's body comes in contact with a cold scale or counter, heat loss results. The transfer of heat between solid objects that are not in contact is radiation. Placing the newborn next to a cold window, despite the room being warm, will cause heat loss through radiation. Evaporative heat loss occurs when water on or in the body changes from a liquid to a gas, and can occur if the infant is not dried thoroughly after a bath.

If the newborn is exposed to temperature variations, multiple physiological responses occur. An increase in environmental temperature may cause vasodilation of the skin arterioles, resulting in increased blood flow from the body core to the periphery in an attempt to dissipate the heat and produce a cooling effect. A decrease in environmental temperature will result in vasoconstriction of the skin arterioles and reduction of heat from the body core. Shivering, a specialized muscular response that increases oxygen consumption and muscle metabolic rate, is limited in the newborn.

The primary form of heat production in the newborn is through brown adipose tissue metabolism. This brown fat is found primarily in the subscapular, axillary, adrenal, and mediastinal regions, and increases cellular metabolic rates and oxygen consumption, resulting in heat. Brown fat cells differ from other adipose tissue because of the fat vacuoles, number of mitochondria, and glycogen stores, and enhance the responsiveness of brown fat to thermal stimuli.

NURSE'S ROLE IN FOSTERING HEALTHY NEWBORNS

Although the time allowed for mothers and newborns to remain in the hospital following delivery has decreased in recent years, nurses can still have an impact on their care, as they are in an excellent position to teach parents about their newborn, and what to expect in the coming months. Education should begin early in the hospital stay not the day of discharge, with frequent reinforcement, and in a variety of formats to accommodate various learning styles. One-on-one or classroom instruction, videotapes, written handouts, and/or demonstration are appropriate methods. Information needs to be individualized for each newborn and caregiver considering cultural and religious beliefs, and educational levels.

The nurse is also in an excellent position to ensure caregivers feel comfortable before the newborn is sent home and are provided with information about community resources that may be helpful. The nurse should also instruct caregivers on the importance of follow-up care including well-baby check-ups and routine immunizations.

REFERENCES

American Academy of Pediatrics. (1997). Breastfeeding and the use of human milk. Policy Statement. *Pediatrics, 100*(6), 1035–1039. Available: www.aap.org/policy/re9729.html.

American Academy of Pediatrics. (1999). *Newborn and infant hearing loss: Detection and intervention* [On-line]. Available: www.medem.com

American Academy of Pediatrics. (2000). *Treating diaper rash* [On-line]. Available: www.medem.com

American Academy of Pediatrics. (2002). Reminding families about the importance of back to sleep. "Kids' Health" supplement in the October 18-20, 2002 weekend edition of *USA Today.* Available: www.aap.org/advocacy/releases/sids.htm (accessed 12/19/02).

American Academy of Pediatrics Joint Committee on Infant Hearing. (1995). Joint committee on infant hearing 1994 position statement. *Pediatrics, 95,* 152–156.

Ballard, J., Khory, J., Wedig, K., Wang, L., Eilers-Walsman, B., & Lipp, R. (1991). New Ballard score: Expanded to include extremely premature infants. *Journal of Pediatrics, 119*(3), 417-423.

Brazelton, T. B. (1994). Behavioral competence. In G. B. Avery, M. A. Fletcher, & M. G. MacDonald (Eds.), *Neonatology: Pathophysiology and Management of the Newborn* (4th ed., pp. 289–300). Philadelphia: Lippincott.

Brion, L. P., Satlin, L. M., & Edelmann, C. M. (1994). Renal disease. In G. B. Avery, M. A. Fletcher, & M. G. MacDonald (Eds.), *Neonatology: Pathophysiology and management of the newborn* (4th ed., pp. 792–836). Philadelphia: Lippincott.

Galvis, S. (2000). *Newborn screening for metabolic disorders* [On-line]. Available: www.neonatology.org

Kalat, J. W. (1993). *Introduction to psychology* (3rd ed.). Pacific Grove, CA: Brooks/Cole Publishing Company.

Maisels, M. J. (1994). Jaundice. In G. B. Avery, M. A. Fletcher, & M. G. MacDonald (Eds.), *Neonatology: Pathophysiology and management of the newborn* (4th ed., pp. 630–725). Philadelphia: Lippincott.

Murray, R. B., & Zentner, J. P. (2001). Assessment and health promotion for the infant. In *Nursing assessment and health promotion: Strategies through the lifespan* (7th ed. pp. 325-383). Upper Saddle River, NJ: Prentice Hall.

Pillitteri, A. (2003). *Maternal and Child Health Nursing* (4th ed.). Philadelphia: Lippincott.

Vanderhoof, J. A., Zach, T. L., & Adrian, T. E. (1994). Gastrointestinal disease. In G. B. Avery, M. A. Fletcher, & M. G. MacDonald (Eds.), *Neonatology: Pathophysiology and management of the newborn* (4th ed., pp. 605–629). Philadelphia: Lippincott.

Walther, F. J., Benders, M. J., & Leighton, J. O. (1993). Early changes in the neonatal circulatory transition. *Journal of Pediatrics, 123*(4), 625–632.

Willinger, M., Hoffman, H., & Hartford, R. (1994). Infant sleep position and risk for sudden infant death syndrome: Report of meeting held January 13 and 14, 1994, National Institutes of Health, Bethesda, MD. *Pediatrics, 93*(5), 814–819.

SUGGESTED READINGS

Alexander, G., de Caunes, F. L., Hulsey, T., Tompkins, M., & Allen, M. (1992). Validity of postnatal assessments of gestational age: A comparison of the method of Ballard et al. and early ultrasonography. *American Journal of Obstetrics & Gynecology, 166*(3), 891–895.

American Academy of Pediatrics. (1999). *Circumcision policy statement.* [On-line]. Available: www.medem.com

Arlotti, J. P., Cottrell, B. H., Lee, S. H., & Curtin, J. J. (1998). Breastfeeding among low-income women with or without peer support. *Journal of Community Health Nursing, 15*(3), 163.

Braveman, P., Egerter, S., Pearl, M., Marchi, K., & Miller, C. (1995). Problems associated with early discharge of newborn infants. *Pediatrics, 96*(4.1), 716.

Brooks, C. (1997). Neonatal hypoglycemia. *Neonatal Network, 16*(2), 15–21.

Cornell, S. (1997). Understanding infant jaundice. A normal but potentially complicated condition. *Advances for Nurse Practitioners, 5*(2), 71–72.

Dodd, V. (1996). Gestational age assessment. *Neonatal Network, 15*(1), 27–36.

Harrison, L. (1997). Research utilization: Handling preterm infants in the NICU. *Neonatal Network 16*(3), 65–69.

Hill, A. S., Kurkowski, T. B., & Garcia, J. (2000). Oral support measures used in feeding the preterm infant. *Nursing Research, 49*(1), 2–10.

Messmer, P. R., Rodriguez, S., Adams, J., Wells-Gentry, J., Washburn, K., Zabaleta, I., & Abreu, S. (1997). Effect of kangaroo care on sleep time for neonates. *Pediatric Nursing, 23,* 408–414.

Neu, M., Browne, J. V., & Vojir, C. (2000). The impact of two transfer techniques used during skin-to-skin care on the physiologic and behavioral responses of preterm infants. *Nursing Research, 49*(4), 215–223.

VandenBerg, K. A. (1997). Basic principles of developmental caregiving. *Neonatal Network, 16*(7), 69–71.

CHAPTER 4

Growth and Development of the Infant

Infant (1 month to 1 year) growth and development is rapid and enables maturation to unfold in a relatively short time. Health status is based on the infant's ability to adapt to these rapid changes. As a health care provider, the nurse must have an understanding of these changes to ensure the infant and his or her family maintain an optimal level of health.

PHYSIOLOGICAL DEVELOPMENT

The rapid changes seen during infancy will never be encountered again throughout the life span. As the body matures, skill development progresses in an orderly fashion to enable the infant to respond to and cope with the world. Gross and fine motor skills develop in a cephalocaudal (head-to-toe) and proximal–distal (central-to-peripheral) fashion; gross motor abilities develop before fine motor abilities.

The infant's physical growth is influenced by genetics, the environment, ethnic background, and biology (Secker, 1999). Physical growth patterns include weight, height, and head circumference changes. The infant's growth measurements should be plotted on a growth chart and, over time, compared to the infant's own growth curve (see Appendix B for growth charts).

Weight and Height

During the first 6 months of life, the infant's birth weight typically doubles. The approximate weight gain is 1.5 lb per month, or 5–7

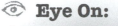

Eye On:
Cultural Weight Differences

Birth weights differ among ethnic groups. For instance, Native American infants are often heavier at birth than European American infants. Infants of Asian descent are typically shorter and lighter than European American infants.

oz per week. In the second 6 months of life, the infant will gain about 3–5 oz per week (less than 1 lb per month). By 12 months of age, the infant's birth weight will have tripled.

Height increases during the first 6 months by approximately 1 inch per month. The rate of growth in height slows to approximately 0.5 inch (1.5 cm) per month by 12 months of age, resulting in almost a 50% increase in height from the birth length.

Head Growth

The size of the head changes rapidly during infancy, reflecting rapid brain growth. By the age of 12 months, the infant's brain will be two-thirds the size of an adult brain. During the first 6 months of life, head circumference will increase by approximately 0.5 inch (1.3 cm) per month. During the second 6 months of life, head circumference will slow to approximately 0.25 inch (0.6 cm) per month. As the head grows, the fontanels gradually close, with the posterior fontanel closing by 2 months of age and the anterior fontanel closing by 12–18 months of age.

Motor Development

Motor development is related to physical, cognitive, and social development. Motor growth includes gross and fine motor development, which provides the infant with the means and freedom to explore the environment. General principles associated with motor development include:

- Voluntary behaviors follow the disappearance of primitive reflexes. To be able to willingly grasp an object, the infant must first lose the involuntary grasp reflex.
- Pronation occurs before supination. The infant must be able to pick up an object (pronation) before being able to put the object in the mouth (supination).
- The ability to grasp an object precedes the ability to release it (Dixon & Stein, 2000).

Gross Motor

Gross motor development is the ability to use large muscle groups to maintain balance and postural control or locomotion. A major task for the infant in obtaining postural control is head control, which is mastered in the prone as well as the upright positions, e.g., standing and sitting.

Infant head control is judged by the presence or absence of head lag. The amount of head lag can be determined when the infant is pulled by the arms from a supine to a sitting position. At 1 month of age, the infant's back is completely rounded while in a sitting position, with the head falling forward. By 2 months, partial head lag is evident, and the infant can hold the head erect with minimal head bobbing while sitting. At 4 months, the infant has no head lag and good head control while sitting (Figure 4-1).

Once head control is established, the infant begins to sit without support.

Locomotion, the ability to move from place to place without assistance, is dependent on head control and sitting without support. A variety of skills such as rolling over, bearing weight, moving forward on all extremities, and standing upright without assistance are also necessary for locomotion.

Critical Thinking

Posterior Fontanel

During 4-month-old Ronnie's assessment, the nurse notes that his posterior fontanel is closed. What would be the most appropriate action for the nurse to take at this time? Why?

Once these skills are developed, the infant will be able to move forward (walk), first with assistance, then alone. A summary of motor skills can be found in Table 4-1.

Fine Motor

As development progresses, the infant begins to utilize the hands and eyes to explore and manipulate the environment. Fine motor development is the ability to coordinate hand–eye movement in an orderly and progressive manner.

A summary of fine motor development can be found in Table 4-2. See Figure 4-2 for development of grasp during the first year.

PSYCHOSEXUAL DEVELOPMENT

According to Freud's theory, the infant is in the oral stage of development (birth to 1 year), during which the need for pleasure dominates life. Since oral stimulation or sucking is the central focus of this stage (Dixon & Stein, 2000), feeding or nutritive sucking becomes the most important source of pleasure and satisfaction.

As development progresses, the infant learns to connect actions with end results. For example, the infant learns that cries of hunger result in being fed, and eventually the caregiver's touch is associated with feeding needs being met as infants learn to delay the need for immediate gratification in anticipation of being fed. Infants not fed within a few minutes of being held will start to cry as a signal that the need for the pleasure or

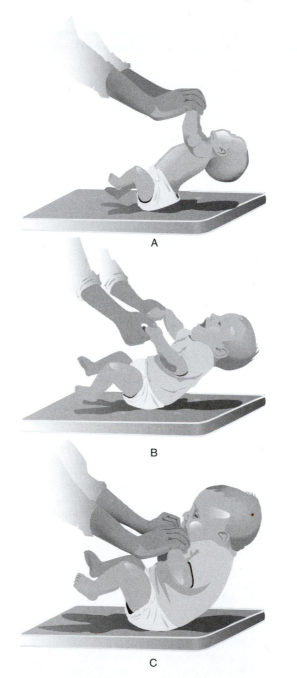

Figure 4-1 Head Lag at (A) 1 Month Old, (B) 2 Months Old, and (C) 4 Months Old

TABLE 4-1 SUMMARY OF GROSS MOTOR SKILLS IN INFANTS

Age	Motor Skill
2–3 Months	Some head lag when pulled to sitting position Holds head up and supports weight on forearms when prone Some head bobbing while supported in sitting position Rolls from abdomen to back Tonic neck and Moro reflexes disappearing
4–6 Months	Good head control with no head lag, holds chest and abdomen up with weight supported by hands while prone Sits with support Rolls from back to abdomen Bears weight in standing position with support
7–8 Months	Sits alone without support Bears weight with some support
9–12 Months	Moves from prone to sitting to standing position without assistance Stands alone without support Goes from crawling to creeping to cruising Attempts to walk alone

TABLE 4-2 SUMMARY OF FINE MOTOR DEVELOPMENT IN INFANTS

Age	Motor Skill
2–3 Months	Follows object past midline Holds hands open Regards own hands and fingers when held in front of face Places hand in mouth Briefly reaches at a dangling object
4–5 Months	Reaches for object beyond grasp Looks from object to hand and back again Places object in mouth Uses whole hand to grasp object Plays actively with hands and feet
6–7 Months	Holds objects securely and bangs them together Actively drops objects Transfers object between hands
8–9 Months	Pincer grasp beginning Releases object at will Dominant hand preference emerging
10–12 Months	True pincer grasp present Can self-feed finger foods Can place small objects into a container Can remove small objects from a container Can hold and mark with a crayon Can turn multiple pages in a book

Grasp of a rattle

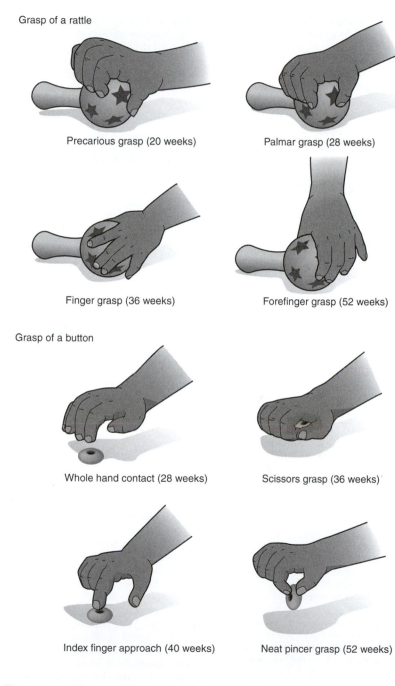

Precarious grasp (20 weeks)

Palmar grasp (28 weeks)

Finger grasp (36 weeks)

Forefinger grasp (52 weeks)

Grasp of a button

Whole hand contact (28 weeks)

Scissors grasp (36 weeks)

Index finger approach (40 weeks)

Neat pincer grasp (52 weeks)

Figure 4-2 Development of Prehension

comfort from the feeding has not been met.

In addition to feeding, another source of pleasure and satisfaction for the infant is obtained through nonnutritive sucking. With the infant's natural tendency to suck, nonnutritive sucking occurs first by accident through the reflex of rooting and then purposefully by actively placing objects, such as toys, fingers, or a pacifier, in the mouth.

PSYCHOSOCIAL DEVELOPMENT

The psychosocial development of an infant, as defined by Erikson (1963), is centered around the concept of trust versus mistrust. According to Erikson, trust is developed when basic needs (feeding, clothing, comforting) are met by caretakers. If these needs are not met, the infant will develop a mistrust of others.

However, trust development involves more than just meeting basic needs. The quality of the caregiver–infant interaction

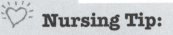

Nursing Tip:

Understanding psychosocial development
To improve your assessment of the infant's psychosocial development, ask yourself:
• Does the infant demonstrate trust in the environment?
• What does the caregiver know about developing the infant's sense of trust?
• Does the caregiver have factors (divorce, financial problems, health problems) that might interfere with the infant's development of a sense of trust?
• Are there any environmental and/or cultural biases that might impede the caregiver's ability to assist the infant in developing a trusting relationship?

while providing care also plays a major role. If the caregiver consistently demonstrates nurturing behaviors (talking, playing, smiling, clothing, comforting), the infant will develop a strong sense of trust. If these behaviors are absent, trust development may be delayed.

COGNITIVE DEVELOPMENT

According to Piaget (1952), an infant is in the sensorimotor stage (birth to 24 months) of cognitive development when knowledge is acquired about an object through interaction with that object and use of the senses. The major task for the infant, according to Piaget, is object permanence, in which the infant learns an object is not an extension of the self and continues to exist even when it cannot be seen. Refer to Table 4-3 for a summary of stages 1–4 of the sensorimotor stage.

HEALTH SCREENING

Health screening provides the opportunity to assess for and detect any problems the infant may have and includes tests to detect phenylketonuria (PKU), iron deficiency anemia, lead poisoning, and hypothyroidism. The infant's health screening actually begins immediately after birth with the first Apgar scoring and physical examination. Once discharged home, the infant's health promotion and maintenance becomes the responsibility of the caregiver, who should be encouraged to contact the health care provider for any health concerns.

In the first year, health screening or well-child visits are usually scheduled when the infant is 2 weeks, and 2, 4, 6, 9, and 12 months old. The screening visit typically includes health assessment, physical examination, growth indicators (weight, height, head circumference), anticipatory guidance, parental concerns, and adminis-

TABLE 4-3 SUMMARY OF PIAGET'S SENSORIMOTOR STAGE OF DEVELOPMENT FOR INFANCY

Name	Stage	Age	Characteristics
Exercising Reflexes	One	0 to 1 month	Newborn uses and gains some control over inborn reflexes. (Suck what is near their mouth, grasp what touches their palm.) Reflexes are practiced and become more proficient, but newborn cannot reach out to deliberately suck/grasp an object.
Primary Circular Reactions	Two	1 to 4 months	Pleasurable behavior is repeated just by chance. (Thumb touches mouth by chance triggering the sucking reflex which results in a pleasurable sensation. Response is repeated.) Is termed *primary* because infant's own body is involved.
Secondary Circular Reactions	Three	4 to 8 months	Infant accidently does something pleasing or interesting (moves a mobile); action is then deliberately repeated so same result is obtained. Is termed *secondary* because it happens outside the infant's body.
Purposeful Coordination of Secondary Schemes	Four	8 to 12 months	Infants coordinate motor activities by using sensory input to become more deliberate and purposeful in their actions. (See a toy they want that is across the room and then crawl so they can obtain it.) Beginning to anticipate events and try out what they have done before to solve problems they currently face.

tration of scheduled immunizations. Table 4-4 provides an outline of typical health screening visits.

During the visit, the caregiver will probably have questions and concerns regarding the infant's ongoing needs and care. The nurse can be instrumental in providing information related to development, nutrition, elimination, hygiene, safety, immunizations, and play.

TABLE 4-4 HEALTH SCREENING VISITS FOR INFANTS

Emphasis of Visit	1 Month	2 Months	4 Months	6 Months	9 Months	12 Months
Assessments: Developmental milestones, hearing and vision, nutritional	✔	✔	✔	✔	✔	✔
Physical examination	✔	✔	✔	✔	✔	✔
Growth measurements: Height, weight, head circumference	✔	✔	✔	✔	✔	✔
Immunizations*						
Anticipatory guidance: Infant care, expected growth, and developmental milestones, safety, dental health	✔	✔	✔	✔	✔	✔
Screenings:						
PKU	✔					
Thyroid	✔					
Hematocrit, Hemoglobin	✔				✔	
Lead					✔ or	✔
Parental concerns	✔	✔	✔	✔	✔	✔

Adapted from: Shelov, S. P. (Ed.), (1998). Caring for your baby and young child. New York: Bantam.
* Refer to Appendix F for latest immunization schedule.

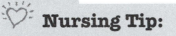

Nursing Tip:

Parental concerns about infant hearing and vision
Be alert to any concerns expressed by the caregiver regarding the infant's lack of response or inability to achieve milestones associated with vision and/or hearing.

Vision Screening

Research has shown that even newborns have full visual array with acuity of 20/100 to 20/200 (Behrman, 2002). Therefore, it is important problems with vision be detected early to prevent significant delays in motor development since visual and auditory abilities have an impact on perception and understanding of the surrounding environment.

Visual development is demonstrated by the infant's ability to follow a light or object placed within the visual field and the cessation of body movements after fixating on the object. Infants prefer the human face, demonstrated by visual attentiveness when

Family Teaching

When to Call Your Health Care Provider

The following signs and symptoms may indicate the need to contact the health care provider:

- Fever: under 2 months 100.2°F (37.9°C); 3 to 6 months 101°F (38.3°C); over 6 months 103°F (39.4°C)

- Feeding poorly: Lack of interest, poor sucking effort, failure to awaken for feeding

- Vomiting

- Decreased activity or alertness: appears listless

- Inconsolable crying

- Abnormal movement: unusual jerking of body

- Unusual skin color: pale or mottled skin color; bluish around the lips

(Reisser, 1998; Shelov, 1998)

Nursing Alert:

Infant Behaviors Related to Visual Problems

- *Absence of blink*
- *Absence of doll's eye reflex (movement of head to the right or left, in which eyes lag behind and do not immediately adjust to the new position; disappears as infant is able to focus)*
- *Does not fixate on objects*
- *Does not follow objects by 1 month of age*
- *Does not watch own hands and feet by 4 months of age*
- *Does not reach for objects by 5 months of age*
- *Absent or poor hand–eye coordination by 7 months of age*
- *Does not watch objects fall when dropped*

Nursing Alert:

Infant Behaviors Related to Hearing Problems

- *Lack of startle reflex or blink with a loud sound*
- *Failure to be awakened by loud noises in the environment*
- *Failure to turn head toward a sound by 6 months of age*
- *Absent babble or voice inflection by 7 months of age*
- *General indifference to sound*
- *Lack of response to the spoken word*
- *Failure to follow verbal direction*
- *Failure to respond to a human voice*

interacting with the caregiver. By 6 months, the infant can recognize familiar faces and may experience stranger anxiety. As visual acuity improves and motor skills develop, the infant begins to respond to the variety of colors and shapes in the environment. Of particular interest to the infant is any object with a black–white contrast (Slusher & McClure, 1992). Any caregiver concern regarding visual responsiveness and/or lack of eye contact in their infant may indicate visual problems.

Hearing Screening

The intensity of the infant's response to auditory stimuli may vary depending on the state of alertness. The human voice is an important and readily available sound stimulus, and infants prefer the human voice to other sounds in their environment. The infant also responds well to musical toys and different sounds.

Hearing problems should be detected early in life to prevent significant delays in speech development. A hearing problem is identified when an infant does not consistently achieve hearing milestones in development (Capute & Accardo, 1978).

HEALTH PROMOTION

Immunizations

The recommended childhood immunization schedule can be found in Appendix F.

Prior to administering any immunization, the nurse assesses for contraindications to

Family Teaching

(Shelov, 1998)
Home Care with Immunizations

- Most common reactions usually last 1–2 days:
  Irritability
  Mild loss of appetite
  Low-grade fever (<102°F)
  Redness, swelling, and tenderness at the injection site

- General treatment of reaction:
  Give acetaminophen at the time of the immunization
  Administer acetaminophen every 4–6 hours for a total of three doses

- Immunization-specific reaction:
  Diphtheria, Tetanus, Pertussis (DTaP)—low-grade fever with redness, swelling, and tenderness at injection site
  Inactivated polio vaccine (IPV)—tenderness at injection site
  Hepatitis B (hep B)—irritability and redness, swelling, and tenderness at injection site
  Measles, mumps, rubella (MMR)—mild rash, low-grade fever, and drowsiness beginning 7–10 days after immunization

- Contact the health care provider immediately if the infant develops any symptoms other than the common reactions or if the mild reactions persist longer than 2 days.

(Shelov, 1998)

administration. However immunizations are usually not contraindicated when a mild illness such as allergic rhinitis, mild diarrhea, or mild respiratory infection is present. The nurse also provides the caregiver with information about the benefits and risks of the immunizations and answers questions about the immunizations. In addition, the caregiver should receive information about possible reactions the infant might experience after receiving the immunizations.

Nutrition

Since the infant experiences rapid changes in growth and development over a relatively short time, a good nutritional foundation is necessary. The responsibility for meeting the infant's nutritional needs falls on the caregiver; needs are normally evaluated during a routine assessment or when the caregiver expresses a concern over the infant's pattern of growth and development.

For the first few months of the child's life, the infant will be either breastfed, formula-fed, or a combination of the two. Both breast and formula feedings are nutritionally sound, easy to digest, and provide the infant with the needed nutrients to grow. They also provide approximately 20 kcal/oz. The infant's nutritional requirements are based on the physical activity and rate of growth needed to support life. At birth, energy requirements are 120 kcal/kg/day. They gradually decrease to 100 kcal/kg/day by 1 year of age (Whitley, Cataldo, DeBruyne, & Rolfes, 1996), because of the gradual decline in metabolic needs as the infant's growth slows. In addition to energy requirements, the infant must have adequate fluid intake, which is based on daily energy expenditure. Infant fluid requirements are 1–1.5 mL/kcal expended per day (Whitley et al., 1996).

The American Academy of Pediatrics recommends introducing semisolid foods, i.e., single-grain infant cereal and applesauce, when the infant can sit well with support, the tongue thrust (extrusion reflex) has decreased, and the infant's hunger seems unsatisfied after nursing or bottle feeding (Arrigo, 1994; Pipes, & Trahms, 1993);

this usually occurs between 4 and 6 months of age. Introduction of solids before this time can contribute to food allergies because food is not completely digested; increased calorie intake, resulting in an overweight infant; and the danger of choking. The decision to introduce solid foods should be individualized. Developmental behaviors related to feeding can be found in Table 4-5 (Arrigo, 1994; Dixon & Stein, 2000).

Usually, the first food introduced is iron-fortified rice cereal, since it is the easiest to digest and the least likely to cause allergies. The cereal can be mixed with formula or expressed breast milk and, later, fruit or juice. Because of the infant's need for iron, iron-fortified cereal should be continued until 18 months of age. Fruits or vegetables are usually the next foods introduced. Vegetables should be introduced before

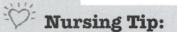 **Nursing Tip:**

Salt and sugar content of strained foods
The caregiver should be cautioned about the salt and sugar content of strained foods. Extra sugar intake can contribute to excessive calorie intake. Salt contributes to an increase in extracellular fluid and a slight rise in blood pressure. Over the past few years, companies that commercially prepare strained foods have made an effort to decrease the salt and sugar content in their baby foods (Dietary Guidelines for Infants, 1997).

TABLE 4-5 DEVELOPMENTAL BEHAVIORS RELATED TO FEEDING

Age	Skill
Newborn–2 Months	Primitive reflexes facilitate feeding Hunger cry initiates feeding interaction
2–4 Months	More alert and interactive during feeding Beginning ability to wait for food Associates caregiver's smell, voice, and cradling with feeding Hand-to-mouth behavior quiets infant
4–6 Months	Readiness for solids Excellent head and trunk control Reaching for objects Loss of extrusion reflex of tongue
6–8 Months	Sits alone with steady head during feedings Chewing mechanism developed Holds bottle Vocal eagerness during meal preparation Much more motor activity during feeding
8–10 Months	Readiness finger foods Grasps spoon but cannot use it effectively Enjoys new textures, tastes Emerging independence
10–12 Months	Increasing determination to feed self Neat pincer grasp Holds cup but frequently spills it More verbal and motor behavior during feeding

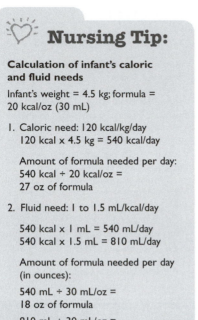

Nursing Tip:

Calculation of infant's caloric and fluid needs

Infant's weight = 4.5 kg; formula = 20 kcal/oz (30 mL)

1. Caloric need: 120 kcal/kg/day
   120 kcal x 4.5 kg = 540 kcal/day

   Amount of formula needed per day:
   540 kcal ÷ 20 kcal/oz =
   27 oz of formula

2. Fluid need: 1 to 1.5 mL/kcal/day

   540 kcal x 1 mL = 540 mL/day
   540 kcal x 1.5 mL = 810 mL/day

   Amount of formula needed per day
   (in ounces):

   540 mL ÷ 30 mL/oz =
   18 oz of formula

   810 mL ÷ 30 mL/oz =
   27 oz of formula

Family Teaching

Common Food Allergies

- Foods to avoid: chocolate, strawberries, citrus fruits, peanut butter, shellfish, egg whites, tomatoes, corn, wheat, nuts

- Common reaction: diarrhea, abdominal pain, nasal congestion, rashes, vomiting

(Reisser, 1998; Shelov, 1998)

Because of cultural variations, it is important to support good nutritional habits that are culturally appropriate.

Due to the potential for an allergic reaction during the infant's first year, certain foods need to avoided until the second half of the first year. (See Family Teaching box.)

When infants can sit steadily, they are usually allowed to drink from a cup. Finger foods are introduced during the second half of the first year as the finger grasp develops, teeth begin to erupt, and hand–eye coordination improves. Table 4-6 is a guide for introducing solid foods.

When discussing the infant's developmental readiness for solid foods, the importance of self-feeding should be stressed. To encourage autonomy, the infant needs to be given the opportunity to explore the texture, smell, color, and taste of food. Refer to Appendix G for information about recommended dietary allowances.

fruits since the infant could become accustomed to the sweet taste of fruits. By 8–10 months of age, most fruits and vegetables should have been introduced and strained meats can be added to the infant's diet. Fruit juices, a good source of vitamin C, which enhances absorption of iron in the cereal, are usually offered the same time as fruits.

TABLE 4-6 GUIDE FOR INTRODUCTION OF SOLID FOODS

Age	Food	Frequency
4–6 months	Cereal	Twice a day
6–8 months	Vegetables	Once a day
	Fruits	Twice a day
	Juices	Between meals (small amounts)
8–10 months	Meats	Once a day
10 months	Egg yolks	Once a day
9–12 months	Finger foods	At least daily

Family Teaching

Feeding Infant Solid Foods

Stress the importance of the infant's need to practice the new skill of eating solids (chewing and swallowing) instead of sucking.

- Introducing one new food at a time at 4–7-day intervals allows for identifying food allergies and gives the infant the chance to become accustomed to the new food.
- Feed solids with a spoon. Put a small amount of food (1 teaspoon) on the spoon and place toward the back of the infant's mouth. This enables the infant to overcome the diminishing extrusion reflex and facilitates the newly acquired skills of chewing and swallowing.
- Give solid foods when the infant is hungry then follow with formula or breast milk. This encourages the infant to eat the solids instead of becoming satiated with fluids.
- Gradually increase solid foods to approximately 4 oz per feeding. As solid food intake advances, the infant's daily intake of milk will decrease to approximately 24 oz at 12 months of age.

(Reisser, 1998; Shelov, 1998)

Family Teaching

Helpful Hints for Infant Self-Feeding

- Place high chair in an area that can be easily cleaned.
- Place infant in a high chair and fasten safety belt.
- Use a large plastic bib.
- Dress infant in easily removable and washable clothes.

Family Teaching

Finger Foods

Rule of thumb: Pieces should be the size of the infant's thumb. Food items that are hard and small should be avoided since they can slip easily into the child's throat and may cause choking.

Foods to avoid:

- Nuts, popcorn, kernel corn, chunks of meat (e.g., hot dogs), chips, pretzels, berries, grapes, cherries, raw fruit and vegetables (e.g., apples, carrots, celery)
- Sticky, stringy, and chewy foods (e.g., peanut butter, caramel)
- Small, hard, or round candy (e.g., jelly beans, peppermints, butterscotch)

(Arrigo, 1994; Martin, 1996; Reisser, 1998)

Weaning is a process of giving up one method of feeding for another, such as the transitions from breast to bottle, and from bottle to cup. Even though there is no right way or time to wean an infant, behaviors consistent with weaning include eating from a spoon, holding the bottle, feeding the self with fingers or a spoon, eating foods that require chewing, and a decreasing desire to be held during feeding. If the infant is weaned too soon from breast milk or formula, iron deficiency anemia could occur (Reisser, 1998). Weaning should be a process in which breastfeeding sessions are gradually replaced by a bottle, and/or the bottle-feeding sessions are gradually replaced by increased amounts of solid foods and drinking from a cup (Reisser, 1998; Shelov, 1998).

Elimination

Since the stomach enlarges during infancy, a greater volume of food can be accommodated and by the end of the first year of life, infants may have one to two bowel movements per day. However, the infant is vulnerable to vomiting, diarrhea, and dehydration if any type of gastric irritation is present. The appearance of the infant's stools reflects gastrointestinal system immaturity. That is why it is not uncommon for solid foods (carrots, corn, peas) to pass incompletely broken down in the stools. In addition, excess fiber in the diet may result in loose, bulky stools.

Breastfed infants are rarely constipated (their stools are usually loose), but formula fed infants may experience constipation if they do not receive adequate fluids. It is not uncommon for infants to grimace, grunt, and have their faces turn red during elimination. This is a normal response to passing a stool as long as the stools do not contain blood or are hard. Stools may become loose with initial introduction of solid foods such as fruits, but this usually dissipates over time.

It is important to teach parents normal elimination patterns for infants. If parents are concerned about an infant's loose stools, it is important to gather information about the number of stools passed per day, their color and consistency, and whether or not they contain mucus or blood. Any accompanying fever, vomiting, abdominal cramping, changes in appetite, weight loss, or decreased voidings may indicate the infant needs to be examined by a health care provider, as these symptoms are indicative of an infectious process.

Hygiene

Infants do not need much bathing during the first year of life. Before bathing, all supplies, including a basin of lukewarm water, a washcloth, towels, baby shampoo, mild soap, and cotton balls should be gathered. While giving a sponge bath, the caregiver should expose only those areas being washed to avoid chilling the infant. A cotton ball can be used to clean the eyes first, moving from the inner to outer areas, before using a washcloth for the remainder of the face. The perineal area is always washed last. It is important to clean all body creases thoroughly, especially the neck folds and perineal area, and wash and dry each body part before moving on to the next area. To prevent cradle cap (seborrhea), a dry, scaly scalp condition, hair should be washed every other day using a mild baby shampoo. If cradle cap does develop, a soft-bristle toothbrush can be used to remove the crusts and mineral oil or petroleum jelly can be used to soften the patches. After the cord falls off, the infant can be bathed in a sink or plastic tub in about 2 inches of warm water. A towel can be placed on the bottom to prevent the infant from slipping. While bathing infants, caregivers should always hold or use a tub ring to stabilize the infant even when able to sit upright without much support. Since bathing can be an important time for bonding and play, it should be unhurried and nonstressful.

Generally, infants do not need lotions or baby powder. If lotions are used, they should be hypoallergenic and initially placed on the hands for warming before being rubbed on the skin. Baby powder, typically a mixture of hydrous magnesium silicate (talc) and other silicates can cause a severe aspiration pneumonia, which can often be fatal. Therefore, its use is discouraged. Nail clippers can be used to keep fingernails and toenails short to prevent infants from scratching themselves. The best time to clip the nails is right after the bath because nails are softer.

Dental Health

Tooth development and eruption are affected by genetics, gender, race, and growth patterns. Deciduous teeth, also referred to as primary or baby teeth, are the first teeth to develop and erupt. The eruption of teeth varies among children, but typically begins around 3–4 months of age. The first teeth to erupt are usually the lower central incisors, followed by the upper central incisors after approximately 4–8 weeks (Shelov, 1998) (Figure 4-3).

Dental hygiene should begin with the eruption of the deciduous teeth by gently cleaning the infant's teeth and gums with a

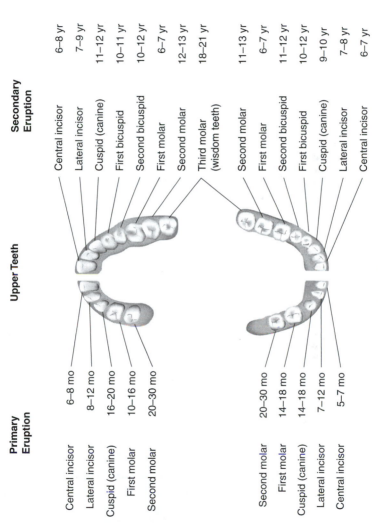

Figure 4-3 Sequence of Tooth Erruption

clean wet cloth using a circular movement or with a small, soft-bristled toothbrush (Jaques, 1993). It is important to establish a routine of dental hygiene early in life to prevent future dental problems.

Fluoride helps prevent dental caries, and may be given as a supplement if drinking water does not contain enough fluoride. The fluoride content of the drinking water system should be investigated by contacting the local water board or company.

An infant who is exclusively breastfed or whose formula is prepared with water that is not fluoridated should receive a daily supplement of sodium fluoride (Jaques, 1993). According to the American Academy of Pediatrics (AAP) (1995), fluoride supplements should be started at 6 months of life. However, when fluoridation is available in the water and exceeds 0.3 ppm concentration, the infant does not need fluoride supplements. The level that protects tooth enamel without causing tooth staining from an excessive amount of fluoride is 0.6 ppm. Refer to Table 4-7 for the dosing of flouride.

Dental caries can also occur in infants who have frequent and/or prolonged exposure to sugars found in milk, formula, or juice. The longer the sugar stays on the tooth enamel, the more opportunity there is for bacteria in the mouth to combine with sugar to form dental caries (Jaques, 1993; Oppenheim, 1996). This type of dental caries, known as nursing or bottle-mouth caries, is commonly seen in infants who receive a bottle filled with formula or juice at nap or bedtime. The problem also occurs in infants who breast-feed for prolonged times or on demand after tooth eruption (Oppenheim, 1996).

Dental hygiene also includes routine visits to the dentist. The first dental visit usually occurs after several teeth have erupted. Most dentists suggest that this first visit occur before the child is 2 years of age (Jaques, 1993; Oppenheim, 1996). The frequency of dental visits is usually based on the child's state of health, family history of dental problems, and the need for fluoride supplements (McDonald & Avery, 1994).

During infancy, the period of eruption of deciduous teeth is called teething and occurs over several months. During eruption, the

periodontal membrane becomes slightly swollen, red, and tender. The infant may have increased drooling and fussiness, mild anorexia, and an increased desire to bite. Other symptoms such as low-grade fever, vomiting, and diarrhea have also been attributed to teething (Shelov, 1998). The accompanying Family Teaching box contains several measures that can be used to soothe the infant during the teething process.

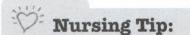

Nursing Tip:

Estimation of deciduous teeth related to child's age
Caregivers are usually concerned about the number of teeth their child should have at a certain age. While each child gets teeth at a different rate, the following formula is used by many clinicians as a guide to determine the expected number of teeth a child should have at a certain age: Subtract 6 from the child's age in months to equal the total number teeth expected. For example: 18 months old − 6 = 12 teeth expected at 18 months.

Family Teaching

Soothing Swollen, Tender Gums

To soothe swollen, red gums, try:

- Frozen teething ring
- Ice cube in a washcloth
- Zwieback
- Hard rubber toy
- Topical application of an oral anesthetic such as Ora-Gel

For irritability and/or a low-grade temperature, give:

- Acetaminophen according to recommended dosage

TABLE 4-7 DAILY FLOURIDE SUPPLEMENTATION*

Child's Age	Fluoride Content of Water		
	< 0.3 ppm	0.3–0.6 ppm	> 0.6 ppm
Birth–6 Months	0	0	0
6 Months–3 Years	0.25	0	0
3–6 Years	0.50	0.25	0
6–12 Years	1.00	0.50	0

* Fluoride dose given in milligrams.
Adapted from the 1995 recommendations of the AAP.

Rest and Sleep

Infants have variable sleep patterns that are influenced by temperament, satisfaction with feedings, caregivers' responses to periodic awakenings, and environmental conditions (Mackin, Medendorp, & Maier, 1989). There is a transition from neonatal sleeping, which is shorter with multiple sleep periods, to the more organized central nervous system maturation after the third month. As the child matures, the sleep–wake cycle evolves into a pattern of being awake during the day and asleep at night (Dixon & Stein, 2000). Refer to Table 4-8.

During the first months of life, infants experience more rapid eye movement (REM) sleep than at any other time in life (Herzog, 1997).

As the infant matures, the amount of REM sleep diminishes, the required hours for sleep gradually decrease, and sleep–wake periods develop into a day/night cycle. These changes develop over time and are termed sleep consolidation (fewer periods of sleep with longer durations) and diurnal cycle (sleeping through the night alternating with daytime wakefulness) (Weissbluth, 1991). By the time the infant is 3 to 4 months of age, the diurnal cycle is well established and a pattern of 9–11 hours of nocturnal sleep has developed. Napping also occurs during this time and the number of naps per day varies with each infant. Generally the infant will take one or two naps by the age of 1 year (Weissbluth, 1991).

After regular sleep patterns develop, the infant may begin to experience periods of awakening during the night, referred to as night wakings. These seem to coincide with the development of separation anxiety. Even though this is a transient phase, night waking can result in a strained caregiver–infant relationship. During this time, it is not uncommon for the infant to have difficulty falling asleep at night and nap times as well as falling back to sleep if awakened. Methods such as soft music, rocking and providing a

TABLE 4-8 INFANT SLEEP TIME

Age	Awake	Day Sleep	Night Sleep
Newborn	7.5 hours	8 hours	8.5 hours
1 Month	8.5 hours	6.75 hours	8.75 hours
4 Months	9 hours	4.5 hours	10.5 hours
6 Months	9.25–9.75 hours	3.25–4 hours	11 hours
1 Year	10.25 hours	2.25 hours	11.5 hours

Adapted from Wright (1994, May). Sleep, little baby. American Baby, 56(5), 75–81.

has both advocates and critics, but no evidence has been presented indicating that this practice is dangerous, psychologically harmful, or even habit forming (Tonnessen, 1996; Wright, 1994).

Part of the nurse's developmental assessment of the infant is the evaluation of sleep patterns related to daily sleep routine, sleeping position, sleeping arrangements, changes in feeding, environmental problems, and occurrence of stressors in the family unit.

The best way to prevent sleep problems is to assist the caregiver in understanding the infant's individual needs, and provide information relevant to healthy sleep patterns and signs of maturation. Cultural practices and personal preferences should be considered as well as measures to foster healthy sleep patterns (Anders, Halpern, & Hua, 1992; Wright, 1995). See Box 4-1 for specific information.

The sleeping position of the infant is also important. Even though some infants may seem to sleep better or more soundly on their stomachs (prone), sudden infant death syndrome has been associated with this sleeping position, and the American Academy of Pediatrics recommends that infants be placed on their back (supine) while sleeping (American Academy of Pediatrics [AAP], 2002). (Refer to Chaper 3.)

pacifier and a dim light (night light) may assist the infant in returning to sleep. Usually, the infant can settle back to sleep if left alone during the awakenings that occur every 2–4 hours during the sleep times.

The infant's sleep state can also be influenced by sleeping arrangements. Sleeping arrangements for an infant vary widely from family to family. For the first few months of the child's life or when the infant is ill, the sleeping arrangement known as co-sleeping is a relatively common practice used by many cultures, especially among African-American, Hispanic, and Asian families (Brazelton, 1990; Wright, 1994). According to Tonnessen (1996), approximately 25%–30% of caregivers co-sleep, or share the family bed, with children. Co-sleeping

Activity and Play

Play for the infant moves rapidly from accidental pleasure-producing activities to purposeful, repetitive activities with an increasing awareness of the surrounding environment. By 6 months to 1 year, the infant engages in repetitive activities involving voices, sounds, music, and a variety of toys, which enhance the development of language and sensorimotor skills.

The caregiver's involvement and responsiveness influence the quality of play; interpersonal contact is essential. The infant needs to be played with, not just allowed to play, because the richest play occurs when the caregiver takes an active role.

Box 4-1   Fostering Healthy Sleep

- Establish a bedtime routine such as giving a bath, reading a book, telling a story, singing, holding, and/or rocking and playing music.
- Provide a quiet, relaxed environment in a cozy, safe crib.
- Maintain a comfortable room temperature.
- Use low-level lighting in the room.
- Do not use the crib as a playpen.
- Place infant in the bed when drowsy but not asleep.
- Place supine or side-lying for sleep.
- Do not feed during the night; if feeding is necessary, make it brief.
- Do not awaken infant to feed or change a diaper.

Caregiver play nurtures the relationship through shared activities, accomplishments, and joys. Suggestions to aid the caregiver in being involved in infant play include (Dixon & Stein, 2000):

- Safety first—be sure toys are developmentally appropriate.
- The infant learns by using all five senses—provide toys accordingly.
- Place the infant in a variety of positions throughout the day, i.e., stomach, side, back.
- Encourage the use of hands and feet in play.
- Offer a few new experiences each day.
- Encourage banging toys together.
- Praise often.

During routine infant assessment, the nurse should ask the caregiver about the nature of the infant's play. With the emergence of voluntary reach and grasp, it is important to investigate the infant's motor competency, visual–motor coordination, and the appropriateness of the environment in exploring the object world. To facilitate the infant's continued development, provide relevant toys and activities appropriate for infants (Dixon & Stein, 2000). Table 4-9 provides a list of developmentally appropriate toys and activities for the infant.

When inquiring about the nature of the infant's play, listen for details about the qual-ity and complexity of play to determine if it is age-appropriate. The description of play behavior can be beneficial in screening for problems such as developmental delays, neurologic problems, delayed social skills, autism, learning disabilities, and emotional disturbances (Dixon & Stein, 2000).

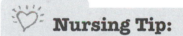 **Nursing Tip:**

Motor skills and coordination
To have a clearer understanding of the infant's motor competency and visual–motor coordination, ask yourself:

- What motor skills does the infant demonstrate?
- Are these motor skills appropriate for the age of the infant?
- How does the infant use hand and mouth in exploration?
- What toy does the infant choose?
- Does the infant use both hands and arms equally?
- Are the infant's movements smooth?
- How does the caregiver facilitate the infant's play?

TABLE 4-9   TOYS AND ACTIVITIES APPROPRIATE FOR THE INFANT

Age	Toys/Activity
Birth–3 Months	Black-and-white or red colored pattern cards Soft, cuddle toys Nonbreakable mirror Rattles Mobiles Music boxes Talking and singing Rocking and holding Gentle massage Interaction with other people
3–6 Months	Crib gyms Squeaky toys Teething rings Different textured toys Noise-making toys Talking and singing Play pat-a-cake, play peek-a-boo Social interaction with other people
6–9 Months	Safe place to creep/crawl Bath tub toys Jack-in-the-box Nested toys Big, soft blocks Drinking cup Toys to bang together Talking and singing Playing hide-n-seek Social interaction with other people
9–12 Months	Continue with toys for 6–9 months Safe place for exploration Push-pull and motion toys Colorful cloth books Paper for tearing Building blocks Metal pots and pans Different shaped and colored toys Social interaction with other people

Safety and Injury Prevention

Infants are in a state of perpetual development and refinement of motor skills. In addition, infants have an insatiable curiosity about the environment. When this perpetual change and curiosity are combined, the infant is at risk for accidental injury, the leading cause of infant deaths, especially between 6 and 12 months of age. To ensure a safe environment, the caregiver must be aware of the safety concerns most associated with each stage of motor development.

Anticipatory guidance, to prevent injury, should include:

- The reason why infants are prone to injury
- The importance of injury prevention
- The importance of setting age appropriate limits
- The importance of always anticipating danger and removing the infant from the danger

A general safety checklist to childproof a home can be found in Box 4-2.

As the infant's ability to explore the environment increases daily, so do the hazards encountered. The caregiver needs to be reminded that the ability to roll and turn makes the infant susceptible to falling if left unattended on the bed, changing table, or counter top. When the infant can reach for and grasp items and bring them to the mouth, the caregiver must be cautious in leaving objects within the infant's reach. With the ability to creep and crawl, the infant can move farther and faster than the caregiver might expect, so the floor should be kept free of small objects and child-proof latches used in cupboards. As locomotion improves, the infant will soon be able to stand and walk (cruise) around objects. Once this occurs, the caregiver must constantly be vigilant since the infant is now susceptible to

falling, suffocating, and drowning. Table 4-10 provides information related to the appropriate infant safety measures associated with specific developmental achievements and type of injury.

ANTICIPATORY GUIDANCE

Use of Pacifiers

Oral stimulation or sucking is one of most important sources of pleasure and satisfaction for the infant, and one of the first coordinated muscular activities. There are two forms of sucking, nutritive and nonnutritive (Turgeon-O'Brien, Lachapelle, Gagnon, Larocque, & Maheu-Robert, 1996). Nutritive sucking enables the infant to obtain essential nutrients necessary for life through either bottle- or breastfeeding. Nonnutritive sucking is used as a source of pleasure and satisfaction, which provides the infant the opportunity to learn self-gratification. Nonnutritive sucking provides the infant with a means of gaining self-control and as a transition from the stages of waking and sleeping (Wagner, 1997).

Since sucking provides the infant with pleasure and satisfaction, caregivers need to understand the difference between nutritive and nonnutritive sucking. If the infant is fussy and crying, the caregiver may offer a pacifier as a soothing method without understanding the infant's true need. If the infant is hungry, however, offering a pacifier will not calm the infant.

In an attempt to understand infant needs, caregivers are encouraged to note the time and circumstances around their infant's distress. Distress may be due to a need for sleep/ food, to be held, or simply to suck (Wagner, 1997). If the infant simply wants to suck, the caregiver may select a pacifier to meet this need, or infants may start sucking on their fingers. As time goes on the infant will decide which method of nonnutritive sucking is the favorite.

If a pacifier is selected, it is important that the caregiver receive appropriate informa-

Family Teaching

Check for Hidden Dangers

To ensure the infant's safety, the caregiver is encouraged to crouch down at what is the child's eye level, close to the floor, to survey the environment for hazards the infant might encounter. It may even be necessary to crawl around to find any hidden dangers. Infants should be placed in appropriate child safety restraints in the back seat whenever riding in automobiles.

Box 4-2 General Safety Checklist

House
- All cleaning supplies, medicines, and cosmetics locked up or out of reach
- All knives or sharp edge objects out of reach
- Poisonous plants in the home removed
- All firearms removed or locked up
- Ammunition stored separately from firearms
- Fans and heaters out of reach
- Carbon monoxide detectors working (Replace batteries every 6 months.)
- All small objects picked up and out of sight
- No removable small parts on toys
- Plastic bags and latex balloons stored out of reach
- Unused large appliances kept locked
- Pool area gated/fenced

Falls
- All unused electrical outlets covered with safety caps
- All electrical wires out of reach or hidden
- Furniture sturdy and in good repair
- Walkways clear of any obstacles
- Stairway gated
- Sturdy handrails on all stairs/steps
- Window screens in good repair
- Nonskid rugs used

Burns
- No smoking around children and all cigarettes and matches out of reach
- Guards on front of heating appliances, furnace, fireplace
- Hot water heater thermostat set at <120°F
- All cooking utensil handles to the back of stove
- No drinking or handling hot liquids around children
- Smoke detectors working correctly (Replace batteries every 6 months.)
- Fire extinguishers easily accessible for adults

Emergency Needs
- Post all emergency numbers by telephones
- House address and phone number by each telephone
- First-aid kit up to date
- Syrup of ipecac in home
- Have and practice an emergency exit plan in case of a fire
- Caregivers know CPR

Adapted from Dixon, S., & Stein, M. (2000). Encounters with children: Pediatric behaviors and development (3rd ed.). St. Louis: Mosby.

TABLE 4-10   INFANT SAFETY

Birth to 4 Months

Places objects in mouth
Reaches for objects
Rolls from side to back

Type of Injury	Safety Checklist
Falls	Keep crib rails up. Never leave infant unattended on a high surface.
Drowning	Never leave infant unattended in bathtub.
Burns	Keep hot water heater temperature <120°F. Always check bath water temperature. Do not hold or drink hot liquids when holding infant. Install smoke and carbon monoxide detectors in home. Avoid sun exposure. Do not use microwave oven for warming formula or food. Always check temperature of formula prior to feeding.
Strangulation	Be sure crib slats are <2⅜ inches apart. Be sure mattress fits tightly against slats. Do not tie anything to crib. Keep infant's crib away from curtain or blind cords. Never tie any string around infant's neck.
Motor vehicle accident	Use only an approved infant-restraint system in the car. Do not leave infant unsecured in car seat. Always put car seat in the back seat facing rear. Never place car seat in front if airbag present or activated.
Choking	Keep small objects out of reach. Never leave infant unattended on the floor.
Suffocation	Do not use pillows in the infant's bed. Keep plastic bags/wrap out of reach.
Ingestion	Do not smoke around infant.

4 to 7 Months

Sits with support
Rolls from back to side
Bears weight in standing position with support
Reaches for object beyond grasp
Actively drops objects

Type of Injury	Safety Checklist (in addition to those listed for birth to 4 months)
Choking and strangulation	Keep floor free of small objects. Never leave infant unattended on the floor. Do not tie toys on infant's crib. Keep infant's crib away from curtain or blind cords.

continues

TABLE 4-10 *Continued*

Type of Injury	Safety Checklist (in addition to those listed for birth to 4 months)
Burns	Cover all unused electrical outlets with safety caps. Put manufacturer-approved protective covering over heaters, furnaces. Never leave infant unattended on the floor.
Falls	Restrain infant in high chair. Do not use walkers. Never leave infant unattended on the floor Gate all stairways.
Ingestion	Use child-proof latches on cupboards/drawers. Never leave infant unattended on the floor. Keep toxic substances/plants out of reach in locked cabinet. Post poison control number by telephone. Keep ipecac syrup handy Do not smoke around infant.

8 to 12 Months
Drops object at will.
Uses pincer grasp.
Can self-feed finger foods.
Places and removes small objects in a container.
Sits alone without support.
Can move from prone to sitting to standing.
Stands alone without support.
Progresses from crawling to creeping to cruising.
Attempts to walk alone.

Type of Injury	Safety Checklist (in addition to those listed for 1–7 months)
Burns	Turn cooking handles toward back of stove. Do not use a dangling tablecloth. Never leave unattended in bathroom. Keep electrical wires or cords out of reach.
Drowning	Never leave unattended in bathroom. Never leave unattended in the yard, pool, or playground.
Falls	Fence all stairways. Be sure furniture is sturdy. Never leave unattended in the yard or playground. Put infant's bed in lowest position.
Ingestion	Keep medicines, cosmetics, toxic substances/plants out of reach. Never leave unattended in the yard or playground. Post poison control number by telephone. Keep ipecac syrup handy. Do not smoke around infant.

continues

TABLE 4-10 *Continued*	
Type of Injury	**Safety Checklist** **(in addition to those listed for birth to 4 months)**
Choking	Use caution with finger foods (i.e., berries, grapes, cherries, carrots, popcorn, hot dogs) and coins.
	Never leave unattended in the yard or playground.
Motor vehicle	Leave infant in the back seat and switch to forward-facing car seat at 20 lb and at least 1 year.

Adapted from American Academy of Pediatrics (1996). Selecting and using the most appropriate care safety seats for growing children: Guidelines for counseling parents. Pediatrics, 97, 761–762; CDC (1995). Air-bag associated fatal injuries to infants and children riding in front passenger seats–United States. Morbidity and Mortality Weekly Report, 44[45], 845–847; and Keeping your child safe. (1994). The parent's almanac. [On-line.] Available: family.starwave.com/resource/pra/bonus27.html.

tion about pacifier use and safety considerations. The pacifier should not be used as a substitute for general caregiving, nor as an attempt to meet needs other than nonnutritive sucking. When the caregiver selects a pacifier, the shape should correspond with the shape of the nipple used for infant feeding. Many lactation consultants stress caution in introducing a pacifier if the infant is being breast fed since nipple confusion and even refusal to breastfeed can occur if a pacifier is introduced before the nursing relationship has been established (Wagner, 1997).

Feeding Problems

Two common feeding problems seen during the infant years are improper feeding techniques and spitting up. Improper feeding techniques include feeding too much or too little food, feeding infrequently or too frequently, especially during the night, selecting inappropriate foods for the infant's motor or physiological development, holding the bottle at such an angle that air rather than liquid flows into the nipple, not being aware of the infant's cues for needing to be burped or being satiated, incorrect preparation of formula, and not placing the breastfed infant on the breast properly. Most times, an explanation of proper feeding positions,

preparations, suggested schedules for feeding, advice on the normal amount and kind of formula/breast milk to feed an infant, as well as a listening ear will alleviate the situation.

Spitting up, the return of small amounts of undigested food after a feeding, is common in many infants, and should not be confused with vomiting which often is associated with disturbances that may need to be evaluated further. Talking to parents about the normal occurrence of this situation and measures to decrease the frequency of spitting up help alleviate concerns. Frequent burping during and after feeding, positioning the child on the right side with the head slightly elevated after a feeding, and minimal handling during or after a feeding can reduce some spitting up.

Although these are easily corrected feeding problems, an infant with a feeding problem can create a stressful situation for parents, whether or not they are first time parents. Patience and concern on the part of the nurse are always important and will be most appreciated.

Communication

Communication enables the infant to express needs, emotions, and attitudes, and involves central nervous system maturation, cognitive abilities, and social interaction. The infant's initial means of communication—crying and smiling—elicit different responses from the caregiver. When the infant cries, the caregiver responds with soothing behaviors such as speaking softly, holding, and establishing eye contact. Caregiver's reactions to an infant's smile include talking, cooing, smiling, and playing. Even though the infant begins smiling as a reflex, by 2 months the infant has a "social" smile used to gain attention and amazement from the caregiver.

The infant's ability to communicate through language follows a predictable course. During infancy, receptive language (the ability to understand words) is greater than expressive language (the ability to speak words). A summary of language development during infancy can be found in Table 4-11.

Awareness of the expected pattern of language development is important during the infant's routine health screening visits. Assessing the infant's language development by using the Denver II screening tool enables the health care provider to detect any potential problems (Frankenberg, 1990) (see Appendix D).

The caregiver should be encouraged to talk to the infant, make eye contact, and smile during feeding and diaper changes. Once the infant starts to vocalize, the caregiver should repeat these sounds in response to the infant's vocalizations. The names of objects or people should be emphasized when talking to the infant, and the caregiver should always be observant of the infant's response to adult vocalization.

TABLE 4-11 SUMMARY OF LANGUAGE DEVELOPMENT IN INFANCY

Age	Expressive Skills	Receptive Skills
Birth–2 Months	Crying	Sounds elicit startle reflex
	Comfort sound with feeding	Turns and looks for sounds
	Coos	Prefers human voice
	Vocalizes to familiar voice	
3–6 Months	Vocalizes during play and pleasure	Watches speaking mouth
	Squeals	Shifts gaze between sounds
	Laughs aloud	Understands own name
	Less crying	Uses sound to get attention
	Uses vowels and consonant sounds that resemble syllables (ma, mu, ba, ga, ah, da)	
7–9 Months	Increases vowel and consonant sounds	Associates words with activity
	Uses two-syllable sounds (baba, dada)	Responds to simple commands ("no-no")
	Talks along with others	Understands familiar words
10–12 Months	Says "mama" and "dada" to identify caregivers	Recognizes family members' names
	Repeats sounds made by others	Recognizes objects by name
	Makes intentional gestures Learns three to five words	Understands simple commands (say "bye-bye")

Temperament

Temperament is the way a child interacts with the surrounding environment. Children are thought to be genetically endowed with specific temperamental characteristics, which, when combined with the caregiver's personality, produce a characteristic pattern of social interaction between the child and the environment.

Temperament characteristics are behavioral tendencies, and can be categorized into nine attributes (Thomas, Chess, & Birch, 1968):

1. *Activity*—intensity and frequency of physical activity

2. *Rhythmicity*—regularity of repetitive physiological functions, i.e., sleep cycle, eating patterns, elimination patterns

3. *Approach–withdrawal*—initial reaction to a given stimulus, i.e., people, situations

4. *Adaptability*—ease or difficulty with which the child reacts or adapts to a given stimulus

5. *Intensity of response*—degree of energy used by the child to react to the stimulus

6. *Threshold of responsiveness*—amount of stimulation needed to evoke a child's response

7. *Mood*—amount of happiness versus unhappiness or pleasant/friendly behavior versus unpleasant/unfriendly behavior exhibited in various situations

8. *Distractibility*—effectiveness of the stimulus to alter the direction of the ongoing behavior

9. *Attention span and persistence*—length of time the child pursues an activity and the continuation of an activity despite the obstacles

The attributes provide a framework for three distinct personality types, as described in Table 4-12. Not all children can be placed into these categories easily; children often exhibit a variety of personality types.

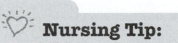

Nursing Tip:

Goodness of fit
The nurse can assist the caregiver by:
• Being aware of the cultural norms of the caregiver
• Taking time to ask about the infant's general behavior characteristics
• Asking how the caregiver interprets the infant's behavior
• Asking questions about areas that may be problematic
• Encouraging the expression of feelings about infant–caregiver interactions

Reflective Thinking

Your Temperament

Recall when you were a child. How would you classify your temperament? Is it similar to how you would classify yourself today? Do others see you the same way?

The knowledge of temperament can be very useful in achieving a goodness-of-fit in the caregiver–infant relationship (Medoff-Cooper, 1995). The nurse can be instrumental in helping the caregiver understand the uniqueness of the child's personality and provide a guide in child-rearing techniques (Medoff-Cooper, 1995). For example, a consistent routine is important for the child who is easily overwhelmed by changes. If the child has problems falling asleep, it may be helpful to provide a calm and quiet environment during the bedtime ritual. For the child who is easily distracted while eating, the caregiver should minimize all distractions by providing a quiet setting during the meal.

By increasing the caregiver's understanding of the child's personality, a more effective plan of care can be developed to meet infant needs. Thus, needs are met, a trusting relationship develops, and the caregiver's frustrations associated with child rearing may be diminished.

TABLE 4-12 SUMMARY OF PERSONALITY TYPES

Personality Type	Characteristics
Easy	Easygoing and adapts rapidly to stimuli Has an overall positive mood Likes to be around people Sleeps and eats well Has regular and predictable behaviors
Difficult	Adapts slowly to stimuli Has an overall negative mood Requires a structured environment Likes people but can do well alone Seems to be in constant motion Has irregular patterns of behavior
Slow-to-warm-up	Adapts slowly to stimuli but is watchful Quietly withdraws and usually moody Primarily a loner and socially shy Oversensitive and slow to mature Primarily inactive Reacts passively to changes in routine

Adapted from Thomas, A., Chess, S., and Birch, H. (1970). The origin of personality. Scientific American 223(2), 106–107.

Colic

Colic, one of the most common health problems seen in infants younger than 3 months of age, describes recurrent episodes of unexplained crying and the inability to be consoled. The onset varies, but usually occurs around 1–2 weeks of age and subsides spontaneously by approximately 16 weeks of age.

Excessive air swallowing, improper feeding techniques, food allergies, infant behaviors, and parental factors have been implicated as causes of colic, but none of these has been supported through research (Keefe, 1996). The colicky episode is characterized by loud, persistent cry and flexing of the hips toward the abdomen. These physical characteristics are thought to be a result of paroxysmal abdominal cramping.

Even though colic usually resolves spontaneously, the episodes are very stressful. The family is usually fatigued, frustrated, and expresses feelings of helplessness; caregivers often blame themselves for not being able to console the infant.

Colic management begins by recognizing a problem exists. First and foremost, it is important for the health care provider to eliminate an infectious or organic cause for the infant's discomfort. Once no underlying medical condition has been identified, colic should be approached in terms of managing the infant's episodes as well as the emotional turmoil experienced by the family.

In managing the infant's episodes, the nurse should assess the infant's daily routine and discuss the infant's normal patterns. Some suggestions for easing the discomfort of colic include (Dixon & Stein, 2000; Keefe, 1996):

1. Feed the infant slowly, burp frequently, and keep in upright position during feeding to decrease the amount of air swallowed. Do not overfeed the infant, which can be determined by calculating the

infant's required calorie needs by body weight.

2. When breastfeeding, avoid eating foods that may contribute to gas formation. Typically these include foods such as onions, cabbage, collards, and dry beans, which cause gas in the caregiver. This is a trial-and-error approach and may take a week before results are seen.

3. Swaddle the infant to decrease self-stimulation by jerky or sudden movements. A front carrier for body contact, swaddling, or gentle movement may be useful.

4. Take the infant for a car ride. Almost all colicky children respond favorably to vibration and movement.

5. Use a swing for at least 20 minutes. This provides movement and allows the family time for a rest period between interactions with the infant.

6. Walk or rock the infant while applying gentle pressure to the infant's abdomen.

7. Gently massage the infant's back while the infant is lying down.

8. Supply background or "white" noise (hair dryer, vacuum cleaner, fan) or play a womb sound tape (known as a "souffle" toy) or some soft music.

9. Place the infant in a quiet, darkened room to reduce environmental stimuli.

10. Let the infant cry it out in the crib when other measures do not work. Sometimes only fatigue will make the infant fall asleep.

The nurse should encourage the caregiver to avoid the tendency to take the episode personally, keep a positive attitude, and remain calm. The caregiver may be encouraged to try breathing techniques to relax, taking some time away from the care of the infant, doing something special when away from the ongoing care of the infant, and/or ask a relative to help in the infant's care.

Nursing Tip:

Care of the infant with colic

To help the caregiver manage colic:

- Stress that no one is to blame!

- Explain the possible reasons for colic.

- Give suggestions for relieving colicky episodes.

- Explain that colic usually disappears by 16 weeks of age.

- Be supportive, and encourage expression of concerns.

- Encourage talking with others who have experienced a colicky infant.

- Encourage brief periods away from the crying infant.

Reflective Thinking

Caring for the Child with Colic

To improve your understanding of colic and the caregiver's situation, ask yourself:

1. How would you personally feel if your infant cried constantly while you provided the care? Would you feel that people thought you were not a good caregiver?

2. What coping techniques would you use?

3. Who would you call when reaching the point of exasperation?

Stranger and Separation Anxiety

Stranger and separation anxiety emerge at approximately 8–12 months of age, peak at 12-15 months and disappear by 24 months. Separation anxiety behaviors are demon-

Family Teaching

Relieving Stranger and Separation Anxiety

Stranger anxiety:

- Encourage friends and relatives to visit often.

- Let the child see the caregiver's expression when a stranger approaches.

- Have the caregiver talk to the stranger first.

- Encourage the stranger to avoid intrusive movements or expressions.

- Have the caregiver maintain a safe distance from the stranger.

- Allow the child to warm up to the stranger.

- Encourage the stranger to approach on the child's level and use a soothing tone of voice.

Separation anxiety:

- Leave the child in a familiar place or with a familiar person.

- Encourage the caregiver to talk to the child before leaving.

- Do not leave the child without saying good-bye.

- Leave a security object with the child, i.e., a familiar toy or an object belonging to the caregiver.

- Encourage the child to explore at own pace.

strated when an infant is separated from the caregiver. Stranger anxiety behaviors are demonstrated by an infant when a stranger appears. Both occur as the infant develops a sense of object permanance.

When these anxieties emerge, developmentally, the infant can produce a mental image of the caregiver and recall that image even after a separation. Separation anxiety occurs because the infant does not understand the caregiver will return. However, as time goes on and with repeated episodes of separation, the infant will be able to cognitively cope with the separation and no longer demonstrate the behaviors (Dixon & Stein, 2000).

The infant's ability to produce a mental image of the caregiver enables the infant to also detect a difference in the appearance of an unfamiliar person.

Typically, the infant who is experiencing stranger and/or separation anxiety will demonstrate overt distress by withdrawing, frowning, whimpering, crying, and clinging. Separation anxiety is more likely to occur if the infant is left in an unfamiliar place or with an unfamiliar person (Mussen, Conger, Kagan, & Huston, 1990). With stranger anxiety, the stranger's approach influences the infant's reaction to the stranger. The infant will usually become anxious if the stranger immediately tries to reach out and touch or pick the child up. When time is provided for adjustment or adaptation to the unknown person, the infant usually reacts with less distress. The caregiver's reaction to the infant's behavior can also either reassure the infant or increase the infant's anxiety (Hoffman, Paris, & Hall, 1994).

Stranger and separation anxieties can be disturbing. Therefore, it is important to help the caregiver understand these anxieties are a normal part of infant development. In addition, information related to the time of occurrence, the rationale for the occurrence, the characteristic behaviors to be expected, and when these anxieties usually disappear should be provided. Suggestions to ease the infant's discomfort can be found in the accompanying Family Teaching box.

Alternative Child Care

When faced with having to leave their infant with another person, caregivers are challenged to find child care that is responsive and developmentally appropriate for young children and provides an environment where the child is safe, nurtured, and challenged to learn (DeBord, 1996). The caregiver must become an informed consumer when searching for quality child care, and the nurse should keep caregivers informed on alternative child care issues such as availability, affordability, and quality.

Table 4-13 provides information on the various types of child care providers available, with advantages and disadvantages of each, and Table 4-14 provides guidelines for choosing quality child care.

While searching for quality child care, the caregiver may inquire about the long-term effects of child care on infant development. Even though this area needs further study, research has shown that quality child care does not seem to have any persistent effect on child development (Scarr, 1998). In fact, most studies report better school achievement, greater social competence, and fewer behavior problems in children who experience quality child care (Bolger & Scarr, 1995). The child who benefits the most from quality child care comes from a socioeconomically disadvantaged environment. Quality care may in fact provide learning opportunities and social and emotional experiences not available for these children at home (Scarr, 1998).

Once equipped with information on quality care, the next step for the caregiver is finding good child care. The Family Teaching box provides some suggestions for locating such a setting.

Lastly, only the caregiver can make the final decision regarding child care. As an informed consumer, it is most important for the caregiver to do the following (Four Steps, 2000):

- Interview the child care provider by calling first and then visiting.
- Check references.
- Make the decision on what is heard and seen.
- Always stay involved.

Family Teaching

Ways to Find Quality Child Care

- Ask friends and neighbors how they found child care.

- Look in the Yellow Pages of the telephone directory under "Child Care Centers."

- Check classified ads in the local newspaper.

- Place an ad in local newspaper.

- Put up notices on community bulletin boards.

- Talk with family child care associations or provider support groups.

- Ask the local affiliate of the National Association for the Education of Young Children.

- Contact the local Human Development Extension agent (usually a person with a college degree in human development or child psychology who works for the county or state).

(DeBord, 1996)

Reflective Thinking

Alternative Child Care

What are your feelings about alternative child care? Provide statements for and against both parents working outside the home and requiring alternative child care.

TABLE 4-13 TYPES OF ALTERNATIVE CHILD CARE

Type	Advantages	Disadvantages
Center-based care	• Group care for two or more children • Located usually in a home, school, church, or building designed for group care • Include nursery school, preschool, parent cooperative • Licensed by local or state agencies • Staff usually trained in child care and development • Structured program of activities • Reliable hours of operation	• Regulations vary from area to area • May be placed on a waiting list for admission • Greater adult:child ratio • Care may not be individualized
Family child care	• Small group care • Good adult:child ratio • Located in provider's home • Special arrangements are easier to make	• Usually includes provider's children • Licensing by local or state agencies usually not required or if required not always licensed • Provider(s) may not be trained in child care and development • Hours of operation may not be reliable
In-home care	• Home care provided by sitter or nanny • Individualized care • Easier to meet special needs (i.e., physical, mental, emotional problem) • Provider may do light home tasks • Do not have to transport child	• Provider may not be trained in child care and development • May infringe on family privacy • Dependent on provider's reliability

Adapted from DeBord, K. (1996). Quality child care: What does it really mean? [On-line]. Available: www.carefinder.com/parents/choose.html; Scarr, S. (1998). American child care today. American Psychologist, 53*(2), 95–108; and Shelov, S. P. (Ed.) (1998). Caring for your baby and young child. New York: Bantam.*

TABLE 4-14   CHOOSING CHILD CARE

Does Provider

Appear warm and friendly?

Seem calm and gentle?

Seem easy to talk with?

Seem to like themselves and the job?

Treat each child as special?

Understand children's stages of development?

Encourage good health habits?

Have previous experience and trained staff?

Accept and respect your family's cultural values?

Seem to enjoy cuddling infants?

Meet infant physical needs?

Provide infant stimulation?

Provide dependable and consistent care?

Provide consistency between home and child care?

Seem to have time for all infants?

Does the Setting Have

Up-to-date license or registration certificate?

A clean and comfortable look?

Enough room to allow children to move freely and safely?

Appropriate staff:child ratio?

Late pick-up policy?

Child-proofed environment?

Enough heat, light?

Enough furnishings for all children?

Furnishings that are safe and in good repair?

Adequate number of clean bathrooms?

Fire safety plan and adequate exits?

Fire extinguishers?

Smoke detectors?

Covered radiators and protected heaters?

Strong screens or bars on windows above first floor?

Nutritious meals and snacks?

A separate place to care for sick children?

A first-aid kit?

Safe gates at top and bottom of stairs?

A clean, safe place to change diapers, sanitized after each use?

Cribs with firm mattresses?

Separate linen for each crib?

Are There Opportunities for the Child to

Play quietly and actively?

Play alone?

Follow a schedule that meets young children's needs?

Learn new developmental skills?

Learn to get along, share, and respect themselves and others?

Learn about their own and others' cultures?

Crawl and explore safely?

Adapted from Labensohn, D. (2000). Parent checklist for child care [On-line]. Available: at www.carefinder.com/parents/choose/html.

REFERENCES

American Academy of Pediatrics. (1995). Fluoride supplementation for children: Interim policy recommendations. *Pediatrics, 95,* 777.

American Academy of Pediatrics. (1996). Selecting and using the most appropriate car safety seats for growing children: Guidelines for counseling parents. *Pediatrics, 97,* 761–762.

American Academy of Pediatrics. (1997). Does bed sharing affect the risks of SIDS? *Pediatrics, 100,* 272.

American Academy of Pediatrics. (2002). Reminding families about the importance of back to sleep. "Kids' Health" supplement in the October 18-20, 2002. weekend edition of *USA Today.* Available: www.aap.org/advocacy/releases/sids.htm (accessed 12/19/02).

Anders, T., Halpern, L., & Hua, J. (1992). Sleeping through the night: A developmental prospective. *Pediatrics, 90,* 554–560.

Arrigo, M. (1994, September). Starting solids. *American Baby, 56*(9), 68–72.

Behrman, R., & Kliegman, R. (2002). *Nelson's essentials of pediatrics* (4h ed.). Philadelphia: Saunders.

Bolger, K. E., & Scarr, S. (1995). Not so far from home: How family characteristics predict child care quality. *Early Development and Parenting, 4*(3), 103–112.

Brazelton, T. B. (1990). Parent-infant co-sleeping revisited. *Ab Initio 2*(1), 1–7.

CDC (1995). Air-bag associated fatal injuries to infants and children riding in front passenger seats—United States. *Morbidity and Mortality Weekly Report,* 44[45], 845–847.

Capute, A., & Accardo, P. (1978). Linguistic and auditory milestones during the first two years of life. *Clinical Pediatrics, 17,* 847–853.

DeBord, K. (1996). *Quality child care: What does it really mean?* [On-line]. Available: www.carefinder.com/parents/choose.html.

Dietary guidelines for infants. (1997). *Current practices in infant feeding.* [On-line]. Available: www.gerber.com/dietguide.html.

Dixon, S., & Stein, M. (2000). *Encounters with children: Pediatric behaviors and development* (3rd ed.). St. Louis: Mosby.

Erikson, E. E. (1963). *Childhood and society* (2nd ed.). New York: Norton.

Four steps to selecting a child care provider. (2000). [On-line]. Available: www.carefinder.com/parents/choose.html.

Frankenberg, W. (1990). *Denver II manual.* Denver: Denver Developmental Materials.

Herzog, J. M. (1997). Birth to two. *Sleep.* [On-line]. Available: www.ctw.org.

Hoffman, L., Paris, S., & Hall, E. (1994). *Developmental psychology* (6th ed.). New York: McGraw-Hill.

Jaques, S. (1993, October). All about your baby's teeth. *American Baby, 55*(10), 92–95.

Keefe, M. R. (1996). Ask the expert. *The Journal of the Society of Pediatric Nurses, 1*(1), 41–42.

Keeping your child safe. (1994). *The parent's almanac.* [On-line.] Available: family.starwave.com/resource/pra/bonus27.html.

Labensohn, D. (2000). *Parent checklist for child care.* [On-line]. Available: www.carefinder.com/parents/choose.html.

Mackin, M. L., Medendorp, S. V., & Maier, M. C. (1989). Infant sleep and bedtime cereal. *American Journal of Diseases of Children, 143,* 1066–1068.

Martin, D. (1996, April). Introducing solid foods to babies. *Foods and Nutrition* [On-line]. Available: ianrwww.unl.edu/ianr/pubs/ extnpubs/foods/g962.html.

McDonald, R. E., & Avery, D. R. (1994). *Dentistry for the child and adolescent* (6th ed.). St. Louis: Mosby.

Medoff-Cooper, B. (1995). Infant temperament: Implications for parenting from birth through 1 year. *Journal of Pediatric Nursing, 3,* 141–145.

Mussen, P. H., Conger, J. J., Kagan, J., & Huston, A. C. (1990). *Child development and personality* (7th ed.). New York: Harper & Row.

Oppenheim, M. N. (1996, February). Early infancy oral health care. *New York State Dental Journal, 62*(2), 22–24.

Piaget, J. (1952). *The origins of intelligence in children.* New York: International Universities Press.

Pipes, P., & Trahms, C. (1993). *Nutrition in infancy and childhood* (5th ed.). St. Louis: Mosby.

Reisser, P. C. (1998). *Baby and child care.* Wheaton, IL: Tyndale.

Scarr, S. (1998). American child care today. *American Psychologist, 53*(2), 95–108.

Secker, D. (1999). Interpreting growth and growth standards. *HINS Articles.* [On-line]. Available: www.hins.org/growth.

Shelov, S. P. (Ed.) (1998). *Caring for your baby and young child.* New York: Bantam.

Slusher, I. L., & McClure, M. J. (1992). Infant stimulation during hospitalization. *Journal of Pediatric Nursing, 7,* 276–279.

Thomas, A., Chess, S., & Birch, H. (1968). *Temperament and behavior disorders in children.* New York: New York University Press.

Thomas, A., Chess, S., & Birch, H. (1970). The origin of personality. *Scientific American, 223*(2), 106–107.

Tonnessen, D. (1996, July). The family bed. *Parents, 71*(7), 47–48.

Turgeon-O'Brien, H., Lachapelle, D., Gagnon, P. F., Larocque, I., & Maheu-Robert, L. (1996). Nutritive and nonnutritive sucking habits: A review. *Journal of Dentistry for Children, 63,* 321–327.

Wagner, H. (1997, February). Pacifier dilemma. *Parents, 72*(2), 80–82.

Weissbluth, M. (1991). Sleep learning: The first four months. *Pediatrics Annuals, 20,* 228–238.

Whitley, E. N., Cataldo, C. B., DeBruyne, L. K., & Rolfes, A. R. (1996). *Nutrition for health and health care.* St. Paul: West.

Wright, J. (1994, May). Sleep, little baby. *American Baby, 56*(5), 75–81.

Wright, J. (1995, May). American baby basics: All about baby's sleep. *American Baby* [On-line]. Available: www.enews.com/da.

SUGGESTED READINGS

Bhavnagri, N. P., & Gonzalez-Mena, J. (1997, Fall). The cultural context of infant caregiving. *Childhood Education, 74*(1), 2–8.

Brenner, R., Simons-Morton, B. G., Bhasker, B., Mehta, N., Melnick, V. L., Revenis, M., Berendes, H. W., & Clemens, J. D. (1998). Prevalence and predictors of the prone sleep position among inner-city infants. *JAMA, 280,* 341–346.

Briggs, S. (1998). Little steps for new parents: A week-by-week guide and journal for baby's first year. Washington, DC: National Association for the Education of Young Children.

Caulfield, R. (1996). Physical and cognitive development in the first two years. *Early Childhood Education Journal, 23,* 239–242.

Denham, S. A. (1995). Continuity and change in emotional components of infant temperament. *Child Study Journal, 25,* 289–308.

Elkind, D. (1994). *A sympathetic understanding of child: Birth to sixteen* (2nd ed.). Needham Heights, MA: Allyn & Bacon.

Fields, T. (1996, July). Carrying position influences infant behavior. *Early Child Development & Care, 121,* 49–54.

Glass, J. (1998). Gender liberation, economic squeeze, or fear of strangers: Why fathers provide infant care in dual-earner families. *Journal of Marriage & Family, 60,* 821–834.

Halpern, L. F. (1995). Infant sleep–wake characteristics: Relationship to neurological status and the prediction of developmental outcomes. *Developmental Review, 15,* 255–291.

Heet, L. M. (1999, January). SIDS a killer for native infants: Aberdeen study points the way to prevention. *American Indian Report, 15*(1), 24–25.

Honig, A. S. (1997). Infant temperament and personality: What do we need to know? *Montessori Life, 9*(3), 18–21.

Miller, K. (1997). Play of infants and toddlers: caring for the little ones. *Child Care Information Exchange, 118,* 41–43

New, R. S. (1999, March). Here, we call it "drop off and pick up": transition to child care, American-style. *Young Children, 54*(2), 34–35.

Potter, K. (1995). Safety checklist. *Childproofing your home.* [On-line]. Available: www.neosoft.com/ ~jrpotter/safety.html.

Potts, N. & Mandleco, B. (Eds). (2002). *Caring for children and their families.* Clifton Park, NY: Delmar Learning.

Ramey, C. T., & Ramey, S. L. (1999). Right from birth: your child's foundation for life: Birth to 18 months. Goddard parenting guides. Beltsville, MD: Gryphon.

Recommendations for reducing the risks for SIDS. (2000). [On-line]. Available: www/sidsallaiance.org/facts/.

Righard, L., & Alade, M. (1997). Breastfeeding and the use of pacifiers. *Birth, 24*(2), 112–120.

Rock-a-bye baby . . . on their backs. (1998). *JAMA, 280,* 396.

Seifer, R. (1996). Attachment, maternal sensitivity, and infant temperament during the first year of life. *Developmental Psychology, 32*(1), 12–25.

Tigges, B. B. (1997). Infant formulas: practical answers for common questions. *The Nurse Practitioner, 22*(8), 70–87.

Weinberger, N. (1998). Making a place for infants in family day care. *Early Education & Development, 9*(1), 79–96.

Wieland, D. (1998). Soothing strategies: successful calming techniques to suit your baby's temperament. *Parents, 73*(7), 28–29.

CHAPTER 5

Growth and Development of the Toddler

During toddlerhood the child begins to seek autonomy, explores the world, learns how things work, begins to tolerate limitations, expresses desires, and develops relationships. However, the toddler's excitement and frustration make this period challenging.

This 24-month-span (12–36 months of age) reflects periods of rapid, unprecedented maturation, and change. The toddler evolves from a dependent infant with limited mobility and communication skills, into a more independent, very mobile, verbal, and inquisitive member of the family.

Promoting toddler health and maintaining wellness involves knowledge of normal growth and developmental processes, an understanding of common significant milestones, and the ability to anticipate deviations.

As the toddler develops autonomy and a sense of identity, increased motor skills combined with a lack of experience and judgment can present innumerable dangers. Strategies to promote and assist the toddler's mastery of major developmental skills, while at the same time protecting the child from environmental dangers, provide structured guidelines and loving discipline, and promote a sense of independence and inquisitiveness should be utilized.

A discussion of toddler physiological, psychosexual, psychosocial, cognitive, and moral development follows. It is always important to remember, however, that development in each area significantly impacts overall growth, development, and maturation, and no area of development can be viewed in isolation.

PHYSIOLOGICAL DEVELOPMENT

The physical changes of toddlerhood occur in a fairly predictable manner; however, no child can be held to a rigid time frame of when those milestones will be reached. While some children initially direct their energy toward accomplishing motor activities first, others initially concentrate on verbal mastery. Generally, this does not mean one toddler is advanced and another delayed; both will accomplish desired developmental tasks within a normal range of time, but at their own pace.

Physical growth slows during toddlerhood, but the toddler should show a steady increase in growth, with an average weight gain of about 5 pounds per year and an increase in height averaging 3 inches per year. This slowed growth rate is evidenced by the toddler's decline in appetite and erratic eating habits. Physical appearance also changes markedly. The head gains a more proportional dimension to the rest of the body, reflecting slower brain growth. Chest circumference increases and soon exceeds the abdominal girth; the top-heavy, wide base (feet spread) pot-bellied stance and toddling gait of young toddlers eventually gives way to a well-balanced appearance and gait as bones lengthen and strengthen and abdominal muscle replaces adipose tissue. Children learn to walk at various ages, with some beginning as early as 12 months; however, most walk by 15 months and climb stairs by 18 months.

Neurological System

Brain growth continues slowly, corresponding to advancing intellectual skills and fine motor development. Improved coordination and equilibrium parallels the almost complete (by 2 years) myelinization of the spinal cord as evidenced by refined walking, jumping, and climbing.

Increasing eye–hand coordination, manual dexterity, and walking/running skills contribute significantly to the toddler's locomotion and socialization. These skills promote throwing and retrieving objects, opening and closing containers with lids, and building objects with blocks before knocking them down (Gemelli, 1996). The neurophysiologic changes that have the greatest impact upon family/child education and suggested nursing interventions are listed in Table 5-1.

Musculoskeletal System

Increased bone length, muscle maturation, and increased muscle strength enable toddlers to develop autonomy. Major advances occurring in the musculoskeletal system during toddlerhood are reflected in Table 5-2.

Gastrointestinal/ Genitourinary System

The gastrointestinal/genitourinary system continues to mature during these years. The stomach enlarges in size, allowing consumption of the traditional three meals per day, all deciduous teeth generally erupt by 30 months of age, and improved eye–hand coordination enables self-feeding. The toddler enjoys a gradual increase in size, accompanied by a decreased appetite and a ritualistic interest in limited types of food. Toddlers also vary in their energy requirements, eating large amounts of food one day and very little food the next. The food likes and dislikes also differ from day to day. This period of decreased appetite as a result of decreased caloric need is often referred to as a time of physiologic anorexia.

Even though caloric needs diminish during this time, protein requirements remain higher than for other age groups. Vitamin and mineral requirements (calcium, phosphorous, iron) increase slightly, creating concern since toddlers often go through food fads or jags and have a decreased food intake. Measures should be taken to help reduce the amount of fat in the toddler's diet by providing low-fat or skim milk, lean meats, and low-fat cheese.

Bladder and bowel control is typically achieved during this time period, and children are able to retain urine up to 4 hours before needing to void. Specific gastrointestinal and genitourinary changes that can be expected and accompanying nursing interventions can be found in Table 5-3.

Cardiorespiratory System

During toddlerhood, the cardiorespiratory system continues to mature; vital signs become more stable and move closer to adult norms. Respiratory and cardiac rates slow, while blood pressure rises. Other significant factors related to cardiopulmonary assessment can be found in Table 5-4.

Sensory System

In addition to the physiologic changes noted in Tables 5-1 to 5-4, the senses of hearing, smell, taste, touch, and vision develop and begin to connect, since toddlers utilize all five senses to explore the world and exert autonomy and independence. Caregivers and health care providers need to be aware of behaviors reflecting hearing and vision difficulties such as failure to develop language, unusual responses to loud sounds, or increased falls. Baseline hearing and vision screening should be performed during toddlerhood and appropriate strategies, if necessary, immediately begun.

Toddler vision should be 20/20 to 20/40, with full binocular capabilities reached shortly after 12 months of age. Depth perception continues to develop throughout the toddler years. This, combined with inquisi-

TABLE 5-1	OVERVIEW OF NEUROLOGICAL CHANGES OF TODDLERHOOD

Significant Changes	Nursing/Caregiver Implications
Anterior cranial fontanel closes at approximately the time of cord myelinization (12–18 months).	Be alert for premature closure as it can impinge on brain growth/function. Prior to closure, a bulging fontanel indicates increased intracranial pressure; sunken fontanel indicates dehydration.
Brain growth continues, reaching 80%–90% of adult size by 3 years.	Increasing head circumference is stimulated by brain growth; small circumference may suggest growth abnormalities, which place child at risk for developmental delay; enlarged size may indicated genetic syndromes or circumference hydrocephalus.
Cognitive development is demonstrated by rapidly expanding vocabulary.	The child begins toddlerhood with a vocabulary of a few words and, by 3 years, uses 300–900 words and 2–3-word phrases.
Control gained over most reflex activity.	Persistence of primitive reflexes may suggest defective cortical development.
Head circumference should approximate chest, with chest enlarging more rapidly after 24 months.	Head circumference should increase 1 inch (2.5 cm) or less per year until school age.
	Always measure head using a paper tape measure placed 1 inch above top of the ears.
Myelinization completed around 24 months of age.	The child is not able to walk well until myelinization has occurred. Walking well is an indication that myelinization has occurred and the child is physiologically capable of bladder/bowel control.
Spinal cord and vertebral column grow at variable rates; cord ends at L3-4 (in adult cord ends L1).	Be alert for positioning of the toddler for lumbar punctures.

TABLE 5-2 OVERVIEW OF MUSCULOSKELETAL CHANGES OF TODDLERHOOD

Specific Changes	Nursing/Caregiver Intervention
Bone length increases due to ossification and long bone growth; by 36 months, the child should be 41 inches (104 cm) in height.	Birth length doubles by 2 years. Gains 4–6 inches (10–12 cm) in height per year until school age. Deviations may indicate endocrine and/or growth hormone abnormalities.
Pot belly appearance is due to lack of abdominal development.	
Between 13–18 months:	Consider safety issues with advancing mobility (stairs, running).
• Walks a few steps without support	
• Walks upstairs with help, creeps downstairs	
• Turns book pages	Toys encouraging use of fine/gross motor skills should be provided.
• Walks and pulls toys	
• Able to remove shoes and socks, tries to put on shoes	Play activities should encourage physical activity.
• Unzips zippers	
• Stacks up to four cubes	
Between 19–30 months:	Encourage use of bike helmet and teach basic safety rules (stop/look before crossing street, etc).
• Goes up and down stairs alone (places both feet on one step before going to next)	
• Kicks ball forward without losing balance	
• Turns doorknobs	Child is interested in pictures and drawing, and is able to copy horizontal/vertical lines and circles.
• Rides tricycle (by 2 years)	
• Builds towers of eight cubes	
• Moves fingers independently, holds crayons with fingers not fist	
• Brushes teeth	
• Dresses self with supervision (buttons, snaps, etc.) but cannot tie shoes	
• Inserts squares into square holes	
• Binocular vision well developed	
By 36 months, large and small muscle groups enlarge, and physically observable actions are refined.	

TABLE 5-3 OVERVIEW OF GASTROINTESTINAL/GENITOURINARY CHANGES OF TODDLERHOOD

Specific Changes	Nursing/Caregiver Intervention
Increased eye coordination: grasps spoon (15 months), drinks from cup without spilling (18 months)	Encourage self-feeding. Finger foods and appropriately shaped cups/utensils are important to foster independence and dexterity.
Gains 4–6 lbs (1.8–2.5 kg) per year, average weight by 3 years = 30–32 lbs (14–15 kg)	Need for protein and calorie intake remains high; toddler needs 1,000–1,500 kcal/day to support growth and 115 mL/kg of liquids per day to maintain fluid balance; weight should reveal a consistent increase on growth chart.
Slowed growth needs produce physiologic anorexia at 18 months; stomach capacity increases to allow for less frequent, larger meals.	Toddlers become "picky" eaters. Do not use food as a disciplinary tool, or cookies and sweets as behavioral rewards.
Poor eating habits and prolonged use of a bottle can create nutritional anemia and tooth decay.	Obtain an accurate food history; teach caregivers alternatives for bottle feeding, especially at bedtime (e.g., sipper cups, finger foods); expand food options; encourage child to make selections as appropriate; add one new food at a time to avoid overlooking food allergies.
Primary dentition (20 deciduous teeth) is completed by 30 months.	Poor nutritional intake and/or constipation can also create a pot-bellied appearance; assess carefully to ascertain cause; encourage tooth brushing after meals. Assess need for adding dietary fluoride to assure dental health if the fluoride level in the water is low.

continues

TABLE 5-3 *Continued*

Specific Changes	Nursing/Caregiver Intervention
Sphincter control enables bladder and bowel training.	Encourage caregivers to develop realistic expectations related to potty training based on child's developmental abilities and physiologic capabilities; encourage food with high-fiber content (such as whole grain cereals, fruits, and vegetables) and adequate fruit juices and fluids to prevent constipation; large quantities of fruit juices, especially apple juice, can produce diarrhea.
Bladder capacity increases, to allow the retention of urine for 2–4 hours; bladder and kidneys reach near-adult functional levels at about 16–24 months, which normally coincides with the ability to walk.	Urinary output should equal or exceed 1 mL/kg/hr.
Urinary bladder is positioned higher in the abdominal cavity than in adults.	Palpate bladder between umbilicus and symphysis pubis.
Urethral structures are short (1–3 inches, versus 4 inches in adult female and 8 inches in adult male). Toddlers are susceptible to urinary tract infections.	Keep perineal area clean, especially during toilet training. Begin teaching child to cleanse self from front to back; encourage child to take breaks while playing to empty bladder, which prevents incontinence and infections from urinary retention.

TABLE 5-4   OVERVIEW OF CARDIORESPIRATORY CHANGES OF TODDLERHOOD

Significant Changes	Nursing/Caregiver Implications
Vessels are easily compressed, obliterating the pulse.	Take pulse apically for 1 full minute. Awake = 70–110; asleep = 60–100 beats/min.; respirations = 25–30 breathes/min.; blood pressure = 90/50 mm Hg.
Circulating blood volume is less than in adult.	Small blood loss, including multiple blood tests, can compromise circulating volume; hypotension is a late sign of circulatory compromise; child may remain normotensive until 25% of blood volume is lost; assess capillary refill as indicator of peripheral circulation status (should refill in 2 seconds).
Lengthening body and decreasing adipose tissues produce thinner chest wall.	Breath sounds are easily heard.
Airway is small and easily compromised.	Asthma and acute allergic reactions may rapidly escalate into respiratory distress; observe for nasal flaring, retractions, and dyspnea.
Cough reflex remains.	Avoid suppressing cough through the use of antitussive medications.
Tracheal diameter approximates size of adult's small finger.	Toddler rapidly reacts with signs of respiratory distress with even small amounts of mucus or obstruction.
Tongue is large in proportion to the size of the mouth.	Airway may become obstructed by tongue if child seizes or loses consciousness.
Larynx cartilage is softer than in adults and is positioned more anteriorly.	Hyperextension of neck may occlude airway, increasing the risk of aspiration/obstruction.
Alveoli are not fully functional.	Watch for rapid onset of respiratory distress due to the tendency for small airways to collapse.
Ear and throat internal structures remain relatively short and straight, tonsils and adenoids are large.	Otitis media, tonsilitis, and upper respiratory infections are common.

tiveness, poor judgment, and occasional lack of coordination, puts the toddler at risk for frequent falls when learning to walk, run, and climb stairs.

PSYCHOSEXUAL DEVELOPMENT

Attitudes related to gender identity, sex roles, and sexuality are mostly determined by the values and morals of the caregiver and the environment. Toddlers are generally able to recognize gender differences by 2 years of age and begin to explore and recognize body parts during toilet training.

According to Freud (1957), toddlers are in the anal stage of development. Freud first pointed out the tension revolving around toddler bowel/bladder training, and viewed toilet training as a possible way of resolving conflict and handling stress. He believed improperly managed toilet training could lead to life-long psychological trauma with accompanying physical bowel/bladder responses (Freud, 1957).

Many thoughts and activities of both the caregiver and the toddler tend to be focused on toilet training, and, because of the close proximity of the genitalia to the urinary and anal orifices, toddlers tend to manually manipulate and inspect these areas. Masturbation is common and should be handled in a matter-of-fact-manner, thereby lessening the child's anxiety and feelings of shame.

Domestic mimicry, or imitation of domestic/role activity, is one way toddlers express their understanding of gender roles. For example, in imaginative play, the child takes the role of "mommy," "daddy," or "baby," and develops life-long attitudes related to gender-specific behavior. Caregiver responses to boys playing with dolls or cooking in the play kitchen, and girls taking a truck apart or building houses in the mud can have a profound influence on later role-related thinking patterns and experiences.

In a similar fashion, the caregiver's response to the toddler's sexually related

Family Teaching

Accomplishing Positive Psychosexual Outcomes with Toddlers

- Avoid using slang, baby talk, or confusing terms. Teach the child correct anatomical names.

- Provide positive reinforcement as the toddler experiments with various gender-related behaviors. Do not confuse the child with statements such as "big boys don't cry" or "only boys play with trucks."

- Accept manipulation of genitalia and masturbation as a natural, private behavior of toddlerhood.

- Respond to questions with age-appropriate language.

- Do not make toilet training a major confrontational issue for the household; try to tie in educational aspects when possible (e.g., always wash hands, wipe front-to-back, etc).

actions and questions can influence future sexual attitudes. Therefore, the caregiver needs to clarify what the child really wants to know before beginning detailed explanations. For example, when the 2 ½-year-old asks, "Where does baby come from?" the child may only want to know that the baby *doll* came from the toy box in the bedroom (Brazelton, 1992).

Since the child's gender identity is formulated during toddlerhood, continual rewards for responding in a manner consistent with a specific gender internalizes that identity. Gender identity is reinforced by observing same and opposite sex caregivers enact their gender roles, attitudes, and values, and by experiencing the way adults treat children of different genders. Refer to Family Teaching for guidelines to encourage appropriate psychosexual development.

PSYCHOSOCIAL DEVELOPMENT

The three major psychosocial tasks of toddlerhood are gaining self-control, developing autonomy, and increasing independence. Progress toward mastery can be judged through observing behaviors listed in Box 5-1.

In the process of mastering self-control, autonomy, and independence, the toddler must also grapple with new, confusing, and frightening situations. The way the child responds to these situations culminates in what Erikson (1963) refers to as autonomy versus shame and doubt. Either the child masters the situation and autonomy and self-concept are strengthened, or he is unsuccessful and doubts his abilities to succeed in such situations in the future. For more information on psycosocial developement, refer to Table 5-5.

Box 5-1   Behaviors Consistent with Psychosocial Development

- Tolerating separation from caregiver (stays with sitter or in day care without prolonged crying/distress)
- Withstanding delayed gratification (waits, without a temper tantrum, until toy is removed from box to play)
- Increasing control over bowel/bladder function (maintains dryness for more than 2 hours)
- Utilizing socially acceptable behavior/language (controls temper tantrums/biting behaviors)
- Walking well and seeking new experiences in the environment
- Interacting with others in a less id-centric/ego-centric manner (shares toys more willingly)

TABLE 5-5   PSYCHOSOCIAL MILESTONES FOR TODDLERS

Age	Description
15 Months	Fears being alone, being abandoned, strangers, objects, and places. Expresses independence by trying to feed/undress self.
18 Months	Negativism predominates; fears water. Temper tantrums and awareness of own gender begins.
24 Months	May resist bedtime and naps, fear the dark and animals; temper tantrums, negativism, and dawdling continue. Bedtime rituals important. Explores genitalia. Shows readiness for bowel/bladder control.
36 Months	Temper tantrums, negativism, and dawdling behaviors subside; self-esteem increases due to increased independence in eating, elimination, and dressing. Explores many emotions in pretend play. Separation fears generally subside; may develop a fear of monsters.

COGNITIVE DEVELOPMENT

During the toddler years, language ability develops rapidly. However, it is dependent upon physical maturity as well as parental encouragement and participation. Although most toddlers' comprehension of words is greater than their ability to verbalize, by 36 months of age, children are able to converse and begin to acknowledge different points of view. These advancements suggest the toddler is more mature than their thinking processes since the meanings of all verbalizations are not always understood. Reasoning skills also remain undeveloped during this time, although an understanding of causal relationships is emerging. Guidelines to enhance communication are found in the Nursing Tip. Refer to Table 5-6 for more information on language development.

Cognitively, toddlers are able to recognize and distinguish between shapes of objects, but they are only beginning to classify objects into categories of use. In the mind of a toddler, all objects that look alike have the same function and are therefore treated equally. For example, a pail is used to collect sand from the sandbox, hold water to scrub the floor, and hold paint. So, in the child's mind, if the toddler is allowed to overturn the pail of sand, then he or she is also allowed to overturn the water pail and the paint pail.

According to Piaget (1952), toddler cognitive development encompasses three major stages divided into two phases: sensorimotor and preoperational. A summary of Piaget's sensorimotor and preconceptual phase of thinking is found in Table 5-7.

Nursing Tip:

How to communicate with toddlers
- Acknowledge use of culturally specific terms/actions/rituals.
- Relate time to familiar activities (after lunch, before bed, after getting up in the morning).
- Speak at the child's eye level.
- Respect the child's personal space; speak before violating this space.
- Touch the child gently on the shoulder to gain attention.
- Use terms that the child understands and that are acceptable to family when adults are introduced (for instance, the family may prefer that all adults be addressed as Mr/Ms, not by a first name).
- Use child's nickname or most familiar name (not necessarily his legal name).
- Use positive reinforcement often ("You've been very helpful").
- Use short, concrete descriptions ("Put the ball into the toy box, please").
- Avoid using literal phrases ("don't cough your head off," or "this will just be a little stick in your arm").
- Use play to project feelings and gain information ("what if you could . . .", "if you had a wish . . .).
- Answer questions simply.
- Set limits firmly, but gently. Reward acceptable behavior (avoid using food as a reward).
- A child's attention span is approximately equal to his age in years (e.g., 3 years old, attention span of 3 minutes).

TABLE 5-6	NORMAL LANGUAGE/SPEECH DEVELOPMENTAL MILESTONES FOR TODDLERS		
Age of Child	Speech	Receptive Language	Expressive Language
12 months to 18 months	• Starts to combine two words • 18–22 words vocabulary	• Recognizes names of body parts • Identifies pictures of familiar objects when named	• Mixes real words with jargon and gestures • Says "ma-ma" and "da-da" • Uses words more than gestures • Announces familiar objects by name
18 months to 2 years	• Articulation lags behind • 270–300 words vocabulary	• Follows two consecutive related directions such as "pick up ball and bring it to me" • Understands more complex sentences	• Refers to self by name • Uses two- and three-word phrases
2 years to 3 years	• Uses consonants and pronouns • Begins to use word endings • 900 words vocabulary	• Learns concepts such as hot/cold, big/little, and so forth • Listens to and identifies sounds	• Begins combining words in short complete phrases • Inverts subject and verb such as "come lunch mommy" • Answers simple yes/no questions

TABLE 5-7 SENSORIMOTOR AND PRECONCEPTUAL PHASES OF TODDLER DEVELOPMENT (PIAGET)

Stage/Age	Cognitive Changes	Behavioral Changes
Sensorimotor Tertiary circular reactions, 12–18 months	Experiences as many new situations as possible to achieve new skills/abilities. Combines new and old knowledge to experiment and begin early reasoning. Enhanced understanding of object permanence. Learns to differentiate self from objects. Develops awareness of spatial and causal concepts.	Inquisitive and curious about "world." Uses all senses to explore and test environment. Increases use of physical skills to increase abilities (e.g., transitions from walking to climbing to reach a higher shelf). Places items in and out of containers; recognizes that items out of sight exist (box of crackers in cupboard). Is comforted by parents' voices, even if they are not visible. Extends separation time from caretakers.
Mental combinations, 18–24 months	Can infer a cause even if only experiencing the effect (threw a toy, child disciplined, toy put out of reach). Beginning to think before acting. Imitation becomes more symbolic. Beginning sense of memory in early problem solving. Better sense of time relationships. Egocentric in actions and thinking.	Follows directions and understands requests (don't run, you will fall; put your toy here). Imitates role model's speaking (words and animal sounds). Demonstrates domestic mimicry. Uses simple words with meaning (sit, go, up, down). Engages in parallel play and senses ownership (my truck). Refers to self by name. Comfort level requires routine schedule and rituals.

continues

TABLE 5-7 *Continued*		
Stage/Age	**Cognitive Changes**	**Behavioral Changes**
Properational Preconceptual, 2–4 years	Thoughts, play, and actions continue to be egocentric.	Increased vocabulary with phrases of 2–3-words.
	Sense of time, space, and causality improves.	Has difficulty sharing and is possessive of toys, family members, and other items (mine or my).
	Uses language as mental representation increases.	Uses vocabulary terms that are future oriented (tomorrow).
	Develops cognitive connection between new experience and things that occurred in the past (refuses to eat food because something before didn't taste good, "icky").	Can follow more complex directions (put this toy in the box behind you).
	Begins trial and error learning.	Can put shoes on even if on wrong foot, repeats procedure again and again.

MORAL DEVELOPMENT

Toddlers have little concept of right and wrong even though Kohlberg's (1976) theory of moral development could be applied to toddlers because of their willful desires to make independent decisions and their increasing cognitive capacities. However, a child's ability to actually make moral decisions is based upon multiple cognitive and social interactions that exceed the abilities of a toddler.

SPIRITUAL DEVELOPMENT

Birth through the toddler years may be termed pre-religious because children at this age do not have the cognitive ability to understand religious convictions of those around them, even though they do have a vague idea of religious teachings and God.

On the other hand, Fowler (1974) does make a strong case for the consideration of early stages of faith development in this age group. Fowler defined faith as a relational phenomenon, an active relationship with another, a commitment, belief, love, and/or hope, which may be directed toward family, religion, God, or friends. As such, undifferentiated faith, as a foundation for other faith development, may occur as early as 2 years of age. Although religious rituals and symbols may not be understood at this time, the child does enjoy interacting with adults and children around simple religious stories.

Therefore, for toddlers, routines such as saying prayers before meals and at bedtime are important and may be comforting. Children at this age also know that imitating or conforming to rituals results in approval of others who are important to the child. Attending religious programs similar to a nursery school that emphasize appropriate behavior and positive self-esteem rather than a lesson is important as well.

HEALTH SCREENING

Routine health visits to a primary health care provider begun in infancy should continue through toddlerhood. Caregivers should be encouraged to schedule well-child visits at 15, 18, 24, and 36 months of age; additional visits should be made if illness occurs. The routine visits are needed for health monitoring and updating or beginning immunizations if not initiated during infancy.

Health screening should always include a complete physical examination (including blood pressure, height, and weight), evaluation of hemoglobin (for iron-deficiency anemia), dental evaluation, and vision and hearing assessment. Before the anterior fontanel closes, the head circumference should be measured. The American Academy of Pediatrics recommends that screening serum lead levels be obtained in children exhibiting poor growth patterns or neurological irritability, or in those living in high-risk areas (AAP, 1998).

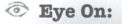

Eye On:

Comparison Standards

Health care providers also need to be sensitive to cultural and ethnic variations when comparing children to preestablished norms. For instance, attention should be given to the height/weight assessment of Asian children. A single evaluation of a child of Asian ancestry, compared to standard U.S. Caucasian norms, may lead to an inaccurate judgment that the child is short in stature or malnourished for age, when actually this should be attributed to genetic makeup.

HEALTH PROMOTION

The nurse's role in toddler health promotion is critical. Education should provide ideas, suggestions, and concepts surrounding growth, development, and parenting skills. This knowledge will allow caregivers to become independent in promoting health with respect to nutrition, elimination, sleep, dental hygiene, care, safety, activity and play, and growth and development. Ideally, the toddler should be seen consistently by the same health care provider since the most accurate clinical judgments are made not on one observation alone, but rather, based on trends over time.

Nurses need to provide assistance and guidance to caretakers for common issues such as nutrition, sleep, dental hygiene, safety and injury prevention, health screening, negativism, ritualism, regression, discipline, sibling rivalry, temper tantrums, toilet training, child (day) care, and play. Each of these topics will be addressed briefly.

Immunizations

The American Academy of Pediatrics (2002) has recently published a revised immunization schedule, which indicates toddlers need boosters of diphtheria, tetanus, and pertussis (DTP, or DtaP), H. influenza (HIB), polio, and hepatitis B (if not received at 6 months of age) by 18 months of age. They also need initial doses of measles, mumps, rubella (MMR) and varicella/chicken pox (Var) vaccines. See Appendix F for the schedule of recommendations for all childhood immunizations. Caregivers should be encouraged to complete the initial immunization series in a timely manner to protect their child and to prevent delayed school entry.

Nutrition

The toddler's ability to chew and swallow as well as use utensils improves during this time. Caretakers who understand these changes will be better able to introduce new foods reflecting the child's abilities. It is also, however, important to avoid foods that may be major choking hazards (pieces of hot dogs, popcorn, nuts, hard candy) (Forgac, 1995; Feeding the Toddler, 2001).

Caregivers should cut food into small bits, offer dipping sauces, and serve small portions. Most adult food can be provided with some modifications; however, toddlers rarely like new food the first time it is introduced. Juice should be limited to 4 ounces per day, because it is a nutrient-dense food that often replaces calories that should come from more nutritious foods. Since there is an increased incidence of severe peanut allergy in young children, any food item containing peanuts should be withheld until 3 years of age.

Mealtimes continue to be messy since toddlers are still becoming proficient with a spoon. Caregivers should be encouraged to provide praise and positive reinforcement since scolding causes tension and stress. Eating habits are established in the first 2–3 years, and forcing food or creating periods of extended tension at mealtime are not healthy.

Caregivers tend to become concerned about the child's decreased food intake and/or the fact that, for weeks, the toddler may eat only cereal (or go on other food jags). Caregivers need to be assured the child will not starve and generally will eat when hungry. A general rule of thumb to use in determining adequacy in the meal is to offer 1 tablespoon of each food group for each year. For example, a 3-year-old would need 3 tablespoons of meat, 3 tablespoons of carbohydrate (rice or potato), 3 tablespoons of vegetable, and 3 tablespoons of fruit.

Different strategies may also be used. Offering smaller amounts of food may encourage the toddler to ask for more. For others, frequent nutritious snacks throughout the day may be more enjoyable. Caretakers should acknowledge ritualistic needs (e.g., same plate, same cup), and encouraging the toddler to explore the world

Family Teaching

The Picky Eater

1. Provide healthy snacks every 1–2 hours; place them where the toddler can independently reach them.

2. Plan snacks for the day; regulate their timing with meals.

3. Allow an occasional junk-food snack.

4. Carry crackers and/or vegetable stick snacks while traveling in the car.

5. Be patient, food jags will pass; the child may eat only grilled cheese sandwiches for a month, but will move on to another favorite food in time.

6. Keep distractions to a minimum; turn off the television during mealtimes.

7. Respect the child's speed of eating.

8. Encourage the child to participate in meal preparation.

9. Use snack time to introduce essential nutrients (a good snack contains two of the five food groups):

If the child . . .	Offer . . .
Isn't a big milk drinker and needs calcium	Yogurt, frozen yogurt, hot cocoa, pudding
Doesn't eat meat and needs iron	Fortified breakfast cereal (not presweetened), raisins, fortified breakfast bars
Eats only white bread and needs more fiber	Fresh fruit and vegetables, bran muffins, bean or pea soup
Doesn't eat vegetables and needs vitamin A	Veggie juice, apricots, sweet potato wedges

of food should be accompanied by clear limits. See Family Teaching box for helpful guidelines in coping with toddlers who are picky eaters.

Elimination

Myelinization of the spinal cord and development of sphincter muscle control occur at approximately 12–18 months of age, and must be complete prior to beginning bowel and bladder training since the average toddler is ready to begin toilet training at approximately 18–24 months. The time to begin toilet training, however, varies from culture to culture and family to family. Nurses should educate parents about the signs of readiness for toilet training, which include the ability to demonstrate cognitive awareness of elimination (diaper is wet), follow directions and communicate understanding of elimination needs to the caregiver (pulls on diaper, asks for diaper change), remain dry for longer periods of time (more than 2 hours), independently dress and undress, and sit, squat, and walk well (Berkowitz, 2001c; Vessey, 2000).

Bladder control is often more difficult to attain than bowel control. The toddler usually has only one to two bowel movements per day, but urinates much more frequently. Often, accidental urinary incontinence occurs because the toddler becomes so involved in play activities that the urge to

Reflective Thinking

Toilet Training

Christine, the mother of a 20-month-old daughter (Jackie), is returning to work in a week and is concerned about placing her daughter in child care. Christine feels that Jackie should be potty trained prior to entering child care, and she wants to know if this can be accomplished during the next week. Considering your understanding of growth and development and the signs of toilet training readiness, what is your response?

urinate is ignored until it is too late to reach the bathroom. When the toddler is attempting to remain dry and learn bowel control, an emotional tug-of-war often develops between the child and the caregivers, leaving both frustrated and angry. Punishment and coercion can lead to shame and feelings of inferiority. A strategy that is often helpful is giving the child control over the process. Telling the child how the body makes "pee" and "poop" daily and helping the toddler succeed as well as using a child-sized potty can encourage participation and responsibility. A relaxed approach, with positive reinforcement and praise, will aid in toilet training, as will avoiding constant reminders and providing incentives for using the toilet correctly. Recording the child's progress and not punishing accidents are also important. Consistent day and night dryness should be achieved by 5 years of age, or further evaluation for physical and/or psychological problems is warranted (Berkowitz, 2001c).

Stress may either interfere with toilet training or precipitate regressive bowel/bladder continence. Caregivers need to be informed that such regressions are usually temporary and understanding, gentle support, reinforcement, and encouragement will assist the toddler regain a sense of independence and success.

Hygiene

Toddlers are usually bathed either every day or every other day, depending on their activity level and state of cleanliness. Their hair can also be washed when they are bathed. Although toddlers may enjoy their bath, they may not enjoy having their hair washed. Using baby shampoo that is less irritating to the eyes, or a wash cloth to cover the eyes may prevent the shampoo from irritating the child's eyes. Bath time for toddlers is often viewed as enjoyable and another time for play. Therefore, it is important to provide plastic toys (boats, ducks, fish) the child can use while in the water. Bubble bath should be avoided because it can cause urethral irritation and has been implicated in urinary tract infections.

The time of the bath should be consistent from day to day. Many toddlers are bathed in the evening before they are put to bed because it has a calming effect and can help the toddler relax after a busy day. Although toddlers may be able to sit well, they should not be left alone in a tub of water as they may turn on the hot water and get burned, or slip, bump their head, and fall under the water. It is always important to check the temperature of the bath water with a thermometer if possible and to keep the child warm after the bath by immediately wrapping a towel around the child afterwards.

Dental Health

In addition to routine health care visits, toddlers should also see a dentist. The child's first visit should be soon after the first teeth erupt at about 1 year of age. An important aspect of the visit is assessment of oral health, education of caretakers regarding correct methods of dental hygiene, and counseling on strategies to prevent caries (Grover, 2001c).

Young children are unable to brush all areas of the mouth, and as a result, caretakers will need to assume some responsibility for effective teeth cleaning. Toddlers may use only water, disliking the taste and foam of toothpaste. There is, however, some danger if fluoridated toothpaste is swallowed and the child also takes flouride supplements. The child may receive too much flouride. Therefore, caregivers should be cautioned that, if toothpaste is used, it be used sparingly. Small toothbrushes that are soft with short, rounded bristles should be used. After cleansing the teeth, flossing is recommended to remove debris below the gum line and prevent gingivitis (Grover, 2001c).

The use of fluoride is an effective method to lessen the extent of tooth decay and promote tooth health (American Academy of Pediatrics Committee on Nutrition, 1986). Tooth enamel resists developing caries when adequate amounts of fluoride are consumed before the teeth erupt. The nurse should educate caregivers regarding correct administration of fluoride supplements if it has been determined that fluoridation of water does not exist in the community (American Academy of Pediatric Dentistry, 1996).

Rest and Sleep

Most 2-year-olds require 12–14 hours of sleep each day with one or two naps a day. Bedtime protests can be reduced by beginning a winding down routine when toddlers are bathed, cuddled, and/or read to prior to being put to bed for the night. Firm consistent limits are needed when the child resists going to bed and dawdles or stalls (asking for water).

Some toddlers wake in the middle of the night and may have trouble returning to sleep. It is important to let the child cry for a short time since this assists the child to learn self-calming and comforting measures. If crying continues, caregivers can offer a hug, backrub, or drink before leaving the room again. A favorite blanket or toy coupled with a calm reassurance can also help facilitate the child's return to sleep. Nightmares are also common in toddlerhood since their dreams seem very real (Grover, 2001a). The toddler will generally respond to gentle reassurances and most often will return to sleep and will not remember the dream the next day.

Activity and Play

Play fulfills three functions for toddlers, including facilitating cognitive development by permitting exploration of the environment, learning about objects, and solving problems. It also advances social development particularly through fantasy play when acting out roles. Finally, it permits problem solving, vents frustrations, uses excess energy, and assists in coping with inner conflicts/anxieties in nonthreatening ways.

Age-appropriate play does not require expensive, shiny, developmentally approved toys. It does, however, require a patient and innovative caregiver who views play activities as major educational and socializing events in the child's life. Table 5-8 suggests toddler play activities.

Safety and Injury Prevention

The coupling of an inquisitive mind and a tottering, but mobile body places toddlers at increased risk for injury through accidents. The types of accidents and injuries experienced are directly related to the child's developmental progression (Table 5-9). Most injuries and deaths to toddlers are due to airway obstruction, poisonings, drowning, falls, burns, and automobiles (Online Safety Project, 2001).

Toddlers should *always* be strapped into a child-safety seat, appropriate for weight and size (Henson, Hadfield, & Cooper, 1999; Thompson & Emslie, 2000). The safety seat should be placed in the *back seat* of the vehicle. Toddlers should *not* ride in the front seat of a vehicle that has an *air bag*, unless they have specific medical conditions (i.e., tracheotomies, uncontrolled seizures, severe respiratory problems) that require constant observation. In these limited cases, the child should be placed in an appropriate front seat car seat and the air bag mechanically disabled (Flaherty & Snyder, 1998). A booster seat (one without side arms) is not appropriate until a child weighs at least 30 pounds. Transition of a child from a booster seat to

TABLE 5-8   TOYS AND PLAY ACTIVITIES FOR TODDLERS

Toy or Play Activity	Development Promoted	Selection Criteria
• Pull toys	• Stimulates gross motor skill and strengths (P) • Stimulates awareness of object when not seen (C)	• Wooden with pull cords • Makes noise indicating their presence (noise may be offensive)
• Picture books	• Teaches page manipulation (P) • Stimulates guided language development (C) • Teaches remembered properties of objects (forms and objects) (C) • Provides social experiences when assisted (S) • Stimulates knowledge and aids in school activities (C)	• Cloth or washable • Nontearable • Facilitates creativity and development of language
• Book of rhymes	• Provides fine distinctions in hearing (P & C) • Social experience and humor (E & S) • Stimulates language development (C & S)	
• Toys as symbols of adult activities • Dress-up kits • Nurse/doctor kits	• Symbols represent actions (e.g., lunch pail equals going to work) (C & S)	• Durable • Nonbreakable
• Scribbling on paper	• Stimulates creativity (C) • Aids in school activities (C) • Stimulates fine motor development (P) • Fosters artistic development (E & C)	• Large nontoxic crayons/markers

Key: C, cognitive development; P, physical development; E, emotional development; S, social development.

continues

TABLE 5-8 Continued		
Toy or Play Activity	**Development Promoted**	**Selection Criteria**
• Small push-pull toys • Cars and trucks	• Stimulates gross motor skills and strength (P) • Provides active experimentation with toys, objects, and movements (C & P) • Stimulates self-expression (E) • Aids in creative expression (C)	• Large • No sharp edges • Durable
• Large, crawl-in box • Trapeze set • Slides • Jungle gym • Teeter-totter	• Teaches gross motor skills (P) • Stimulates creativity (C) • Creates own environment (P & C) • Fosters social development (S)	• Durable • Adult supervision with trapeze, jungle gym equipment, and slides
• Stuffed animals • Dolls • Blanket • Blanket surrogate	• Comforts and provides security through familiarity (C, E, & S) • Promotes creativity (C) • Promotes imitative behaviors (C & S)	• No pieces that can be removed and swallowed
• Filling and emptying toys • Take-apart toys • Large size Legos • Loc-blocks • Block set • Hammer and nail sets	• Provides self satisfaction with repetition (P, C, & E) • Provides outlet for emotional expression (E) • Promotes gross motor skill and strength (P) • Promotes creativity (C)	• Durable • Nonbreakable

Key: C, cognitive development; P, physical development; E, emotional development; S, social development.

continues

TABLE 5-8 *Continued*

Toy or Play Activity	Development Promoted	Selection Criteria
• Puzzles • Tinker Toys	• Provides awareness of simple shapes (C)	• Nontoxic substances • No sharp edges
• Balls • Sandbox • Wagons • Hobbyhorse	• Provides awareness of shapes/textures (C) • Promotes gross/fine motor development (P) • Promotes social development (S)	
• Finger paints • Drums • Modeling clay	• Promotes awareness of textures, colors, shapes (C) • Promotes artistic development (E & C)	

Key: C, cognitive development; P, physical development; E, emotional development; S, social development.

Adapted from Lee, J., & Fowler, M. (1986). Merely child's play and developmental work and playthings. Journal of Pediatric Nursing, 1(4), 260-269; Florey, L. (1971). An approach to play and play development. American Journal of Occupational Therapy, 25(6), 275-280; Betz, C. (1983). Teaching children through play therapy. Journal of Association of Operating Room Nurses, 88(4), 709, 712-713, 716-717; and Betz, C., & Poster, E. (1984). Incorporating play into the care of the hospitalized child. Issues in Comprehensive Pediatric Nursing, 7(6), 343-355.

TABLE 5-9 DEVELOPMENTAL SPECIFIC INJURY PREVENTION FOR TODDLERS

Developmental Characteristics of Toddler (1-3 years)	Prevention Strategies
Walks, runs, may dart into street	Prevent injuries from motor vehicle accidents (as passenger, cyclist, or pedestrian):
More independent and developing autonomy	• Begin teaching stop–look both ways at curbside; stay off streets with riding toys and tricycle.
Not aware of dangers but is intent on exploring	• Use appropriate car seat.
Will stray from caregiver	• Do not allow child in front seat of vehicle with air bags.
Walks with unsteady gait	• Supervise—toddler acts impulsively!
Explores with mouth	• Provide fenced play area.
Can reach, climb, open lids, turn doorknobs	• Teach toddler not to enter the car of strangers.
Uses all senses to explore environment	Prevent fall-related injury:
	• Don't run with anything protruding from mouth (e.g., popsicle or lollipop sticks).
	• Use gates in stairways until child is very stable in walking and climbing stairs.
	• Remove scatter rugs, which may slide with child.
	• Remove electrical cords from walkway.
	• Keep child away from machinery and lawn mowers.
	• Teach child to wear bike helmets when on tricycle or on back of adult bicycle.
	• Secure screens in all open windows; use secure window guards.
	• Keep door to stairwells closed or gates in place.
	• Remove objects from crib that could be used to climb out of crib or window.
	• If child climbs out of crib, place in different bed.
	Prevent aspiration:
	• Check all toys for small, removable parts (buttons, eyes).
	• Use Mylar balloons only.
	• Avoid popcorn, nuts, hard candy, and other small, hard foods or large chunks of meat or hard vegetables.

continues

TABLE 5-9 *Continued*

Prevention Strategies

Prevent suffocation:

- Keep all plastic bags and similar objects out of reach.
- Do not use a plastic bag as liner for trash can in child's room.

Prevent burns:

- Set water heater at less than 49°C (120°F).
- Keep curling iron and cords out of reach.
- Turn handles of pans toward center/back of stove.
- Do not place containers of hot liquid on table cloth or scarf, which can be pulled.
- Use safety covers on electrical outlets.
- Keep child away from fireplaces and space heaters.
- Keep cigarettes, lighters, and matches out of sight and reach.

Prevent ingestion/poisoning:

- Store poisonous substances in original containers.
- Lock or remove medications and poisonous substances out of reach.
- Never refer to medication as candy.
- Do not keep medication, including vitamins, on counter, on table top, or in purse or diaper bag.
- Discuss meaning of poison with child.
- Use Mr. Yuck or similar designation for items that are off limits for child.
- Keep syrup of ipecac in home to be used *only* when directed by Poison Control Center.
- Post phone number of Poison Control Center by each telephone in house.

continues

TABLE 5-9 *Continued*

Prevention Strategies

Promote gun safety; if gun in house:
- Keep gun locked up and unloaded.
- Store bullets away from the gun.

Prevent drowning:
- Supervise child while in bathtub.
- Instruct child to never go near water alone.
- Provide close supervision around water.
- Instruct child never to run around pool or other bodies of water.
- Standing water should not be left in small wading pools unless a cover is applied.
- A child-approved life vest should be on child whenever on a boat or near water.
- Surround pools with locked fences.
- Teach child to swim but supervise—*closely*.

Miscellaneous:
- Teach child caution when approaching unknown animals (dogs, cats, raccoons).
- Do not expect young children to supervise toddlers.
- Use sun screen.
- Eliminate passive smoke in environment.
- Keep alcohol out of sight and reach.

lap-shoulder belts should not occur until the child reaches at least 4 years of age, 40 pounds, and/or 40 inches in height.

The Child-Occupant Safety Checklist (Table 5-10) should become a routine part of your teaching approach.

By 3 years of age, the child should begin to understand the concept of stopping and looking both ways before moving into a street. Even if toddlers do not understand the concept of oncoming danger, repetition of the stop–look sequence helps build the concept of safety.

Homes and surrounding play areas need to be childproofed to prevent drowning, falls, poisonings and accidents. Even when caregivers make a conscious effort to protect toddlers, toddlers need to learn what they may and may not play with in a home. All medications and toxic substances (e.g., gasoline, pesticides, household cleaning products) must be kept out of the child's reach and preferably locked away. These items should never be stored in familiar containers (such as soft drink bottles) and should have a "Mr. Yuck" or similar poison alert symbol affixed. Never tell a child that medication is candy, and never leave medications (including vitamins) sitting on tables or in the diaper bag or purse. Homes where toddlers live or frequently visit should have a bottle of syrup of ipecac in case a child accidentally ingests a toxic substance. However, caregivers should be instructed to administer syrup of ipecac *only after* consulting a Poison Control Center.

Alertness to water safety issues continues from infancy. The toddler's anatomical configuration (larger head/shorter lower extremities) creates a higher center of gravity and, when combined with an unsteady gait and insatiable curiosity, increases the risk of injury near bodies of water. Toddlers should *never* be left alone in a bathtub or pool since the child's attempts to stand may result in a fall, injured bones, fractured skulls, cause unconsciousness, and/or precipitate drowning. Being alone in the tub may also encourage the inquisitive toddler to turn on the hot water faucet, producing scalding water burns. Standing water should never be left in uncovered kiddie pools, and a locked fence should surround larger outdoor pools. Toddlers should not be allowed to go near any standing water without adult supervision; life jackets are recommended at poolside and required whenever the toddler is on any boat.

Injuries related to the toys children play with are central to toddler safety. Toys must be strong, safe, and large enough to prevent swallowing. Popped balloons are a major culprit, and for this reason, the use of latex balloons should be discouraged. Mylar, foil-type balloons are the only ones recommended as safe for young children.

It is impossible to teach toddlers the differences between toy guns and real guns since their cognitive abilities are not well enough developed to comprehend gun safety. Therefore, if guns are in the house, they must always be kept locked away from the inquisitive toddler (Society of Pediatric Nurses, 1998).

ANTICIPATORY GUIDANCE

Negativism

Negativism is an expression of the toddler's constant search for autonomy. The toddler resents being given directions and/or not being allowed to explore what is desired in an expanding environment. Characteristically, the toddler seems to delight in doing the opposite of what is asked and responding "no" to all requests. Caregivers are frequently frustrated when trying to deal with toddler negativism and are delighted to learn that this period typically passes by about 30 months of age.

As with any attention-seeking behavior, it is best to ignore the negativism.

Ritualism and Regression

As disrupting as negativism can be, another characteristic developing simultaneously is ritualism, or the need to maintain sameness (same cup, same spoon). The toddler needs stability within the expanding environment and to know, when in a new play area, familiar people and places will still be available.

TABLE 5-10 CHILD-OCCUPANT SAFETY CHECKLIST

Criteria	Yes	No
Child in restraint device	❑	❑
In the back seat (middle preferable)*	❑	❑
If more than 20 pounds, child faces forward in auto; if less than 20 pounds, child faces rear.*	❑	❑
Proper position (less than 20 pounds, at approximately a 45 degree recline; more than 20 pounds, upright)	❑	❑
Infant's or child's back firmly against back of safety seat	❑	❑
Head contained within the seat or, if in booster, within automobile seat back	❑	❑
Child car seat intact (no cracks in shell, no frays in straps, straps not torn, no exposed foam, no bent frames)	❑	❑
Car seat straps straight (not twisted)	❑	❑
Shoulder harness on shoulders	❑	❑
Shoulder harness taut (not more than 2 inches from shoulders)	❑	❑
Harness in slots below shoulders for rear-facing position, above shoulders for facing front	❑	❑
Infant/child not wearing bulky clothing or blanket under harness	❑	❑
Auto seat belt across chest (not across face, neck, or under arm)	❑	❑
Auto seat belt used with child car seat	❑	❑
Auto seat belt routed correctly through child car seat	❑	❑
Auto seat belt tight (doesn't slide and has locking clip if sliding type)	❑	❑
Restraint latch releases without difficulty (but doesn't pull out without pressing latch release)	❑	❑
Child car seat stable (can't be pulled forward away from auto seat or side to side)	❑	❑
Child car seat within edges of auto seat (doesn't extend over)	❑	❑
Child car seat made after 1981	❑	❑
Child car seat not on recall list	❑	❑
One infant/child in a restraint device (no sharing a restraint device)	❑	❑
In proper restraint for age and size	❑	❑
Booster seat used with shield/lap belt or lap/shoulder belt	❑	❑

* If there are no adults other than the driver in the car, the child can be placed in the front seat facing the rear, which is safer than back seat facing front. However, if car is equipped with air bags, young children must ride in the rear seat.

Data from Gaines, S., Benjamin, H., & Deforest, M. (1998). Promoting automobile safety for young children. MCN, 23(3), 148–151.

Rituals, such as mealtime and bedtime routines, provide repetition where the child may gain comfort and security. When rituals are disrupted, as when a child is ill or hospitalized, the child experiences stress, responds by exerting autonomy, and frequently regresses (returns to a earlier, safer, more familiar behavior) to dependence and negativism.

The best initial approach is to ignore regression while complimenting the child on positive attributes and behaviors. Since the loss of a newly acquired skill is frightening to the toddler, regression should be disciplined cautiously.

It not uncommon for toddlers to demonstrate a variety of behaviors when stressed.

Family Teaching

Handling "No!"

- Reduce the opportunity to say "no." Don't give the child an option if one doesn't really exist. **Don't ask:** "Do you want lunch now?" **Ask:** "Do you want peanut butter or bologna for lunch?"

- Avoid complex requests or overstimulating situations (such as trips to the grocery store) when the toddler is tired or hungry.

- Don't draw attention to negative behaviors, but if you are going to deal with them, do it immediately; otherwise, the child will have forgotten why reprimanding occurred.

- Do not threaten the child, especially as a reaction of frustration or anger. State disciplinary guidelines briefly, in simple terms. Be sure the child understands the consequence. The toddler may not remember both the terms and the consequence with a lengthy explanation. Example: "You need to brush your teeth so we can read your bedtime story," *not* "If you don't hurry up and brush your teeth there will be no story tonight."

Family Teaching

Routines That Work

1. Set a schedule that fits both the caregiver's lifestyle and the child's personality whenever possible. For example, if the caregiver works the night shift and the child is an early riser, plan enjoyable activities early in the day (e.g., playing outside, going shopping, doing the bath time routine), so that both can rest in the early afternoon.

2. Stick to a schedule, since routines provide security for toddlers. Establish a bedtime and bedtime routine (e.g., change clothes, brush teeth, read story). Adhere to these unless exceptional circumstances arise.

3. Use a consistent alternate caregiver. It is much easier to develop trust and separate from the primary caregiver if the same person cares for the toddler in the caregivers' absence.

Family Teaching

Avoiding or Managing Regression

- Do *not* introduce new foods, activities, and/or expectations at stressful times (birth of a sibling, illness).

- Attempt to identify the stressor, and consider various options to help the toddler manage the situation (i.e., care for a doll; help with new baby).

- Alternate activities and provide more caregiver attention and interaction to help prevent regression.

- Remind that regression is normal and generally does not have long-lasting effects.

These behaviors include aggression, avoidance, distraction, isolation, seeking information, self-consoling activities, and emotional expression. That is why toddlers may use a security blanket, have a favorite teddy bear, ask many questions, argue, cry, or have temper tantrums (Ryan-Wenger, 1992).

Discipline

Self-control develops best by consistently applied discipline. Regardless of the methods used, teaching the reasons for the discipline is essential (Blum & Williams, 1995).

Limit setting (letting the child know what they are able to do and not do in a situation) is an important part of discipline. These limits may be established by the child, adult caregivers, or the external environment.

Caregivers who provide clear and concise limits facilitate autonomy development and help the child gain a sense of order, control, and security (Gottesman, 2000).

Caregivers should agree upon both the limits not to be exceeded and the type of discipline used when established boundaries are pushed. The American Academy of Pediatrics Committee on Psychological Aspects of Child and Family Health (1998) identifies three essential components of successful and effective discipline: (1) a supportive and loving relationship between parent(s) and child, (2) use of positive reinforcement to promote desired behaviors, and (3) removing reinforcement to reduce and eliminate undesired behaviors.

Refer to the Family Teaching box for more information.

Family Teaching

Appropriate Toddler Discipline

- Predetermine and communicate limits.
- Allow limit testing.
- Assist in achieving mastery of socially acceptable behavior. (How to accept disappointments.)
- Provide ways for channeling undesirable feelings into constructive activities. (If angry, allow to use a toy hammer and nails.)
- Provide assurance child is loved even when certain behaviors are inappropriate. (Tell child he/she is loved, even though the behavior displayed is not approved of.)

Reflective Thinking

Corporal Punishment

You see a parent spanking a child in public. How do you feel about corporal punishment? What would you do?

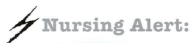

Nursing Alert:

Toddler Discipline

1. Nurses should never physically discipline a child. (Physical punishment may legally be administered only by a parent or legal guardian and the type and degrees of such punishment are currently under scrutiny.) The American Academy of Pediatrics' (1998) statements related to spanking, discipline, and punishment are accepted as the professional standard and can be found on their website.

2. If the child is hospitalized, discuss with caregivers how you may support their methods of discipline. Explain that hospitalized children frequently display regressive behavioral patterns, and carefully think before implementing any disciplinary measures related to regressive behavior.

3. If you observe inappropriate verbal or physical discipline, as a professional you are mandated to report it. The reporting mechanism will differ from state to state, but your responsibility does not change.

Family Teaching

Discipline

1. The sooner discipline is incorporated into the child's life, the more readily it will be respected.

2. Discuss discipline philosophies with other cardgivers behind closed doors, but when disciplining a child, be unified and supportive of each other.

3. Avoid disciplining in the wrong place, with the wrong motives, or with wrong timing; the child will rebel every time.

4. Avoid threatening to discipline and then not following through.

5. If a rule is broken, corrective actions should follow.

6. Expect respect in all interactions.

7. Follow discipline with love and positive encouragement.

8. Allow crying, but not screaming.

The type of discipline utilized will vary from family to family and culture to culture; however, approximately 90% of parents in the United States use corporal punishment (physical punishment) in disciplining their children (APA, 1998). Corporal punishment may bring about an immediate change in behavior, but the long-term effect is questionable for toddlers. Use of caregiver role modeling (Bandura, 1986) has been successful in disciplining toddlers, but requires the child to (1) see the correct behavior enacted, (2) remember what the role model did, (3) be physically able to repeat the role model's action and (4) be motivated to engage in the modeled behavior. This works especially well where a strong trust relationship exists with the role model. Role modeling, use of the teaching process, scolding, ignoring, and/or time out (placing the child in a nonstimulating environment) seem to be among the most widely used methods of achieving behavioral change with toddlers (Berkowitz, 2001a).

Sibling Rivalry

Sibling rivalry, defined as intense feelings of jealousy between siblings, often is seen when an infant is born into a family with a toddler. The arrival of this new baby can be devastating to toddlers since now they must compete for a caregiver's attention and fear loss of love or abandonment (Berkowitz, 2001b; O'Brien, 1996; Steelsmith, 1997).

See the Family Teaching boxes for some suggestions for handling this common problem.

Temper Tantrums

Temper tantrums are outward explosive reactions to inward stressful or frustrating situations that are a normal part of toddler life. Between 2 and 3 years of age, the child is faced with new environments, new rules, and new fears. Toddlers need to express their feelings, wishes, and frustrations, but lack the language skills to do this. All of these new experiences, coupled with the child's quest for autonomy, may create tension and erupt into a tantrum. Tantrums are ways toddlers say, "I have needs, I am important, I need to have some control." A typical temper tantrum—occurring when the toddler can't control his or her emotions, feels overwhelmed, or does not get what is wanted when it is wanted—may involve crying, screaming, falling onto the floor, kicking the feet, flailing the arms, banging the head, and breath holding (Grover, 2001b). Head banging requires intervention if it is continuous and/or unsafe, and to prevent injury, the caregiver should hold the child's head, make few comments, and/or provide a protective mat or pillow. Beyond this, as with any attention-seeking behavior, the tantrum should be ignored. Speaking softly and calmly, recognizing the child's feelings, and holding can help.

At the conclusion of the tantrum, the caregiver should offer a toy or option not related to the incident-producing difficulty. ("Why don't we play with your new tea set?") Disciplining a child after a tantrum usually is of little value. However, if the caregivers have told the child there would be a consequence to this behavior, they should follow through as promised.

Family Teaching

Tips for Dealing with Sibling Rivalry

- Establish a time frame when attention is focused exclusively on the toddler.
- Maintain the toddler's rituals as long as needed.
- Do not introduce new developmental tasks (e.g., toilet training or weaning from nighttime bottle) near the time when a new baby is expected.
- Have the toddler "sleep over" in the home of grandparent or individual who will be caring for him/her when the mother is in the hospital several times before the birth occurs. Reassure the child that his or her mother will return.
- If the toddler will be moved out of a nursery or crib to make room for a new baby, make the move several months in advance, and do not announce the real purpose of the move. Emphasize positive aspects: "you're getting to be so big."
- Do not tell the toddler that the new brother or sister is a playmate. This encourages the toddler to have unrealistic expectations of the neonate and can intensify negative behaviors.
- Be alert for subtle responses (not all sibling rivalry is overt) of sibling jealousy, such as taking the baby's bottle, pacifier, toys.
- After the new baby arrives, encourage visitors to spend time talking to the toddler. Keep small "gifts," which can be given to the toddler when presents are given to the neonate.
- When toddlers demonstrate rivalry, set limits and consistently administer discipline with love.
- Plan joint time with children, equalizing attention as much as possible.
- Encourage participation in the play-time and care of the new sibling; praise positive interactions.

Tantrums cannot always be controlled, but caretakers can take measures to lessen their frequency and/or intensity, including developing a regular schedule for the toddler, reducing the need to say "no," allowing choices, rewarding good behavior, and staying calm. Tantrums can sometimes be avoided by using time-outs or by placing a child in a bedroom before the behavior escalates. Temper tantrums are considered a normal developmental response of toddlerhood but should disappear by 4 years of age.

Child Care

Placing the toddler in a child care setting if both parents are employed outside the home is becoming more common today. Caregivers might seek support from professionals that use of such facilities is perfectly acceptable in today's society. Refer to Infant Chapter for more information on the use of child care.

REFERENCES

American Academy of Pediatric Dentistry. (1996). Reference manual 1996–97. *Pediatric Dentistry 18*(6), 24–77.

American Academy of Pediatrics. (1998).

Screening for elevated blood lead levels (RE 9815). *Pediatrics, 101,* 1072–1078.

American Academy of Pediatrics Committee on Nutrition. (1986). Fluoride supplements. *Pediatrics, 77,* 58–761.

American Academy of Pediatrics Committee on Infectious Diseases. (2002). *Recommended childhood immunization schedule—United States, January–December, 2002* [On-line]. Available: http://www.aap.org/family/parents/immunize.htm

American Academy of Pediatrics Committee on Psychosocial Aspects of Child and Family Health. (1998). Guidance for effective discipline: A policy statement. *Pediatrics, 101*(4), 723–728.

Bandura, A. (1986). *Social foundation of thought and actions: A social cognitive theory.* Englewood Cliffs, NJ: Prentice Hall.

Berkowitz, C. (2001a). Discipline. In C. Berkowitz (Ed.), *Pediatrics: A primary care approach* (pp. 114–118). Philadelphia: Saunders.

Berkowitz, C. (2001b). Sibling rivalry. In C. Berkowitz (Ed.), *Pediatrics: A primary care approach* (pp. 105–107). Philadelphia: Saunders.

Berkowitz, C. (2001c). Toilet training. In C. Berkowitz (Ed.), *Pediatrics: A primary care approach* (pp. 108–111). Philadelphia: Saunders.

Betz, C. (1983). Teaching children through play therapy. *Journal of Association of Operating Room Nurses, 88*(4), 709, 712-713, 716-717.

Betz, C., & Poster, E. (1984). Incorporating play into the care of the hospitalized child. *Issues in Comprehensive Pediatric Nursing, 7*(6), 343-355.

Blum, N. J., & Williams, G. E. (1995), Disciplining young children: The role of verbal instructions and reasoning. *Pediatrics, 96*(2), 336.

Brazelton, T. B. (1992). *Touchpoints, the essential reference: Your child's emotional and behavioral development.* Reading, MA: Addison-Wesley.

Erikson, E. (1963). *Childhood and society.* New York: Norton.

Feeding the toddler [On-line]. (2001). Available: www.uri.edu/coopext/efnep/toddlers/toddler.p2.html.

Flaherty, L., & Snyder, J. (1998). National Highway Safety Administration: final air bag ruling. *Journal of Emergency Nursing, 24*(3), 260–261.

Florey, L. (1971). An approach to play and play development. *American Journal of Occupational Therapy, 25*(6), 275-280.

Forgac, M. T. (1995). Timely statement of the American Dietetic Association: dietary guidance for healthy children. *Journal of American Dietetic Association, 95*(3), 370.

Fowler, J. (1974).Toward a developmental perspective of faith. *Religious Education, 69,* 207–219.

Freud, S. (1957). In J. Strachey (Ed.), *The standard edition of the complete psychological works of Sigmund Freud* (Vol. 18). London: Hogarth.

Gaines, S., Benjamin, H., & DeForest, M. (1998). Promoting automobile safety for young children. *MCN, 23*(3), 148–151.

Gemelli, R. (1996). *Normal child and adolescent development.* Washington, DC: American Psychiatric Press.

Gottesman, M. M. (2000). Patient education review. Nurturing the social and emotional development of children, a.k.a. discipline. *Journal of Pediatric Health Care, 14*(2), 81–84.

Grover, G. (2001a). Sleep: Normal patterns and common disorders. In C. Berkowitz (Ed.), *Pediatrics: A primary care approach* (pp. 39–44). Philadelphia: Saunders.

Grover, G. (2001b). Temper tantrums. In C. Berkowitz (Ed.), *Pediatrics: A primary care approach* (pp. 118–121). Philadelphia: Saunders.

Grover, G. (2001c). Dental care. In C. Berkowitz (Ed.), *Pediatrics: A primary care approach* (pp. 44–48). Philadelphia: Saunders.

Henson, R., Hadfield, J. M., & Cooper, S. (1999). Injury control strategies: Extending the quality and quantity of data relted to road traffic accidents in children. *Journal of Accident & Emergency Medicine, 16*(2), 87–90.

Kohlberg, L. (1976). Moral stages and moralization: The cognitive-developmental approach. In Likona, T. (Ed.), *Moral development and behavior.* New York: Holt, Rinehart, & Winston.

Lee, J., & Fowler, M. (1986). Merely child's play and developmental work and playthings. *Journal of Pediatric Nursing,* 1(4), 260-269.

O'Brien, M. (1996), Child-rearing difficulties reported by parents of infants and toddlers, *Journal of Pediatric Psychology,* 21(3), 443–446.

Online Safety Project [On-line]. (2001). Available: http://www. safekids.com

Piaget, J. (1952). *The origin of intelligence in children.* New York: International University Press.

Ryan-Wenger, N. (1992). A taxonomy of children's coping strategies: a step toward theory development. *Amercian Journal of Orthopsychiatry,* 62(2), 256–263.

Society of Pediatric Nurses. (1998). Policy statement for prevention of pediatric firearm injuries. In *SPN policy manual.* Denver: Author.

Steelsmith, S. (1997). *Helping young children adjust to a new baby* [On-line]. Available: www.parentingpress.com /t_970705.html.

Thompson, R., & Emslie, A. (2000). Young children and the risk of accidental injury: running an audit at nine months. *Community Practitioner,* 73(10), 799–800.

Vessey, J. A. (2000). Toilet training methods, clinical interventions, and recommendations. *Journal of Child and Family Nursing,* 3(1), 33.

SUGGESTED READINGS

American Academy of Pediatrics, Committee on Injury and Poison Prevention (1996). Selecting and using the most appropriate car safety seats for growing children: Guidelines for counseling parents. *Pediatrics,* 97(5), 761–763.

Benasich, A., & Brooks-Gunn, J. (1996). Maternal attitudes and knowledge of child-rearing: Associations with family and child outcomes. *Child Development,* 67, 1186–1205.

Bennetts, L. (1996). Raising intelligent kids: Part 2—Emotional savvy. *Child, March,* 56–64.

Berkowitz, C. (2001). Thumbsucking and other habits. In C. Berkowitz (Ed.), *Pediatrics: A primary care approach* (pp. 127–130). Philadelphia: Saunders.

Berkowitz, C. (Ed.). (2001). *Pediatrics: A primary care approach.* Philadelphia: Saunders.

Faber, A., & Mazlish, E. (1997). *Siblings without rivalry: How to help your children live together so you can live too.* New York: Norton.

Gellin, B. G. (2000). Do parents understand immunizations? A national telephone survey. *Pediatrics,* 106(5), 1097–1102.

Green, M. (Ed.). (1994) *Bright futures: Guidelines for health supervision of infants, children and adolescents.* Arlington, VA: National Center for

Education in Maternal and Child Health.

Gronlick, W., Bridges, L., & Connell, J. (1996). Emotion regulation in two-year olds: Strategies and emotional expression in four contexts. *Child Development,* 67, 928–941.

Heller, L. (1996, June). The magic of make-believe. *Parents,* 76–78.

Occupant protection law across the nation. (1997). Washington, DC: National Safe Kids Campaign.

O'Flaherty, J. E., & Pirie, P. L. (1997). Prevention of pediatric drowning and near-drowning: A survey of members of the American Academy of Pediatrics. *Pediatrics,* 99(2), 169–174.

Pendrys, D. G. (1995). Risk of fluorosis in a fluoridated population: Implications for the dentist and hygienist. *Journal of the American Dental Association,* 126(12), 1617–1624.

Reid, M. J. (1999). Treatment of young children's bedtime refusal and nighttime wakings: A comparison of "standard" and graduated ignoring procedures. *Journal of Abnormal Child Psychology,* February 1999.

Youngblut, J. M., Singer, L. T., Boyer, C., & Wheatley, M. A. (2000). Effects of pediatric trauma for children, parents, and families. *Critical Care Nursing Clinics of North America,* 12(2), 227–235.

CHAPTER 6

Growth and Development of the Preschooler

The preschool years span ages 3 to 6. Although physical growth slows, this is a time characterized by refinement of the cognitive and social skills begun during the toddler years. The preschooler establishes control of body systems as indicated by the ability to toilet, dress, and feed self, and is also able to tolerate longer periods of separation from caregivers, and interact cooperatively with adults and other children. In addition, the preschooler can use language in a sophisticated manner and has an increased attention span and memory. The refinement of these skills prepares the child for entrance into school.

Body systems also continue to mature and stabilize. All the senses mature, and visual acuity reaches 20/20 with intact color vision. (Berry, Simons, Siatkowski, Schiffman, Flynn, & Duthie, 2001). Tonsils may grow and levels of antibodies may increase to assist the preschooler in better fighting infection. Children generally have all 20 of their deciduous teeth by 3 years of age. By the end of the preschool years, the eruption of permanent teeth may begin.

Handedness is established by the end of the preschool years. Muscle and bone growth continues, but maturity is not reached yet.

PHYSIOLOGICAL DEVELOPMENT

Physical Growth

During the preschool years, the rate of physical growth and change slows as compared to the rate experienced during the infant and toddler years. Generally, children will gain an average of 2 pounds per year in weight and 3 inches per year in height. By 5 years of age, half the adult height will be reached (Brazelton, 1994).

The preschooler's body contour also changes. The prominent abdomen, lordosis, and wide-legged gait characteristic of the toddler years gives way to a slimmer, taller, more posturally erect contour.

Gross and Fine Motor Skills

The preschool period is a time of refinement of eye–hand coordination and muscle coordination. Walking, running, and jumping are well established and fine motor skills develop at an advanced rate. Both fine and gross motor skills can be tested through the use of the Denver Developmental Screening Test (DDST), a standardized development test in wide use throughout the United States.

The refinement and mastery of gross and fine motor skills encourage expression and independence, which leads to a greater sense of self-achievement and success as the child gets ready to enter school. Table 6-1 summarizes the preschooler's physiological development.

TABLE 6-1	PHYSIOLOGICAL DEVELOPMENT OF THE PRESCHOOLER		
	3rd Year	**4th Year**	**5th Year**
Growth	Weight increases 4–6 lb (1.8–2.7 kg) per year. Average weight is 32 lb (14.6 kg). Height increases 3 in (7.5 cm) per year. Average height is 37½ inches (95 cm). Visual acuity is 20/20. Color vision is fully intact. May have achieved night-time control of bowel and bladder.	Weight increases at a rate similar to the prior year. Average weight is 37 lb (16.7 kg) Height increases at same rate. Average height is 40½ inches (103 cm). Birth length is doubled. Maximum potential for development of amblyopia. Cooperates with Snellen test.	Weight increases at a similar rate. Pulse and respiration rates decrease slightly. Average weight is 41½ lb (18.7 kg). Height increases at same rate. Average height is 43¾ inches (110 cm). Half of adult height. Handedness is established. Eruption of permanent teeth may begin. Pulse and respiration rates decrease slightly.
Gross motor	Walking, running, and jumping are well established. Rides tricycle. Jumps off bottom step. Balances on one foot for a few seconds. Alternates feet going up stairs.	Skips and hops on one foot. Alternates feet going up and down stairs. Able to walk forward heel-to-toe, climbs jungle gym, and catches ball with both arms.	Skips on alternate feet and jumps rope. Jumps from height of 12 inches and lands on toes. Begins to skate and swim. Throws and catches ball well. Rides bike with training wheels. Able to walk backwards heel-to-toe and run on toes. Arms are coordinated with legs when running. Proficient climber.
Fine motor	Builds towers of 9–10 cubes. Cannot draw a stick figure but may make a circle with facial features. Copies circle and can build a bridge. Dresses and undresses self.	Uses scissors successfully. Draws stick figures with 3 parts. Can lace shoes but may not be able to tie shoes. Copies a square and traces a cross or diamond. Shows hand preference.	Begins to tie shoelaces. Improved cutting with scissors. Uses a pencil very well. Copies square and triangle. Draws person with at least 6 parts.

PSYCHOSEXUAL DEVELOPMENT

During the preschool years, the child is curious about his or her body, and learns about the physical differences between boys and girls. Freud described this period of time as the Oedipal, or phallic, stage of psychosexual development (Freud, 1959), when the child experiences subconscious conflicts and an intense attraction and love for the parent of the opposite sex. In turn, the child feels competition with the parent of the same sex for the attraction/affection of the other parent. This is termed the Oedipus (preschool boy to his mother) or Electra (preschool girl to her father) complex. Caregivers can be reassured that this phenomenon of competition and romance is normal, but may need help handling feelings of anger and jealousy that may arise. The resolution of the Oedipus or Electra complex comes as the child identifies with the parent of the same sex (Freud, 1959).

During this stage, the child becomes aware of himself or herself as a male and female, and begins to take on the behavior of the same sex caregiver (Charlesworth, 2000). For example, a young girl sees her mother putting make-up on and wants to do the same. Or a young boy sees his father vacuuming and wants to help.

Children will display sexual curiosity and interest in bodily differences according to gender. They may explore these differences through play such as "doctor" and "nurse," or ask many questions. If these questions are not answered by an adult, the children might come up with their own answers, which often are inaccurate (Brazelton, 1994). Therefore, caregivers should answer questions simply, by using correct terms for all body parts, including genitalia. Caregivers should be cautioned to only answer questions asked, since often the child is curious only about one aspect of sexuality and not interested in hearing a complete description. This is also an optimum time to teach children that certain body parts are private and should not be touched by "strangers." Table 6-2 summarizes preschooler psychosexual development.

PSYCHOSOCIAL DEVELOPMENT

The development of a sense of initiative versus guilt is the chief psychosocial task described by Erikson (1963). This is a time of very energetic learning, as the child participates in play and work with energy and enthusiasm, and develops a sense of accomplishment and satisfaction in activities. This increases the child's ability to use initiative, but as established limits are overstepped, feelings of guilt for not behaving appropriately may appear. A feeling of conflict may also arise as the child realizes actions were not appropriate. Feelings of guilt may also arise from thoughts the child has that are different from expected behaviors. Refer to Table 6-3 for a summary of psychosocial development.

COGNITIVE DEVELOPMENT

During the preschool years, many changes in the child's cognitive ability, or the capacity to understand and use information are occuring (Piaget, 1969).

During Piaget's preoperational stage, between the ages of 2 and 6 years (Piaget, 1969), the child develops the ability to perform mental operations governed by personal perceptions and linkage to events previously experienced. The preschool child can understand experiences only from his or her own point of view, and cannot imagine that another person would have a different perspective (egocentrism). There is no separation of internal and external reality. The preschooler uses a personal system for organizing objects and events in his or her mind (idiosyncratic) and reasons from one particular to another, often by unrelated events (transductive reasoning), when in reality the particulars are not linked at all. Animism (belief that objects have human qualities) is also a part of the preschooler's thinking (Dixon & Stein, 2000). See Table 6-4 for examples of preoperational thinking.

TABLE 6-2 PSYCHOSEXUAL DEVELOPMENT OF THE PRESCHOOLER

	3rd Year	4th Year	5th Year
Sexuality	Knows own and others' gender. Begins to adopt culturally prescribed behavior, and roles.	Masturbation may increase. Displays sexual curiosity and interest in bodily differences between girls and boys. May explore differences in gender through play ("doctor" and "nurse"). May have own ideas to explain sexual differences and reproduction.	Displays gender stereotypic roles. Curiosity and sexual exploration continues. Able to understand potential for sexual abuse.

TABLE 6-3 PSYCHOSOCIAL DEVELOPMENT OF THE PRESCHOOLER

	3rd Year	4th Year	5th Year
Psychosocial		Developing a sense of Initiative vs. Guilt (Erikson). This is a period of very energetic play and the child can develop a sense of accomplishment and satisfaction in his/her activities. As the child oversteps his/her limits he/she experiences a feeling of guilt for not having behaved appropriately. This is the beginning of the development of a conscience (superego). The child has mostly overcome stranger anxiety and separation anxiety. More sociable and willing to please. Likes being a helper.	
Family relations	Likes to please parents and conform with their wishes. Is less jealous of younger siblings (may be an opportune time for birth of additional sibling). Is aware of family relationships and sex-role functions.	Takes aggression and frustrations out on parents or siblings. "Dos" and "Don'ts" become important. Rivalry with older and younger siblings increases. May "run away" from home. Is able to run simple errands outside the home.	Gets along well with parents. May seek out parent for reassurance and security, especially when starting school. Begins to question parent's thinking and principles. Enjoys activities such as sports, cooking, shopping, or working.

continues

TABLE 6-3 *Continued*

	3rd Year	4th Year	5th Year
Social	Feeds self completely and dresses with minimal help. Has increased attention span. Can help to set the table and/or do the dishes.	Very independent in dressing and feeding. Tends to be selfish, impatient, and physically aggressive. Has mood swings. Shows off dramatically to entertain others. Tells family stories to others without restraint.	Less rebellious and quarrelsome. More settled and eager to please. Tries to live by the rules. Trustworthy and can take on responsibilities. Has fewer fears. Has better manners.
Coping	Temper tantrums, negativism, ritualism begin to decrease. Coping behaviors may include regression, denial, projection, displacement, attack, rationalization, and sublimation. Active imagination (may have an imaginary friend).	Begins to verbalize fears about body integrity, animals, or the dark. Uses play and fantasy.	Verbalizes feelings in later preschool years, may temporarily regress. May display independence through non-compliance or express confusion over inconsistent limits.
Play	Learns through play and imitation of adult behaviors. Will play cooperatively with other children and share toys. Plays group games with simple rules. Also likes dramatic play and is very imaginative and creative.		

TABLE 6-4 PREOPERATIONAL THINKING OF THE PRESCHOOLER

Question	Conclusion
Egocentrism	
Why do cars go?	Cars go to take me to the park.
Why does the sun shine?	The sun shines to see me when I play outside.
Why did I get sick?	I hit my sister.
Animism	
How did you get hurt?	The bike threw me off.
Why did you hit the door?	The door hit me in the head.
Transductive Reasoning	
Daddy is home.	It must be time for dinner.
The doctor put that thing in my ear.	I have an earache.
I ate cookies right before dinner.	The cookies made me get sick.

The 3-year-old child's attention span is increasing, but it lasts for a short time. Learning occurs through observation and imitation, as the 3-year-old asks many questions about the world around them, has a beginning concept of time, and begins to recognize colors and numbers. Due to the 3-year-old's active imagination, fears, including fears of bodily harm, may be experienced at this time (Charlesworth, 2000).

The 4-year-old child is less self-centered and has an increasing awareness of others and can comprehend simple analogies, for example, "if fire is hot, ice is cold." The child can also understand time better as well as the concept of opposites, for example, heavy/light and long/short. Finally, the 4-year-old can sort objects into like piles (Charlesworth, 2000).

The 5-year-old is busy learning the values and acceptable behavior of the culture, will question parent's thinking by comparing with peers and other adults, and has a fairly good estimate of time. In addition, the 5-year-old begins to see other perspectives but only tolerates differences, rather than understanding them. The 5-year-old also demonstrates a more realistic understanding of cause and effect (Charlesworth, 2000).

Refer to Table 6-5 for a summary of cognitive and language development.

MORAL DEVELOPMENT

Children of preschool age are in the preconventional or premoral stage of moral development as described by Kohlberg (Kohlberg, 1981). The child's moral judgment is at the most basic level, and right and wrong are determined from rules parents have established. Additionally, right and wrong are determined through rewards or punishments the child receives in response to an action. However, the preschool child has little understanding of why something is right or wrong, and if questioned, will often say "because my mother says so." Young preschoolers may have difficulty applying known rules to a different situation. For example, if a parent says "there is no jumping on the couch in our house," the preschooler may jump on the couch in a friend's house. Later, the child is able to direct actions toward satisfying personal needs rather than the needs of others, and develops a concrete sense of justice and fairness.

TABLE 6-5 COGNITIVE AND LANGUAGE DEVELOPMENT OF THE PRESCHOOLER

	3rd Year	4th Year	5th Year
Cognition	Preoperational thinking characterized by egocentrism, concrete/tangible thinking, transductive reasoning, magical thinking, and the inability to distinguish between one's own perception and that of someone else. This is a period of magical thinking and the inability to reason logically. Concepts of time, space, and causality are primitive.		
	Attention span is still short but is increasing. Learns through observing and imitating. Continues to be very self-centered. Believes that objects have human qualities (animism). Begins to learn concepts of time. Asks questions about environment. Fears are more specific, including fear of bodily harm. Active imagination! Color and number recognition begins.	Less self-centered and developing social awareness. Comprehends some simple analogies such as "if fire is hot, ice is cold." Better understanding of time. Understands concepts of long/short, light/heavy, etc. Can sort objects into like categories. Usually separates from family easily. Starts, but may not complete projects.	Questions parents' thinking and principles by comparing to peers and other adults. Learns the "rules" of the culture (values and acceptable behavior). Beginning to see other perspectives but tolerates differences rather than understanding them. Very curious about factual information about the world. Shows more realistic sense of causality. Classifies objects according to similarities. Personality qualities are noticeable.
Language	Knows name and age. Forms sentences of 3–4 words. Asks many questions. Uses mainly "telegraphic" speech. Correct use of plurals and pronouns. May use personal, made-up words and may carry on conversation with self. Vocabulary of about 900 words.	Use of longer sentences (4–5 words). Tells exaggerated stories. Questioning is at peak. Correct use of some prepositions. Names one or more colors. Vocabulary of about 1,500 words.	Use of longer sentences (6–8 words) and uses prepositions, past verb tenses, adjectives, etc. correctly. Vocabulary of about 2,100 words by the end of the 5th year of age. Names four or more colors. Knows names of days of week, months, and other time-associated words. Follows three commands in succession.

SPIRITUAL DEVELOPMENT

During the preschool years, children's knowledge of religion and faith continues to be learned from significant others (usually parents). They often have a concrete conception of God, who has physical characteristics, and can understand simple religious stories. Even though they may participate in some religious rituals, their understanding of the meaning of these rituals is limited. Children accept the religion of their parents because for them, parents are omnipotent and powerful. Some children will ask questions such as: How come we go to church on Sunday but Luke and Sarah go on Saturday? What is God? What is heaven? Does God push the clouds? Is thunder God hammering? Simple explanations that match daily practices and religious ceremonies, rituals, and pictures are important. If questions arise as to religious holidays, the spirit of the holiday and ceremonies associated with it should be explained.

HEALTH SCREENING

A preschooler should see a health care provider yearly, including a physical examination with care taken to assess growth parameters, and vision, hearing, and blood pressure screening. If the young child is uncooperative with the vision screening, another appointment should be scheduled 6 months later (Green, 1994).

The health screening should also include an assessment for the risk for hyperlipidemia, high-dose exposure to lead, and a tuberculin (TB) test. The TB test is required only once prior to school entrance unless there are risk factors present; then the test can be done annually with the health screening (Green, 1994; Dixon & Stein, 2000).

The common health problems of the preschool years include mostly minor illnesses such as otitis media, colds, or gastrointestinal disturbances. In fact, during the preschool years, minor illnesses are more common than at any other age. This is probably because this is when most children start playing together more frequently, attend child care, or start preschool/school activities resulting in more exposure to illness. Therefore, teaching children hand washing principles (after using the bathroom and before eating) may decrease the incidence of illnesses.

HEALTH PROMOTION

As with any age group, it is important to look at the ways normal growth and development impact daily activities and the health of the child. In the preschool period, families play a major role in ensuring health and preventing injury and illness. The following sections explore the unique issues a preschooler may encounter related to health promotion and injury prevention.

Immunizations

Preschoolers' immunizations need to be kept current, especially upon entering school. If the child has received all recommended immunizations according to the schedule recommended by the CDC during infancy and toddlerhood, only booster doses of diphtheria, tetanus, acellular pertussis, inactivated polio vaccine, measles, mumps, and rubella will be needed during the preschool years. Refer to Appendix F for the current schedule of immunizations.

Nutrition

Nutritional health is important in the preschool years because of the impact good nutrition has on growth and also for the value of establishing good health habits for the rest of one's life. By 3 years of age, a child should be eating table foods. The diet of a preschool child should revolve around the principles of the U.S. Department of Agriculture's food pyramid, which suggests six to 11 servings of breads and cereals; three to five servings of vegetables; two to four servings of fruit; three servings of milk products; two to three servings of meat; and sparse use of fats and sweets every day. In addition, this is a good time to switch the preschooler to low-fat or skim milk to decrease the amount of fat intake, since total fat intake should be no more than 30% of total caloric intake per day (American Academy of Pediatrics [AAP], 1999).

Planning meals and snacks around the pyramid will give the child a well-balanced diet and provide all the nutrients necessary to maintain health. If the child is eating a well-balanced diet, it shouldn't be necessary to supplement the diet with vitamins or minerals. If the child does not get a balanced diet, it may be necessary to start vitamins.

It is overwhelming to a preschooler to be served too much of any one food. Because of the decreased rate of growth during the preschool years, the appetite will also be decreased and the child may not be able to eat a large serving at one time. Serving 1 tablespoon of food per every year of age is as appropriate for preschoolers as it is for toddlers. It is also a good idea to vary the types of foods offered (Brazelton, 1994). Some children may be labeled "picky eaters," but this is an age of exploration, and something the child refuses one day may be eaten another day. Experimenting with various ways of preparing foods, as well as letting the child help prepare the foods may also increase intake (Green, 1994).

Some preschoolers will go on a "feeding strike" where they will refuse to eat much for a few days. This is normal, since children will often self-regulate their needs and eat when hungry. Others may continue to have "food jags" or go through a period of time when they will only eat one food or only foods of one color. Once again it is all right for children to make these choices. Caregivers should not fall into the trap of making eating and mealtimes a power struggle. Instead, they should be happy and enjoyable times for the family.

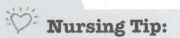

Nursing Tip:

Vitamins
Children's vitamins look fun and taste good, so children may be tempted to take more than the one per day. Be sure all vitamins are stored with other medications in a locked cupboard so the preschooler cannot "get into" the vitamins and take too many.

Elimination

Bowel and bladder control, including nighttime control, is generally achieved during the preschool years. However, accidents may still occur if the child becomes absorbed in an activity. If accidents do occur, it is best to maintain a matter of fact attitude and help the child clean himself or herself up.

Hygiene

Even though preschoolers are able to sit alone in the bathtub, they should always be supervised. It is not uncommon for children of this age to be scalded by turning on the hot water, or slip and fall under the water while playing. Many preschoolers enjoy their bath time, but the use of bubble bath (as with toddlers) is discouraged, because it might increase the incidence of urinary tract infections. Parental assistance may be needed for hair washing and cleaning fingernails and ears, as with toddlers. Often during preschool, children begin taking showers rather than baths. If this is the case, parental supervision is also necessary. Although children are capable of washing their hands independently when they become dirty from playing outside, the hands may not get as clean as they would if parents supervised the child. Turning the water heater temperature down to below 120 degrees will help prevent burns as these children become more independent in their hygiene.

Dental Health

By the beginning of the preschool period, the eruption of the deciduous (primary) teeth is complete. It is essential to preserve these primary/temporary teeth so the permanent teeth will have room to form correctly and the dental arch will not be narrowed. Since the preschooler is also very willing to be involved in brushing his or her teeth, this is an appropriate time to establish good dental habits that will last a lifetime.

The number one dental problem during this time is dental caries, which may cause the premature loss of teeth and a consequent alteration of the dental arch, compromising development of the permanent teeth. Prevention of dental caries is accomplished through daily brushing and flossing. If toothpaste containing fluoride is used, only a pea-sized amount of toothpaste should be used (AAP, 1988; Centers for Disease Control and Prevention [CDC], 1991). The preschool-aged child will also need assistance flossing because motor skills are lacking.

The preschool child should visit a dentist at least every 6 months. The first time the child visits the dentist, the child should not be told there will be no pain because, if pain is felt, trust will be lost and the child will become frightened (Hauck, 1991). Most dentists prepare children according to their developmental level before any work begins. The dentist will determine if the child needs to take fluoride supplements depending on the amount of fluoride in the drinking water.

Lastly, children should avoid sugary snacks that may predispose them to dental caries. Instead, parents should provide healthy snacks such as fruit, vegetables, or cheese. Gum should be sugar-free, and when the child does have a sugary treat, the child should brush or at least rinse the mouth out with plain water (Green, 1994).

Some children grind their teeth at night. This is common during the preschool years and may be a way to release tension and calm oneself in order to fall asleep. Generally, tooth grinding lasts for a short time as the child slips into sleep. Children with cerebral palsy, however, often grind their teeth due to jaw muscle spasticity. If tooth grinding is excessive, the child should be referred to a health care provider.

Rest and Sleep

Sleep patterns begin to change during the preschool years, and may vary from child to child. Generally, the preschooler will sleep a total of 12 hours every day. Some children sleep 10.5 hours a night and another 1.5 hours during an afternoon nap. Others will sleep for 12 hours every night. If children participate in preschool or day care centers, they will generally have a nap time. Even though many preschoolers will not sleep during this nap time, it is important to have the children at least rest (Stanford Sleep Center, 2000).

It is critical to establish a bedtime routine for the child, and hopefully, those rituals started during the infant and toddler years can be continued. If bedtime rituals have not been started earlier, this is the time to establish routines that prepare the child for sleep. By participating in the routine consistently, the child will enjoy bedtime and the household will not be disturbed as much (Stanford Sleep Center, 2000).

It is also important to help the child relax and prepare for sleep. Some children like to take a bath, play a quiet game, read a bedtime story, have a chat, say "goodnight moon," listen to soothing music, or have a light left on. All of these can help the child relax, learn how to be calm, and fall asleep.

The Family Teaching box offers suggestions on establishing a bedtime routine.

Activity and Play

The preschool child is refining both gross and fine motor coordination and skill which allows participation in more physical games and sports where motor activity is used. An emphasis on physical fitness has emerged in the last few years, and regular physical activity can benefit a child in many ways—for

Family Teaching

Establishing a Bedtime Routine

The bedtime routine should include various components:

- Establishing a bedtime and sticking to it
- Establishing a wake-up time and sticking to it
- Avoiding stimulants such as sugar or caffeine, or roughhousing near bedtime
- Making the bedroom cozy and inviting
- Avoiding nonsleep activities in bed, for example, watching television
- Maintaining quiet in and near the bedroom
- Making bedtime a fun time to be with the child
- Providing a quiet activity (reading a story) prior to going to bed

👁 Eye On:

Toys that Teach

Through advertisements, some toys are promoted as "toys that teach," meaning they teach, for example, "cause and effect" and "manual dexterity." While these toys are safe and attractive, the nurse must caution caregivers to be cognizant of deceptive advertising. For instance, an advertisement may imply that, if children do not have this toy, they will be developmentally delayed or that this toy is an adequate substitute for caregiver–child interaction. These claims are not true.

example, improved ability to perform motor skills; enhanced self-confidence and body image; development of lifetime habits; and prevention of disease processes associated with inactivity (Roberts, 2000). Physical activity can also help get rid of tension and excess energy.

By introducing the preschooler to sports, physical fitness can improve. Therefore, the main goal of sports for this age is to have fun, get exercise, and learn to enjoy the activity. However, since not all children will enjoy every sport, it is important to find the right sport for each child in order to make it a positive experience. The American Academy of Pediatrics suggests that caregivers encourage a variety of physical activities in a noncompetitive environment, with an emphasis on fun and safety. Some sports meeting this criteria are T-ball, karate, gymnastics, bicycling, or dance.

Preschoolers enjoy group play. They engage in imitative, dramatic, and imaginative play.

A 3-year-old still plays in an egocentric manner but is developing more tolerance of playmates. Appropriate toys and activities for this age may include a tricycle, pounding bench, big blocks, musical/rhythm toys, show and tell, guessing games, and puzzles.

A 4-year-old's play is interactive. The child can also obey limits and often has an imaginary friend. This imaginary friend is often given up by the time the child enters school. Toys and activities may include construction toys, puzzles, memory games, fantasy play, books, and music.

A 5-year-old has achieved impulse control and plays well in groups, so this is an optimal time to introduce the child to group sports and games. The 5-year-old child enjoys pretend play, puppets, dress-up, books, and art activities (Lytle & Lytle, 2000). Refer to Table 6-6 for activities stimulating development.

The child's love of reading and interest in obtaining the skill is established during this time period when caregivers spend time reading to young children. The child will show early literacy skills by reciting the name of the books they want to read; retelling the stories in the book; asking questions about the story; pretending to read a favorite book; correcting the reader if a page is skipped; and paying attention through the entire story (USOE Family Literacy Program, 2000).

Preschoolers will also enjoy books with more words that tell stories, especially if the book has lots of pictures. Books about children with similar experiences, including going to the doctor, going to the park, and going to school, or books about friends and families are also appropriate for children this age. Lastly, books with a predictable story

TABLE 6-6	TOYS AND ACTIVITIES THAT STIMULATE DEVELOPMENT OF THE PRESCHOOLER
Skill	**Toy/Activity**
Hand–eye–mouth coordination	Bubbles Coloring books Scissors Video games Large beads to string Stickers Markers or paint Large building set
Small motor	Crayons Sewing cards Art projects Play dough
Gross motor	Playing catch Kicking a ball Riding a tricycle Building blocks
Dramatic play	Play tools Kitchenette with dishes Dolls Magic wand Dress-up supplies Action figures Cars, trucks, trains Play people and animals
Cognitive	Books Puzzles Educational videos
Problem-solving	Puzzles Shape sorter Board games
Socialization	Group games such as London Bridge and Red Rover Board games Pretend play

line and repeated phrases help keep the child's attention.

Safety and Injury Prevention

With the increase in motor skills and coordination, the preschool-aged child is less prone to falls common during the toddler years. However, due to their increased mobility and skills, there are other dangers. One of the greatest areas of concern is playing near the street or driveway since preschool children still need close, constant supervision by adults to remain safe.

It is also important to remember that the preschool-aged child is less reckless, will listen more to rules, and is aware of potential dangers such as hot objects, sharp instruments, or dangerous heights. This makes it easier for the adults who are supervising preschoolers to set limits and expect obedience. However, as this is a time when the child likes to imitate whatever adults do, it is critical that adults also abide by the same rules, for example, putting on a seat belt before the car moves (Murphy, 1999).

Box 6-1 gives guidelines for injury prevention.

ANTICIPATORY GUIDANCE

Preparation for School

During the preschool years, many children attend some type of early childhood program (child care, preschool), which provides an excellent opportunity to encourage development. The experience can bring increased time for interaction with other children of the same age, teach group cooperation skills, stimulate language, physical, and social development, and help them cope with frustration and dissatisfaction (Brazelton, 1994; Dixon & Stein, 2000).

Most early childhood programs include quiet play; active, outdoor activities; group activities and games; art projects; creative or free play; snack time; and rest time. All activities are tailored to provide mastery of skills and to give the child an increased sense of achievement, confidence, and success.

Caregivers often ask health care providers for advice on knowing when the child is ready to attend preschool or school. Even though there are no absolute indicators of school success, the child's social maturity (age, physical abilities, and ability to play with other children) and potential to participate in learning (can follow instructions and has an attention span that is long enough to be able to participate in activities) can provide an indication of readiness (Dixon & Stein, 2000).

Preparation for attending preschool/school can help the transition. Since there will be separation issues when the child initially starts school, this can be lessened by helping the child understand what will happen at school if the experience is presented as fun and exciting. If the child thinks school

Family Teaching

Preparation for the First Day of School

- Send detailed information about the child to the school, including familiar routines, favorite activities, food preferences, and names of siblings and parents.

- Put the child on a "school" schedule a few weeks before school actually starts. This will assist the child to feel comfortable with the routine before school actually begins.

- Practice school-type activities: ride the bus, have school lunch at home (play cafeteria), sit in chair at table to color, practice printing name, tie shoes, and have rest.

- Introduce child to the school, surroundings, and the teacher.

- Stay with the child on the first day if possible. Be available but not conspicuous.

Box 6-1   Injury prevention guidelines

Home safety—Refer to information in infant and toddler chapters.

Play safety
- Ensure that playgrounds are safe. Check for impact- or energy-absorbing surfaces under playground equipment.
- Teach the child about playground safety.
- Teach the child about sports safety, including the need to wear protective sports gear.

Water safety
- Ensure that home and neighborhood swimming pools are enclosed by a four-sided fence with a self-closing, self-latching gate. Children should be supervised by an adult whenever they are in or around water.
- Ensure that the child wears a life vest if boating.
- Teach the child how to swim.
- Teach the child safety rules for swimming pools.

Car safety
- Continue to use a car seat or a properly secured booster seat until the child's head is higher than the back of the seat. When the child moves out of a booster seat, ensure that the seat belt is always fastened when the car is moving.
- The child should always ride in the back seat.
- Never leave the child alone in the car or in the house.

Safety with others
- Keep the child away from cigarette smoke. Do not allow smoking in the home.
- Choose sitters carefully. Discuss with them their attitudes about behavior in relation to discipline.
- Teach the child safety rules regarding interacting with strangers.
- Ensure that the child is supervised before and after school in a safe environment.
- Teach the child his phone number and address in case he/she becomes lost.

Outdoor safety
- Put sunscreen on before going outside to play.
- Supervise all play near streets or driveways.
- Teach the child pedestrian and neighborhood safety skills.
- Teach the child about safety rules for getting to and from school.
- Teach the child about safety rules for bicycles. Teach the correct signals for traffic safety.
- Ensure that the child wears a bicycle helmet when riding a bicycle, tricycle, or scooter.

Emergency preparedness
- Keep your address and phone number posted near the phone.
- Keep your list of emergency numbers (doctor, hospital, nearest neighbor, poison control center, etc.) near the phone.
- Keep a 1-oz. bottle of syrup of ipecac in the home and use as directed by the poison control center or health care provider.

Adapted from Green, M. (Ed.) (1994). Bright futures: Guidelines for health supervision of infants, children, and adolescents. *Arlington, VA: National Center of Education in Maternal and Child Health.*

is an adventure and learning can be fun, the change will be embraced quicker.

Discipline and Limit Setting

Limits are needed to help the child learn acceptable behavior. Initially, the child will test limits, but in the end, the child will welcome the limits because they define expected behaviors. If the child crosses over these boundaries, disciplinary action must be taken, and the child's behavior redirected in as positive a manner as possible (Green, 1994).

Time-outs can also be an effective method of discipline. No longer than 1 minute per each year of age, time-outs teach the child how to calm down and will give the child enough time to calm down but not too much time to become resentful (Brazelton, 1994).

One of the challenges of working with preschoolers is diverting aggressive behavior. Preschoolers tend to engage in instrumental aggression, that is, aggression designed to unblock a blocked goal such as a getting back an object, territory, or privilege. The caregiver needs to encourage sharing and nonaggressive ways of resolving conflict. Preschoolers engage in modeling, which is imitating behavior that they witness. It is important for caregivers to not only model positive behavior but reward for positive behavior (Charlesworth, 2000).

Childhood Obesity

Today, there is an increasing incidence of childhood obesity. This might relate to the growing number of obese adults since studies have shown, prior to 3 years of age, that parental obesity is the biggest predictor of a child's risk of developing obesity in adulthood (Buiten & Metzger, 2000). Childhood obesity has both immediate and long-term physical and psychosocial effects. The physical effects may be hyperlipidemia, obstructive apnea, pancreatitis, gallbladder disease, maturity onset diabetes of the young, and hypertension, which often lead to long-term cardiovasular diseases. The obese child also often has lower self-esteem and may find it hard to "fit in" with a group of peers (Buiten & Metzger, 2000).

The prevention and treatment of childhood obesity includes three components: (1) nutritional diets—with a decreased amount of foods with poor nutritional value, for example, candy, chips, and soda pop, and an appropriate serving size for age; (2) increased amounts of physical activity/exercise; and (3) behavior modification to teach the child appropriate ways to lead a healthy life (Roberts, 2000).

Sleep Disturbances

An increase in the number and kind of sleep problems are common and normal during the preschool years. They should resolve and diminish, however, as the child gets older, since many are related to irregular sleep habits and/or anxiety about going to bed and falling asleep. By following a bedtime routine and teaching the child ways to become calm and relaxed before bed, the caregiver can minimize the incidence of these problems. Other children suffer from bedtime fears, which may be helped by using a night light and by having an open discussion to resolve those fears (Stanford Sleep Center, 2000).

Nightmares, which are also fairly common, often involve a major threat to the child who wakes up crying because of being scared. If nightmares awaken a child, the parent should comfort and reassure the child that the nightmares are not real, and help the child remain in bed and fall back to sleep (Brazelton, 1994).

Sleep terrors, talking in the sleep, and sleepwalking are other sleep disturbances occurring during the preschool years. In these situations, the child may appear to be awake but in actuality is confused and can't communicate clearly. Most often, children will just experience a single or an occasional episode of sleep disturbance. If the episodes occur several times a night or nightly, the child should be seen by a health care provider. Fortunately, as children mature, these sleep problems should diminish (Stanford Sleep Center, 2000).

Television/Media

The influence of television and other media on children has become controversial since both can be constructive and positive, as well as inappropriate and negative. Television, however, is not a substitute for education and play, but some programs can reinforce learning, promote creativity, and encourage cognitive growth by teaching colors, numbers, the alphabet, and social skills in a creative and stimulating manner. On the other hand, some programs are inappropriate for young children (Leland, 1999). Since preschoolers often believe that what they see is real, they cannot differentiate between reality and fantasy in television programs. Inappropriate programs give children a distorted view of how to deal with problems, which often is with violence (AAP, 1999).

While the television should not be used as a babysitter, it is virtually impossible to "ban" television viewing. Instead, caregivers should closely monitor and control what a child watches. The AAP recommends a preschooler only watch 1–2 hours of television per day. See Box 6-2.

Fears

Preschoolers can become fearful of real or imagined things (bugs, the dark, animals), and it is best to tackle the problem directly. Instruct caregivers to find realistic ways to overcome or deal with the fear. For instance, keep a night light on at night. In some cases, continuous exposure to the fear stimulus may diminish the fear. However, it is important to not force a child. For example, if a child has a fear of swimming, the caregiver should encourage the child to put on a swimsuit and life-saving gear, and sit by the edge of the pool. As the child witnesses the safe fun that other children and caregivers are experiencing, they may realize that there is nothing to be afraid of.

Box 6-2   Guidelines for television and video viewing

- Limit child's viewing time to no more than 1–2 hours per day.
- Control what the child watches.
- Watch television with children, especially if the child is viewing a new show or a new video.
- If the child is allowed to watch a program while the parent is occupied with another activity and cannot supervise appropriately, encourage the child to select a video with known content.
- Provide feedback to the networks regarding the quality of children's programming.
- Avoid putting a television in a child's bedroom.

Adapted from AAP, Committee on Public Education. (1999). Media Education. Pediatrics, *104(2), 341–343.*

REFERENCES

American Academy of Pediatrics, Committee on Nutrition. (1988). Fluoride supplementation for children. *Pediatrics, 95*(5), 800.

American Academy of Pediatrics, Committee on Public Education. (1999).

Media education. *Pediatrics, 104*(2), 341–343.

Berry, B. E., Simons, B. D., Siatkowski, R. M., Schiffman, J. C., Flynn, J. T., & Duthie, M. J. (2001). Preschool vision screening using the MTIphotoscreener™. *Pediatric Nursing, 27*(1), 27–34.

Brazelton, T. B. (1994). *Touchpoints.* New York: Perseus Press.

Buiten, C., & Metzger, B. (2000). Childhood obesity and risk of cardiovascular disease: A review of the science. *Pediatric Nursing, 26*(1), 13–18.

Centers for Disease Control and Prevention. (1991). Public Health Service report on fluoride benefits and risks. *Morbidity and Mortality Weekly Report, 40*(RR-7): 1–8.

Charlesworth, R. (2000). *Understanding child development.* (5th ed.). Clifton Park, NY: Delmar.

Dixon, S. D., & Stein, M. T. (2000). *Encounters with children: Pediatric behavior and development* (3rd ed.). St. Louis, MO: Mosby.

Erikson, E. H. (1963). *Childhood and society.* New York: Norton.

Freud, S. (1959). *Collected papers.* New York: Basic Books.

Green, M. (Ed.) (1994). *Bright futures: Guidelines for health supervision of infants, children, and adolescents.* Arlington, VA: National Center of Education in Maternal and Child Health.

Hauck, M. R. (1991). Cognitive abilities of preschool children: Implications for nurses working with young children. *Journal of Pediatric Nursing, 6*(4), 230–235.

Kohlberg, L. (1981). *The philosophy of moral development, moral states, and the idea of justice.* New York: Harper & Row.

Leland, J. (1999, June 19). The magnetic tube. *Newsweek, Special Issue,* 89–90.

Lytle, R., & Lytle, D. (2000, December). Play, playfulness, and expressive activities. *Exceptional Parent Magazine,* pp. 64–70.

Murphy, J. M. (1999). Pediatric occupant car safety: Clinical implications based on recent literature. *Pediatric Nursing, 25*(2), 137–148.

Piaget, J. (1969). *The theory of stages in cognitive development.* New York: McGraw-Hill.

Roberts, S. (2000). The role of physical activity in the prevention and treatment of childhood obesity. *Pediatric Nursing, 26*(1), 33–41.

Stanford Sleep Center. (2000). *Children's sleep problems* [On-line]. Available: www.stanford.edu/~dement

USOE Family Literacy Program. (2000, October). *Early literacy development.* Paper presented at Seminar, Salt Lake City, UT.

SUGGESTED READINGS

Chen, J., & Kennedy, C. M. (2001). Ask the expert: Television viewing and children's health. *Journal of the Society of Pediatric Nurses, 6*(1), 35–38.

Cohen, S. M. (2001). Lead poisoning: A summary of treatment and prevention. *Pediatric Nursing, 27*(3), 125–130.

Davidhizar, R., Havens, R., & Bechtel, G. A. (1999). Assessing culturally diverse pediatric clients. *Pediatric Nursing, 25*(4), 371–375.

Dokken, D., & Sydnor-Greenberg, N. (2000). Exploring complementary and alternative medicine in pediatrics: Parents and professionals working together for new understanding. *Pediatric Nursing, 26*(4), 383–390.

Hall-Long, B. A., Schell, K., & Corrigan, V. (2001). Youth safety education and injury prevention program. *Pediatric Nursing, 27*(3), 141–146.

Kennedy, C. M. (2000). Television and young Hispanic children's health behaviors. *Pediatric Nursing, 26*(3), 283–291.

Knestrick, J., & Milstead, J. A. (1998). Public policy and child lead poisoning: Implementation of title X. *Pediatric Nursing, 24*(1), 37–41.

Manworren, R. C. B., & Woodring, B. (1998). Evaluating children's literature as a source for patient education. *Pediatric Nursing, 24*(6), 548–553.

Sawicki, J. A. (1997). Sibling rivalry and the new baby: Anticipatory guidance and management strategies. *Pediatric Nursing, 23*(3), 298–302.

Selekman, J. (1998). Infectious diseases and the immunizations of today and tomorrow. *Pediatric Nursing, 24*(4), 309–315.

Strasburger, V. C., & Donnerstein, E. (1999). Children, adolescents and the media: Issues and solutions. *Pediatrics, 103*(1), 129–139.

Vessey, J. A. (1995). Developmental approaches to examining young children. *Pediatric Nursing, 21*(1), 53–56.

CHAPTER 7

Growth and Development of the School-aged Child

The phase of development from 6 to 12 years, the school-age years, is crucial to establishing positive self-esteem, a sense of belonging, and feelings of competence. During this time the child moves from egocentric thought to experiencing the world through peers and the school environment. Today's child can experience the world beyond the classroom with the help of the Internet, electronic mail, educational videotapes and cable television.

PHYSIOLOGICAL DEVELOPMENT

The school-age years are marked by a steady rate of physical growth. However, keep in mind that each child is unique and growth is affected by genetics, gender, the presence of acute or chronic illness, and the environment (Rudolph & Kamei, 1998).

During the school-age years, the child's weight increases by 5 to 6 pounds per year and height increases by 2 inches per year (Schor, 1999). At 6 years, the average boy weighs 45 pounds and is 46 inches tall; the average girl weighs 43 pounds and is 45 inches tall. At 12 years, the average male weighs 88 pounds and is 59 inches tall; the average female weighs 91 pounds and is 60 inches tall. Skeletal growth is particularly noticeable in the long bones of the extremities. Growing pains, which occur because the long bones grow faster than the attached muscles, affect up to 15% of school-aged children (Rudolph & Kamei, 1998).

Muscle strength and size also increase at a gradual rate during school-age years and six basic gross motor skills (balancing, catching, throwing, running, jumping, climbing) continue to be refined. At the same time, improved balance and coordination enable the school-aged child to explore new physical activities, such as bike riding and rollerblading. However, muscles can be easily injured so physical activities should be selected according to the abilities of the child.

Boys have a greater number of muscle cells than girls, so it is common to find they do well with gross motor activities such as throwing and running. In contrast, girls tend to have better dexterity of fingers and hands, so they are more adept at fine motor skills. As eye–hand coordination and motor skills improve, the school-aged child is able to

Critical Thinking

Physiological Development

Eight-year-old Ryan and ten-year-old Wally have come to the office for a physical. Ryan weighs 43 pounds and is 45 inches tall. Wally weighs 68 pounds and is 50 inches tall. The boys are accompanied by their mother; she is worried about their weight and height. Why is she showing concern? What does the nurse need to consider when answering the mother?

write, tie shoes, and become autonomous in dressing. Motor development progresses in a cephalocaudal and proximal to distal direction, with refinement of both gross motor and fine motor skills occurring as the central nervous system matures (Rudolph & Kamei, 1998).

To meet the increased activity levels during the school-age years, the cardiovascular and respiratory systems develop in size and capacity. The heart growth slows and assumes a more vertical position in the chest as the diaphragm descends to allow for lung expansion. As the cardiac and respiratory systems become more efficient, the pulse and respiratory rates slow. The average apical pulse rate for the school-aged child is 90 to 95 beats per minute while at rest. The average respiratory rate for the school-aged child is 20 breaths per minute while at rest. In addition, the tidal volume doubles (Stedman's Medical Dictionary, 2000).

It is during the school-age years that the 20 deciduous teeth are shed and the permanent teeth appear. This process usually starts at age 5 years and is complete before adolescence, except for the third molars (wisdom teeth). The first permanent teeth appear by age 6 years and are called the central incisors and first molars. Over the next five years, the deciduous teeth are replaced at a rate of 4 teeth per year. When children start to lose their teeth, the rate of loss is determined by genetics and gender. It is common for girls to lose their teeth earlier than boys. However, for both boys and girls, by the end of the school-age years, the 20 deciduous teeth are replaced by 28 of the 32 permanent teeth (Stedman's Medical Dictionary, 2000). Often the permanent front teeth seem too large for the face giving the child an odd look.

During the preschool years, children are exposed to and develop immunity to a variety of microorganisms. Therefore, the school-age years are often one of the healthiest phases of life. Antibodies are produced by the lymphatic system and reach their peak by age 7 years. Because of the increase in body size and maturity of the immune system, school-aged children are able to respond to illnesses similar to adults.

Family Teaching

Heart Murmur

- Explain to caregivers that an "innocent" murmur is created from the sound of the blood flowing through the heart and can be heard because of the child's thin chest wall.

- Reassure the child and caregiver that the murmur is not associated with heart disease and will no longer be heard when the child reaches adolescence.

- Provide the school nurse with medical documentation confirming the presence of an innocent heart murmur.

- Provide coaches with medical documentation confirming the presence of an innocent heart murmur.

The last years of the school-age period are called prepubescence, meaning the two years before puberty. The first physiological signs of prepubescence, such as breast tissue development, and body odor changes can appear as early as 9 years of age in females. However, in the United States, the average age of puberty is 12 years for females and 14 years for males (Santrock, 1998).

PSYCHOSEXUAL DEVELOPMENT

Freud (1923) believed that, starting at age 6 years and throughout school-age, the child enters a calm period in the development of their sexuality, called latency. Freud theorized the school-aged child identified with the same-sex parent by modeling the behaviors and emotions of this parent and learned about sex-role behavior and identity by observing caregiver interactions, the media, and friendships with children of the same gender.

PSYCHOSOCIAL DEVELOPMENT

The school-age years introduce the child to the world of peers and school. As each child interacts within this new context, a more realistic sense of self and place in this world evolves. A newfound independence from caregivers is discovered and peers become a major socializing agent. Because they are the major socializing agents at this time, children behave according to what they deem is acceptable to their friends. Although school-aged children need the love and support provided by caregivers, peers provide the support needed to gain independence from family as increased amounts of time are spent with peers of the same gender.

The developmental theory of Erik Erikson (1963) identified the major task of the school-age period as industry (the ability to be useful or productive) versus inferiority. During this time, energy is channeled into activities such as school projects, sports, and hobbies. These concrete endeavors become the child's work and bring a sense of accomplishment and worth. The school-aged child also develops the ability to work with others on school projects and athletic teams in preparation for becoming a citizen of the world.

Erikson (1963) believed development is a continual process based on prior success, and if children are not able to realize a sense of industry, feelings of inferiority may develop. This occurs when children feel they cannot live up to the expectations of caregivers or teachers, or when they feel different from peers. In order for school-aged children to feel a sense of competence, it is imperative that they have a positive relationship with an affirming adult.

COGNITIVE DEVELOPMENT

Piaget (1962) suggested that around 6 years of age, children start to move from the egocentric view of the preschool age to the more open and flexible thought of the school-aged child. As children learn about the ideas of their peers and adults, they are able to see things from another's point of view.

The expanded cognitive abilities enable the child to imagine the world without having to experience it. However, because abstract thought has not been developed, the child is limited to thinking concretely and in the present time frame. During these concrete operations, the child gains the skills of classification (the ability to group items according to common characteristics), conservation (the ability to acknowledge that a change in shape does not mean a change in amount), and reversibility (the ability to recognize that actions can move in reverse order). For example, the child who has mastered classification can group animals according to the dog, cat, or horse family, and often collects baseball cards, coins, and rocks. Conservation emerges as the child's egocentric thinking is replaced by cognitive reasoning, develops over time, and begins with the conservation of numbers, followed by mass, weight, and volume. Reversibility is important when learning addition and subtraction, and is seen when a child can reassemble a toy or play a game in reverse order. Refer to Figure 7-1.

> ### ♡ Nursing Tip:
>
> **Understanding the concepts of time, height, weight, and volume**
> Because of the child's skill in concrete operations, more detail can be included when preparing the child for new health care experiences. For example, in preparing a child for a medical procedure, the nurse can explain the scheduled date and time of the procedure, how the procedure will be performed, and what the child will have to do. This kind of explanation, as well as the child's increased participation in self-care and treatment are important when caring for the school-aged child.

Original	Physical Change	Question	Nonconserving Response	Conserving Response
Child agrees that the same amount of drink is contained in each glass.		Is there still the same amount of drink in each glass, or does one glass have more?	No, they are not the same; there is more in the tall glass.	Yes, they have the same amount; you just put the drink in a different size glass. It is taller, but it is also thinner.
Child agrees each ball contains the same amount of clay.		Is there still the same amount of clay in the ball and the snake, ordoes one have more?	No, there is more clay in the snake because it is longer (or more in the ball because it is fatter).	Yes, they have the same amount. You just rolled one ball out in a different shape.

Figure 7-1 Physical Changes in Conservation Tasks. Source: Charlesworth, R. (2000). *Understanding child development* (5th ed.). Clifton Park, NY: Delmar.

During the school-age years, the child's ability to use language is enhanced and vocabulary expands from 2,000 to 50,000 words (Click, 1998). By six, the school-aged child uses six-word sentences and can follow a story without the use of pictures. By seven, the school-aged child understands time and the difference between right and left and by eight, the child can use language as a tool for reasoning (Dixon & Stein, 2000). School-aged children also can learn the literal meaning of words and are beginning to understand a word's nonliteral meaning. By 11 years of age, metaphors are understood and used in conversation, such as when describing a headache as "drums pounding in my head." However, temperament, social and cultural factors, and verbal and language environment affect language acquisition. This is especially true of expressive verbal skills (Rudolph & Kamei, 1998).

Besides a tool for communication, language becomes a tool for socialization as the school-aged child's language becomes less egocentric. Adults need to use words school-aged children can understand and carefully assess their comprehension because their mental capacity and control of language is not fully developed.

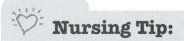

Nursing Tip:

Explain medical terms
Language unites groups and cultures. Medicine has a distinct language from mainstream society. Therefore, when caring for school-aged children, it is important to use correct terminology they will understand. Since children of this age may interpret each word literally, avoid using terms such as "taking a CAT scan" or "being put to sleep." Instead, explain the sequence of events the child will experience and exactly what will happen.

During the school-age years children begin to acquire the ability to read, through letter identification, telling a story from looking at the pictures, and being read to. Reading should be encouraged by choosing books the child enjoys, being read to by an adult, and reading alone.

MORAL DEVELOPMENT

The school-aged child is at the conventional level (Stages 3 and 4) of moral development, when the conscience develops an internal set of "rules" that must be followed in order to "be good" (Kohlberg, 1969). During Stage 3 (ages 6 to 10 years), the child's morality is based on avoiding the disapproval of others, and maintaining a positive relationship with friends, family, and teachers. Accidents can be viewed as punishment for disobeying. For instance, a toy breaking may be punishment for spilling milk in the family room where drinking is prohibited. During Stage 4 (ages 11 and 12 years), the child is concerned with doing the "right" thing and showing respect for authority figures. Children at this level can also demonstrate rigid behavior in an effort to obey the law. These children can take into account circumstances surrounding an incident rather than just looking at the result. Older school-aged children understand the need to treat others as they would like to be treated.

Table 7-1 describes key milestones for school-aged children.

SPIRITUAL DEVELOPMENT

During school age, the child moves from thinking of God as being a fairy tale-like giant to thinking of God as like a human being. Family, friends, teachers, church, books, and the media teach ideas that help the child develop a religious philosophy used in interpreting and understanding the world. The concepts of Allah, God, Jesus, religious rites, ancestor worship, life after death,

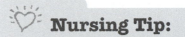

Nursing Tip:

Modeling moral behavior
It is imperative that nurses model moral behavior and use sound moral judgment in caring for school-aged children and families. Nurses need to assist these youngsters in making decisions regarding their health care, keeping in mind they may agree with suggestions in order to do the "right thing." Nurses also need to present good health care options and encourage school-agers to choose the option that works best for them.

heaven, hell, and reincarnation are developed during this time as well, and often, children picture God as a "loving" and "helping" human. Coles (1990) says most children, even those with an atheistic background, are able to develop a concept of God and likely to believe in God even though they may not discuss this with others. During these years, children can be taught through stories emphasizing moral traits, and they continue to ask questions about religious teachings and God. It is not unusual for school-aged children to pray for recovery from illness and protection from danger for others as well as the self. Children of this age believe in a Supreme Being that loves and gives to others. As the child enters preadolescence, he or she realizes self-centered prayers are not always answered and there is no magic involved in religious beliefs. Blind faith that previously existed in the younger child is replaced by reason.

HEALTH SCREENING

When compared to traditional standards, school-aged children enjoy excellent health (Prescott, 1999); when school-aged children are sick, it is typically for a minor illness. School-aged children average two health

TABLE 7-1 SCHOOL-AGE MILESTONES

6 to 7 Years

Gross and Fine Motor Skill	Cognitive Development	Social Development
Legibly prints letters.	Learning to tell time.	Able to bathe and dress self.
Uses knife, fork, and spoon.	Learning to read. Can read from memory.	Able to fix own hair.
Rides 2-wheel bike.	Understands right and left.	Enjoys games with peers of same gender.
Masters all skills on the DDST.	Knows value of currency.	Shares and cooperates.
Improved dexterity.	Interested in magic and fantasy.	May be jealous of younger siblings.
Cuts, pastes, folds paper.	Defines common objects according to their use.	Needs praise and recognition.
Ties shoe laces.	Understands concept of numbers.	Fewer mood swings.
Throws overhand.	Attention span increasing.	Enjoys helping around the house.
Copies a diamond.	Enjoys word and spelling games.	Participates in school and community activities.
Walks a straight line.	Obeys three commands.	Attentive listener.
	Likes to help.	Demonstrates independence.
	Knows right and left hand.	Spends time in quiet play.
	Concrete, animistic thinking	
	Attends first and second grades.	
	Reflective.	

continues

TABLE 7-1 *Continued*

8 to 9 Years

Gross and Fine Motor Skill	Cognitive Development	Social Development
Developing eye-hand coordination.	Understands concept of time.	Likes competitive games and sports.
More fluid movement.	Knows the date and month.	Runs errands.
Plays team sports. Body becomes flexible.	Collects and classifies objects.	Social, well behaved.
Able to use household tools.	Increased ability to read.	Modest.
Writes using cursive.	Learning fractions.	Demanding and critical of others.
Dresses self completely.	Understands space, cause, effect, conservation.	Compares self with others.
Jumps, skips, draws three-dimensional figures.	Knows similarities and differences of objects.	Looks up to adults.
	Counts backward from 20.	Dependable, responsible.
	Shows interest in music lessons.	Rules are important.
	Can make change (small currency).	Able to do household chores.
	Helps around the house.	Best friends are important.
	Can be critical of accomplishment and failure.	Tolerant and accepting of others.
	Learns from experiences.	
	Punctual.	
	Improvises simple activities.	
	Less animistic in thinking.	
	Attends third and fourth grades.	

continues

TABLE 7-1 *Continued*

10 to 12 Years

Gross and Fine Motor Skill	Cognitive Development	Social Development
Eye-hand coordination well developed.	Developing ability for abstract thought.	Rules are important.
Fine motor skills well developed.	Able to write stories.	Interest in opposite sex.
Gross motor skills may become awkward with growth spurt.	Drawings are detailed.	Quarrelsome with siblings.
Balances on one foot for 15 seconds.	Easily distracted.	Developing social competence.
Catches a fly ball.	Knows death is irreversible.	Self-disciplined.
Cooks and sews.	More realistic than idealistic.	Easy to please.
	Truthful.	Obedient.
	Reads for enjoyment; reads well.	May have best friend.
	Knows limits.	Becoming diplomatic.
	Interested in the future.	Affectionate, sensitive.
	Likes to memorize and identify facts.	Respects parents.
	Likes to discuss and debate.	Self-directed and independent.
	Unaware of effect on others.	Can stay at home alone for short periods of time.
	Beginning formal operations.	Increased interest in family.

care visits each year, with dental problems being the most frequent reason to visit a health care provider (Schor, 1998). The American Academy of Pediatrics (AAP) recommends routine medical exams for the school-aged child at least every 2 years, and suggests they occur at ages 5, 6, 8, 10, 11, and 12 years. These exams should include height, weight, vital signs, physical exam, vision and hearing screening, and assessment of dietary intake and use of tobacco/alcohol/ drugs (Schor, 1999). Scoliosis screening is also recommended. In addition, annual TB testing is recommended for any high-risk children.

HEALTH PROMOTION

Immunizations

By the time they enter kindergarten, most children have received all the recommended immunizations. For the school-aged child, booster shots of diphtheria, tetanus, and pertussis (DTP), and measles, mumps, and rubella vaccine (MMR) are recommended between the ages of 4 and 6 years. If the MMR booster is not given at this time, it is given at ages 11 to 12 years, as is the Td (tetanus and diphtheria) booster. Td is then repeated every 10 years as well. Refer to Appendix F for the current Immunization schedule.

Nutrition

The nutritional needs of the school-aged child should remain relatively steady and children should be encouraged to make independent food choices. Eating a healthy breakfast before school is encouraged as a means to provide the essential nutrients needed for academic and physical performance. While at school, it is imperative that nutrition education be a part of the curriculum so the school-aged child will have the knowledge to select the most nutritious and appropriate quantities of food.

Although school-aged children are more independent in making food choices, the influences of culture and caregivers cannot be ignored as eating habits established during childhood may be difficult to alter later in life. Leading a fast-paced life is common for many families today, so nutritious foods like fruits and vegetables must be readily available in order to avoid the temptation to live on fast-foods, which are often high in calories, fat, and sodium, and low in vitamins and minerals. If consumed on a regular basis, fast-foods can lead to obesity, a fact that probably contributes to the increase in obesity in children during the past three decades (Luder & Bonforte, 1996). Childhood obesity is a problem because it is associated with social isolation, lowered self-esteem, impaired potential for athletics, health problems, and long-range proclivity for heart disease, cancer, and diabetes (Covington, 1996). See Family Teaching box for steps in preventing childhood obesity.

Caregivers may be hesitant to limit the dietary intake of their school-aged child because of their concern regarding nutrients needed for physical growth. However, careful meal planning, setting a schedule for snacks and meals, and physical activity are crucial for the physical and emotional health of the school-aged child. Table 7-2 includes the nutritional needs of the school-aged child.

Family Teaching

Steps in Preventing Childhood Obesity

1. Offer a variety of foods that are healthy.

2. Encourage your school-aged child to help with meal preparation.

3. Respect your child's ability to decide how much to eat.

4. Consult your physician if you are concerned about your child's weight.

5. Encourage physical activity and discourage sedentary activities such as watching television.

(Evers, 1997)

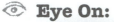

Eye On:

Dietary Differences

The diet of children raised in a traditional Native American household is usually high (35–50%) in fat and carbohydrates. The diet of children raised in traditional Hispanic American households usually consists of beans, salsa, tortillas, and rice with hot spices, and there is a tendency for these children to be heavier than their counterparts. Nurses need to be cognizant of family and ethnic traditions when counseling on nutrition and try to work these traditions into dietary planning.

TABLE 7-2 NUTRITIONAL NEEDS OF THE SCHOOL-AGED CHILD	
Food	**Daily Servings**
Milk (Milk, cheese, yogurt)	2–3
Meat (Lean meat, chicken, fish, beans, eggs, peanut butter)	2
Bread (Bread, cereal, rice, pasta)	6–9
Vegetables	3–4
Fruit	2-3

USDA Dietary Guidelines for Americans (2000)

Elimination

By the time children are old enough to attend school all day, they have learned to control and independently care for their own elimination patterns. Usually stools are well formed and school-aged children have one to two stools per day. The amount of urine passed is dependent on intake, temperature, time of day, and the child's emotional state. It is always a good idea to suggest to school aged-children that they use the bathroom prior to beginning their play or returning to the classroom so their activities are not disrupted.

Hygiene

Children older than 6 or 7 years of age are capable of carrying out their own personal hygiene practices daily, and by the time they are 8 or 9 can be held responsible for independently bathing, grooming, dressing, and properly discarding their soiled clothing. However, many young school-aged children continue to need help cleansing hard to reach places (ears, back, fingernails) and in regulating the bath water temperature. Because many school-aged children are busy with activities, they may not want to take the time to bathe daily. Taking a shower instead of taking a bath may be appealing to many, as it can be less time consuming, yet is still an effective method of maintaining cleanliness. As children become more aware of changes in their bodies as they reach late school age, they begin to take more interest in and are more reliable in their own grooming and cleanliness.

Dental Health

School-aged children should be encouraged to brush at least twice a day and to floss before bedtime, to help prevent cavities. Because of the lack of manual dexterity, it is important to monitor and assist the younger school-aged child with tooth brushing and flossing. Caregivers need to be advised to provide fluoride toothpaste and keep regular dental check-ups in order to ensure healthy teeth. The child's first visits to the dentist can greatly influence future visits, so it is important to seek a pediatric dentist.

During the school-age period, malocclusion or an abnormality of the coming together of the teeth can occur when the permanent upper and lower teeth do not approximate, leaving them crowded or uneven and requiring a referral to an orthodontist. If braces are needed, frequent brushing and flossing are critical in preventing dental caries. An evulsed tooth (tooth that is knocked out) should be picked up, rinsed gently under water, and placed back in its socket. The child should hold the tooth in place. A dentist should be contacted immediately. If the tooth cannot be held in place, it should be put in cold milk or held in the mouth, under child's or caregiver's tongue until seen by a dentist.

Rest and Sleep

By the time children reach school-age, most do not need to nap. Although nighttime sleep habits may vary, at 6 years children require at least 10 hours of sleep, and at 12 years children require 8 to 9 hours of sleep. Sleep is essential during the school-age years to foster physical growth and academic performance, and failure to receive adequate rest can lead to irritability and lack of attention span at school, which may lead to falling asleep and the potential of failing grades.

Nightmares and night terrors are less common during the school-age years. However, it is estimated that somnambulism or sleep walking, occurs in 15% of all school-aged children and is not uncommon between 4 and 8 years of age (Rudolph & Kamei, 1998). The sleepwalking event is usually not remembered in the morning, occurs more frequently in boys, and can be associated with nocturnal enuresis. Most children outgrow sleepwalking by adolescence. Somniloquy or sleep talking can occur at any age across the life span and does not indicate a health concern (Rudolph & Kamei, 1998).

Activity and Play

Piaget (1962) described play during the school-age years as games with rules as the child is able to think more objectively, thus making group activities a possibility. Socially, school-aged children are beginning to understand the concept of cooperation and reflect this in their play as they work together for the good of their team. Strict adherence to rules provides the framework for playing the

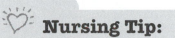

Nursing Tip:

Encouraging play
During play children enact that which they cannot verbalize or physically demonstrate. As nurses, we can incorporate play into health care experiences as a way of helping children express needs and actively cope with experiences. Scribbling, finger painting, coloring, and drawing are useful tension-reducing methods, which are inexpensive and can foster a child's creativity (Ryan-Wenger, 1998).

game and creating a sense of security.

Play also provides the opportunity to learn what the body is physically capable of as gross and fine motor development are stimulated. By the time the school-aged child is 6 years old, the physical strength and stamina for team sports have developed, contributing to physical health and release of frustrations. Children enjoy playing board games, starting collections, participating in, listening to, or playing music.

Physical activity is important in maintaining a healthy lifestyle (Long & Williams, 1998). Although most school-aged children are physically active, a concern remains related to their decreased physical activity and increased sedentary activities (watching television, playing computer games). Physical activity for school-aged children can take many forms and includes hiking, spontaneous sports activities, or being a member of an organized community team. It is important for the child to find something enjoyable. This will foster future participation.

As the child's skeleton and muscle size continue to grow at a gradual rate, the gross motor skills of jumping, running, throwing, and catching continue to be refined. However, muscles and bones are easily injured because of immaturity so athletic activities must be selected according to the child's physical development and not the caregiver's wishes. Careful attention must also be paid to limiting activities that stress the child's physical development and endurance, such a contact sports and long distance running.

As the child seeks cooperative play with rules, team sports become interesting. Team play can contribute to not only physical, but also social development as the youngsters learn to play as team members and work for common goals. Sports should encourage everyone to participate and recognize all team members for their contributions, not just a select few. However, during the school-age years, the child is also exposed to the high value placed on winning and competing, and should learn a healthy balance between playing for the sake of playing and always winning or competing.

Safety and Injury Prevention

The leading cause of death in this age group is accidents, so health care should be focused on accident prevention (Prescott, 1999). Factors contributing to the high incidence of accidents for this group are their increased independence, desire to have peer approval, and increased involvement in physically challenging activities. Most accidents are related to motor vehicles, but firearm injuries continue to increase in incidence (Children's Defense Fund, 2002). During the 1980s, violent crime for children ages 10 to 14 continued to steadily increase and by 1990, 1 of 8 deaths among children ages 10 to 14 years was caused by a firearm (Fingerhut, 1993). One out of every 18 victims of violent crimes and 1 out of 3 victims of sexual assault is under age 12. (Children's Defense Fund, 2002).

Because school-aged children may understand but resist rules in an effort to gain independence and peer approval, safety rules must be clearly defined through education and enforced with discipline. Rules related to motor vehicle, bike, skateboard, and swimming safety, and avoidance of firearms and strangers are critical. The Family Teaching box offers examples of important rules that need to be established and enforced by caregivers, nurses, and teachers.

⚡ **Nursing Alert:**

Children, Pickup Trucks, and Automobiles

- Children riding in the cargo area of pickup trucks are at risk for death or injury if the vehicle is involved in an accident. Caregivers should be reminded not to allow their children to ride in that area.
- Children seated in the front seats of vehicles are at increased risk of death and injury in crashes. This holds especially true in vehicles with passenger-side airbags. Almost all children killed by airbags were either unrestrained or improperly restrained at the time of the crash. Children under 12 years of age should sit in the back seat.
- Seat belts fit correctly when the lap portion of the belt rides low over the hips. The well-fit shoulder belt crosses the sternum and shoulder. Correct seat belt fit is usually not achieved until the child is 9 years old.

ANTICIPATORY GUIDANCE

School and Homework

School is an exciting new world because it provides the arena for physical, intellectual, and social development. Schools do affect the evolving character of the school-aged child and every school has the potential to actively encourage prosocial behavior. The teacher can guide and provide a structured environment where learning can take place, regulate what is being learned, how it is being learned, with whom it is being learned, and in what context the learning occurs.

Teachers serve as role models: they strive to stimulate intellectual development; are in a position to influence the child's attitudes and values; and can be an important factor in determining school success. The child facing extreme difficulties of poverty, abuse, and violence may find safe haven at school and learn to cope with life stressors because of a

Family Teaching

Safety Rules for School-aged Children

Motor vehicle	Always wear a seat belt, sit in backseat, especially in car with airbags.
Bike/skateboard/Rollerblades	Wear helmet, elbow and knee pads.
Pedestrian	Use caution when crossing streets, obey traffic lights.
Trampolines	Use should be discouraged.
Swimming	Learn how to swim, never swim alone.
	Wear a life jacket while in a boat.
	Do not dive in shallow water.
Firearms	Avoid guns, do not assume a gun is not loaded.
Strangers	Do not talk to strangers or accept rides from strangers.
	Learn home address and telephone number.
	Use 911 if needed and know how to call a safe neighbor.
Medicines	Should be kept out of reach; explain consequences of taking the drugs.
Drug use/Smoking	Teach about illicit drugs; counsel on why and how to avoid their use.
Burns	Teach escape route; cook/bake under supervision of adult.

teacher's positive influence. Dedicated teachers must be credited with keeping students' performance at a steady pace when considering the conditions many children and families have faced over the past decades (Children's Defense Fund, 2002).

As social interaction and communication develop between school-aged children, so does their role in facilitating the transmission of knowledge. Vygotsky (1962) suggested that when a child of one stage of development helps another child of the same level of development, both benefit. Nurses can also use cooperative learning as an effective method of teaching the school-aged child in the health care setting.

School-aged children may occassionally have homework assignments, although many teachers try to allow time within the school day to complete assignments. If children do have school work that needs to be completed at home, the AAP (2001) suggests that caregivers:

1. Provide a positive atmosphere where children can work without being distracted. This means no television and an area that is free of clutter.

2. Show interest in the child's work. Check to see that the homework is complete and be prepared to explain the assignment if the child does not understand what the teacher has asked the child to do.

3. Be prepared to help the child in a particular subject that is difficult, or consider using a tutor.

4. Re-evaluate the after-school activities the child is involved in, especially if these activities leave little time to complete the homework assignment.

Peers

During the school-age years, children transition from the central focus of their home and caregivers, to a world of school and peers. As school-aged children become older, gain more independence, and spend more time with peers of the same gender, friendships develop that may influence them for the rest of their life. Peers help each other learn about the world and all its possibilities, influence self-esteem and self-confidence, and are important sounding boards for issues needing to be discussed. Child–child interactions provide opportunities to learn a wide variety of social behaviors and how to cope in situations such as cooperation, competition, aggression, disagreement, and negotiation (Charlesworth, 2000).

Self-Concept

The development of a positive self-concept and self-esteem are critical at this time. Self-concept is influenced by physical appearance, athletic ability, academic achievement, approval from caregivers, and is shaped by comparisons with peers (Overbay & Purath, 1997). Caregivers and peers also play a role in determining self-esteem, a global evaluation of self also known as self-image or self-worth. The closer the perceived self is to the ideal self (how the child would like to be) the higher the child's self-esteem. Acceptance by peers also influences a child's sense of self-worth and healthy body image. Examples of positive self-esteem include the ability to express an opinion, work cooperatively with others, and initiate a conversation. A child with poor self-esteem may feel shame, inadequacy, and the inability to gain respect from others (Schor, 1999).

Body Image

School-aged children are knowledgeable about their bodies and often will compare how they look to how their peers or adults look. Children also are acutely aware of physical differences related to height or weight, and know if they are not as coordinated as their friends. School-aged children who are especially sensitive about these differences may be uncomfortable in a swimming suit or shorts, and not participate in activities where their "differences" may become apparent. If the child has a physical disability, it is not uncommon for other children to call attention to the disabililty, exclude them from activities and, at the same time, worry that they themselves have a similar disability. Children who call attention to physical disabilities in others need to realize such comments may have lasting effects and should be discouraged from making hurtful comments.

Bullying

Developing social skills is one of the primary tasks of the school-age years (Schor, 1998). For children who lack such skills, one of the ways to express their anger is the act of bullying (inflicting verbal or physical harm on another). Usually, boys are more likely to engage in bullying than girls, and reasons given for bullying include to get even; others do it; for fun; because the other child annoys me; to show how tough the child is; because the other child was a wimp; and for money (Rigby, 1998). Reactions to bullying can include sadness, reduced self-esteem, having fewer friends, being less popular or absent from school, as well as complaining of headache, sleep disturbances, and stomachache (Rigby, 1998). Identifying both the victims and perpetrators of bullying behavior and taking action for the safety and well-being of all involved is important. Some of the recent incidences of school violence and shootings were carried out by students who were bullied by peers.

Dealing With Bullying Behavior

Consider the following situation: You are a school nurse in a large urban school. Over the past month, 11-year-old Chad, who is new to your school, has been stopping in your office on a weekly basis with complaints of headache and stomachache. You noticed at this visit that he has a number of bruises on his face. Chad reluctantly responds to your question about the bruises and admits that a group of bullies have been "beating him up" because he would not steal for them. He tells you he is scared to tell his mother, as she can not afford to send him to another school.

1. Determine the approach you should use with Spencer.

2. Discuss ways you could intervene to prevent future harm.

3. Describe how would you address Spencer's concern about notifying of his mother.

4. Would you notify school administrators? If so, how would you do this?

5. Identify school and community resources that could help this family.

feels resources and supports are available it may be viewed as a positive challenge instead of a negative threat. If stress is viewed as a negative threat and beyond their ability to handle, children may exhibit some of the signs listed in Table 7-3 and need assistance in working through the experience.

TABLE 7-3 SIGNS OF STRESS

1. Frequent fatigue
2. Irritability
3. Change in sleep or eating pattern
4. Complaints of headaches or stomachaches
5. Substance abuse
6. Drop in academic performance

Nursing Tip:

Stress reduction strategies
Nurses need to work in partnership with the child and family to determine effective methods of stress reduction. Since school-aged children often enjoy writing, they can be encouraged to write about their experiences in order to cope. Additional stress reducing techniques such as relaxation, guided imagery, or distraction may also help some children.

Stress

The school-aged child in today's world is constantly exposed to stress. Like never before, children are subjected to the effects of a high divorce rate, peer pressure, and use of illicit drugs and alcohol. A situation is considered stressful for a child when there is a discrepancy between demands placed on the child and the child's perceived ability to meet these demands (Menke, 1981). However, what is stressful for one school-aged child may not be stressful for another; if the child

Latchkey Children

Today, in both single- and two-caregiver families, more caregivers are working outside the home. As a result, many children come home after school to an empty house and are home alone for a period of time without adult supervision (latchkey children). The current number of latchkey children in this country is difficult to determine, but it is estmated over 40% of children are left home at some time during the day (American Academy of Child and Adolescent Pyschiatry, 2000). An even greater number of children whose caregivers work are cared for by an older sibling. Because of this lack of adult supervision, latchkey children are at risk for developing physical and social problems, and anxiety (Schor, 1999).

Family Teaching

Tips for Latchkey Children

Nurses must take a proactive role in promoting quality after-school programs in their communities. School nurses can encourage students who go home to an empty house to discuss with their caregivers safe rules to abide by while they are alone. The following tips for latchkey children can be reinforced by the school nurse:

1. Do not open the door to anyone you do not know.

2. Do not tell a telephone caller you are home without a caregiver.

3. Make a list of emergency phone numbers and the phone number for a neighbor who can be trusted. Keep this list in a safe place near the phone.

4. Create an after-school routine such as homework, household chores, or caring for pets.

Reflective Thinking

Caring for a Latchkey Child

1. How would you feel if a 7-year-old boy you are caring for in a health care setting told you that he was left alone for many hours every day without adult supervision?

2. How would you feel about his caregivers and what actions would be appropriate?

Dishonesty

It is not uncommon for school-aged children to steal, cheat, or lie. Although these behaviors may be upsetting for caregivers, they are often just a phase the child goes through, and may be related to immature cognitive development, or on the other hand, indicate a more serious problem. Young children may steal because they want something another person has, feel they were treated unfairly and want revenge, or want to be able to bribe other children. Other children may observe family members take things from one another (money out of a purse, clothes from a drawer) and see nothing wrong in doing the same thing. Children may cheat because they want to win a game they are playing, or do well on an examination. If winning or being the best is important to their caregivers, or if they see caregivers cheat, children are more likely to model that same behavior. Young school-aged children may also lie to cover up misbehavior or avoid being punished, whereas older children lie because they may not meet expectations of teachers or caregivers.

Limit Setting and Discipline

Nurturant caregivers are warm, supportive, and empathetic. By providing clear limits of behavior and positive reinforcement for good behavior, the caregiver is better able to help the child develop self-confidence.

Implicit in discipline approaches is a fundamental attitude toward the child. Taking the child seriously and treating the child as a person whose feelings and questions matter is critical. The child's preference, however, cannot always be accommodated but should be considered and never dismissed. The school-aged child is someone with a distinctive point of view and a unique set of needs. The child needs not only warm and empathetic caregiving but also models of honesty and prosocial behavior (helping, sharing, and caring). Reasoning capabilities of the school-aged child are being developed, so talking about and explaining a negative behavior or act should be encouraged. Withdrawing privileges is often a satisfying method of discipline.

Sexuality

School-aged children may engage in some form of sex play during the late school-age years. This is normal behavior, and it is important to avoid drawing attention to it or making them feel guilty. Unless adults are honest and open about sexual issues, children will seek answers to their questions from peers. All too often the information from peers is inaccurate; therefore, it is imperative to provide education regarding sexuality to children and caregivers. In providing education, it is important to use the appropriate anatomical terms and encourage open discussion.

REFERENCES

American Academy of Child and Adolescent Psychiatry. (2000). *Home alone children* (#46) www.aacap.org/publications/factsfam/homealone.htm (accessed 12/19/02).

American Acadamy of Pediatrics. (2001). *Back to school tips* [On-line]. Available: www.aap.org/advocacy/release/augschool.htm.

Charlesworth, R. (2000). *Understanding child development* (5th ed.). Clifton Park, NY: Delmar.

Children's Defense Fund. (2002). *The state of America's children yearbook.* Washington, DC: Author.

Click, P. (1998). *Caring for school-age children* (2nd ed.). Clifton Park, NY: Delmar.

Coles, R. (1990). *The spiritual life of children.* Boston: Houghton Mifflin.

Covington, C. (1996). Childhood obesity: Too much, too little, too late. *Issues in Comprehensive Pediatric Nursing. 19*(4), iii–v.

Dixon, S., & Stein, M. (2000). *Encounters with children: Pediatric behavior and development.* St. Louis, MO: Mosby.

Erikson, E. (1963). *Childhood and society.* New York: Norton.

Evers, C. (1997). Empower children to develop healthful eating habits. *Journal of the American Dietetic Association 97*(10), S116.

Fingerhut, L. (1993). *Firearm mortality among children, youth, and young adults 1–34 years of age: Trends and current status.* United States Department of Health and Human Services. CDC, No. 231.

Freud, S. (1923). *The ego and the id.* London: Hogarth Press.

Kohlberg, L. (1969). *Stages in development of moral thought and action.* New York: Holt, Rinehart, & Winston.

Long, K., & Williams, D. (1998). Health care for the school age child. In *Annual review of nursing research* (pp. 39–61). New York: Springer.

Luder, E., & Bonforte, R. (1996). Health and nutrition issues during childhood years. *Topics in Clinical Nutrition, 11*(3), 47–55.

Menke, E. (1981). School-aged children's perception of stress in the hospital. *Journal of the Association for the Care of Children's Health, 9*(3), 80–86.

Overbay, J., & Purath, J. (1997). Self-concept and health status in elementary school-age children. *Issues in Comprehensive Pediatric Nursing, 20,* 89–101.

Piaget, J. (1962). *Play, dreams and imitation in childhood.* New York: Norton.

Prescott, B. (1999). Health care of the school age child. *Montana Nurses Association Pulse, 36*(1), 18.

Rigby, K. (1998). Gender and bullying in schools. In P. Slee & K. Rigby (Eds.), *Children's peer relations* (pp. 47–59). London: Routledge.

Rudolph, A., & Kamei, R. (1998). *Rudolph's fundamentals of pediatrics* (2nd ed.). Stamford, CT: Appleton & Lange.

Ryan-Wegner, N. (1998). Children's drawings: An invaluable source of information for nurses. *Journal of Pediatric Health Care, 12*(3), 109–110.

Santrock, J. (1998). *Adolescence* (7th ed.). New York: McGraw-Hill.

Schor, E. (1998). Guiding the family of the school-age child. *Contemporary pediatrics, 15*(3), 75–84.

Schor, E. (Ed.). (1999). *The complete and authoritative guide: Caring for your school-age child.* New York: Bantam Books.

Stedman's Medical Dictionary (27th ed.). (2000). Philadelphia: Lippincott, Williams, & Wilkins.

USDA Dietary Guidelines for Americans. (2000). *Nutrition and your health: Dietary guidelines for americans,* 2000, 5th edition, www.nal.usda.gov/fnic/dga/index.html (accessed 12/19/02)

Vygotsky, L. (1962). *Thought and language.* New York: Wiley.

SUGGESTED READINGS

Colizza, D., & Colvin, S. (1995). Food choices of healthy school-age children. *Journal of School Nursing 11*(4), 17–20.

Cowell, J., Warren, J., & Montgomery, A. (1999). Cardiovascular risk prevalence among diverse school-age children. *Journal of School Nursing, 15*(2), 8–12.

Davidson, L. (1999). School age prostitution: An issue for children's nurses. *Journal of Child Health Care, 3*(2), 5–10.

Finan, S. (1997). Promoting healthy sexuality: Guidelines for the school-age child and adolescent. *The Nurse Practitioner, 22*(11), 62–72.

Ginsburg, H., & Opper, S. (1988). *Piaget's theory of intellectual development.* Englewood Cliffs, NJ: Prentice Hall.

Hoffert, M. (1997). Weaving the fabric of a life: A phenomenological inquiry of solitude experienced by school age children. *Prairie Rose, 66*(1), 4–6.

Jones, F., & Selder, F. (1996). Psychoeducational groups to promote effective coping in school-age children living in violent communities. *Issues in Mental Health, 17,* 559–571.

Kohlberg, L. (1981). *The philosophy of moral development.* San Francisco: Harper & Row.

Leonard, K. (1999). Firearm safety courses for elementary school-age children. *Canadian Journal of Public Health, 90*(1), 35–36.

Lightfoot, J., & Bines, W. (1997). Meeting the health needs of the school-age child. *Health Visitor, 70*(2), 58–61.

Long, K., & Williams, D. (1998). Health care for the school-age child. In *Annual review of nursing research* (pp. 39–61).

New York: Springer.

MacBriar, B., Burgess, M., Kottke, S., & Maddox, K. (1995). Development of a health concerns inventory for school-age children. *Journal of School Health, 11*(3), 25–29.

McClowry, S. (1995). The influence of temperament on development during middle childhood. *Journal of Pediatric Nursing, 10,* 160–165.

Menke, E. (1998). The mental health of homeless school-age children. *Journal of Child and Adolescent Psychiatric Nursing, 11*(3), 87–98.

Neff, E., & Dale, J. (1996). Worries of school-age children. *Journal of the Society of Pediatric Nurses, 1* (1), 27–32.

Rodgers, G. (1996). Bicycle helmet use patterns among children. *Pediatrics, 97,* 166–173.

Schwartz, D., Dodge, K., Pettit, G., & Bates, J. (1997). The early socialization of aggressive victims of bullying. *Child Development, 68*(4), 665–675.

Sharrer, V., & Ryan-Wenger, N. (1995). A longitudinal study of age and gender differences of stressors and coping: Strategies in school-age children. *Journal of Pediatric Health Care, 9,* 123–130.

Wilson, A., & Yorker, B. (1997). Fears of medical events among school-age children with emotional disorder, parents, and health care providers. *Issues in Mental Health Nursing, 18*(1), 57–71.

Wood, L., & Masterson, J. (1999). Use of technology to facilitate language skills in school-age children. *Seminars in Speech and Language, 20*(3), 219–232.

CHAPTER 8

Growth and Development of the Adolescent

Between childhood and adulthood, individuals experience the unique developmental period known as adolescence (ages 12–21), when young people begin to focus on who they are, how they are similar to or different from those around them, and what they want to become when they reach adulthood. It is a time of exploration, excitement and discovery, and sometimes confusion and despair.

Adolescence is second only to infancy in the amount of change individuals encounter physiologically and psychosocially. In order to effectively identify issues and problems commonly seen in adolescence, it is important to consider the physiological, psychosexual, psychosocial, cognitive, and moral transformations occurring during this time, as well as changes in adolescents' rapidly expanding social context, including the family, school, and peers.

Adolescence consists of early, middle, and late periods. Each is distinguished by several different aspects of adolescents' lives and constitute the ages of 12–14, 15–17, and 18–21 years. Another way to differentiate these periods relates to physiological development: prepubertal (early), pubertal (middle), and postpubertal (late adolescence).

PHYSIOLOGICAL DEVELOPMENT

The physiological changes occurring during adolescence are extensive, do not occur in isolation, and have an impact on the adolescent's psychosexual, psychosocial, and cognitive development. These changes also affect the experiences adolescents have with family members, peers, and others in their social world, as well as their own body image and self-esteem.

Musculoskeletal System

During the adolescent growth spurt (AGS), which lasts about 4.5 years (Gallahue & Ozmun, 1995), the body assumes an adult appearance. Girls may begin their spurt as early as 7.5 or as late as 12 years of age, whereas boys typically begin their growth spurt by age 13. During the AGS, there is rapid acceleration in weight and height gain: boys gain 12–14 lb and grow 3–6 inches; girls gain 8–10 lb and grow 2.5–5 inches.

The AGS is not uniform; weight begins to increase first, followed in 4–6 months by a rapid increase in height (Tanner, 1990). The age of onset, intensity, and duration of the AGS varies from individual to individual, and differs for boys and girls.

Typically, height begins increasing in early adolescence for females and in midadolescence for males. Females achieve peak height velocity (PHV), the maximum annual rate of growth in height during the AGS, at about 11 years of age, or 6–12 months before menarche. Very few females grow more than 2 inches after menarche. Males reach PHV at about age 13, after axillary and mature pubic hair appears, and growth of the penis and testes begins (Malina & Bouchard, 1991). Most males do not grow in height after 18 or 20 years of age.

Weight increases for adolescents tend to follow the same growth curve as height. Peak weight velocity (PWV), the period when weight gain is the most rapid, is greater for males than females, and occurs simultaneously with PHV (Malina & Bouchard, 1991). PWV for females occurs about 6 months after PHV. Females frequently are heavier than their male counterparts during the AGS and tend to weigh more than males until about age 14, when their weight gain begins to level off. Weight gain in adolescent males is due primarily to increases in muscle mass and height, whereas in females, it is due primarily to increases in fat and height (Gallahue & Ozmun, 1995). Diet, gastric motility, exercise, socioeconomic status, lifestyle, and hereditary factors affect adolescent weight gain.

Significant changes also occur in skeletal size, muscle mass, skin, and adipose tissue. Full bone length is first reached in the extremities and moves inward. Trunk growth begins with lengthening and widening of the hips, especially in females, then involves broadening of the chest and shoulders, especially in males. Males have greater arm and leg length relative to trunk size and delayed skeletal ossification as compared with females. Supporting muscles grow more slowly than the skeletal system, and large muscles develop faster than small muscles.

The period of greatest muscular development does not occur until a year after the PHV, and in males it continues into late adolescence. Endurance increases for both genders, especially with fitness training. Subcutaneous fat decreases in males and increases in females. In males, fat is deposited more commonly on the trunk, whereas in females, it is deposited over the thighs, buttocks, and breasts.

Sebaceous glands increase in size as they become active for both genders (Murray & Zentner, 2001; Steinberg, 2001). Eccrine and apocrine glands mature as well. The skin becomes darker, and the texture thickens and toughens in males. Females, on the other hand, develop soft, smooth-textured skin, with fine hair growing on the cheeks and upper lip (Katchadourian, 1977).

Genitourinary System

Secretion of neurohormonal releasing factors by the hypothalamus stimulate the anterior pituitary gland to release follicle-stimulating hormone (FSH) and luteinizing hormone (LH). In females, FSH stimulates ovarian follicle growth and estrogen production. Estrogen causes breast changes, including enlargement and darkening of the nipple, growth and development of the reproductive organs (vagina, uterus, ovaries), and growth and darkening of pubic and axillary hair. Estrogen also promotes epiphyseal maturation, which in turn inhibits long bone growth. LH initiates ovulation and formation of the corpus luteum, which then produces progesterone. Progesterone prepares the uterus to accept a fetus and maintain a pregnancy (Katchadourian, 1977).

In males, FSH is responsible for sperm production and maturation of the seminiferous tubules. LH promotes testicular maturation and testosterone production. Testosterone causes the musculoskeletal system changes discussed earlier and promotes growth and development of the male reproductive system. It also stimulates epiphyseal maturation, which then inhibits long bone growth (Katchadourian, 1977).

These reproductive hormones are also responsible for secondary sexual characteristics, that occur during puberty. The age when the changes occur and the rate of progression through the sequence varies.

Nursing Tip:

Breast self-examination
Adolescence is a good time to begin teaching breast self-examination (BSE). It is important to remind the adolescent to perform BSE once per month, 8 days following menses or on a given fixed date each month. BSE should be avoided when breasts are tender due to menstruation or ovulation.

Cross-cultural studies show the onset of these secondary sexual changes varies with environmental conditions, race and ethnicity, geographical location, and nutrition (Eveleth & Tanner, 1990).

This sequence of secondary sexual characteristics has been divided into five stages, called the Tanner stages. For females, the stages describe breast and pubic hair growth. For males, the stages describe growth of the testes, penis, scrotum, and pubic hair.

The first visible sign of female sexual maturation is breast development, which may not be symmetrical. This is followed by growth of pubic hair, which begins on average between 11 and 12 years of age, and is complete by about age 14 (Katchadourian, 1977; Marshall & Tanner, 1969). Breast development and pubic hair growth for females is described in Appendix H.

In females, menarche (first menstrual period) indicates puberty and sexual maturity.

Even though regular menstrual cycles and ovulation typically begin 6–14 months after menarche, adolescent females can become pregnant after their first menstrual period. Menarche occurs about 2 years after breast development starts and after the AGS peaks. The exact time menarche begins, however, varies among populations and is influenced by nutrition, exercise, weight, breast development, health, metabolism, heredity, stress, depressive affect, family relations, and other environmental influences (Brooks-Gunn, 1988; Gallahue & Ozmun, 1995; Graber, Brooks-Gunn, & Warren, 1995; Moffitt, Caspi, Belsky, & Silva, 1992; Warren, Brooks-Gunn, Fox, Lancelot, Newman, & Hamilton, 1991).

For males, puberty and sexual maturity are initially indicated by growth of the penis and testes, spermatogenesis, and seminal emissions. The first ejaculate, however, usually does not contain mature sperm, and occurs about 1 year after the penis begins its adolescent growth. Testicular enlargement begins between 10 and 13 years of age and is usually complete by age 18 (Katchadourian, 1977; Marshall & Tanner, 1970). A description of male external genitalia development and pubic hair growth is found in Appendix H.

Family Teaching

Physiological Development

Teach caregivers and teens that physiological development may vary among individuals, and even though development may be early or late, these are "normal" and temporary situations. However, if females do not begin breast development by age 13 and males do not demonstrate testicular enlargement of 2.5 cm by age 14, referral may be warranted.

Avoid ridiculing and blaming adolescents about their hygiene; they are trying to gain acceptance from peers and control over their changing body at a time in life when self-esteem is fragile.

Teachers need to be aware of different maturity levels of their students and realize late maturers may not feel comfortable showering in front of their early maturing peers. Allow ample opportunity for showering after physical education classes.

Coaches need to be aware of physiological development of their athletes.

Critical Thinking

Physiological Development

How can nurses help adolescents struggling with the physiological changes their body undergoes when they have not received correct information from their parents or peers or when they are slower than their age-mates? How can nurses help parents explain correct physiological development to their teenagers?

During this time, it is not uncommon for one side of the scrotum to grow faster than the other; 60% of males experience transient breast enlargement (gynecomastia), and many after the age of 14 experience nocturnal emissions (loss of seminal fluid during sleep).

Cardiorespiratory System

The heart almost doubles in weight and increases in size by about one half during adolescence (Malina & Bouchard, 1991). Although the heart continues to enlarge until age 17 or 18, the rate of growth is slower in comparison with other body systems and the pumping mechanism is somewhat ineffi-cient. This may be one cause of fatigue and symptoms of inadequate oxygenation that some adolescents complain about (Murray & Zentner, 2001). Systolic blood pressure accelerates during puberty, before achieving adult values by the end of adolescence. Average blood pressure is 100–120/50–70 mm Hg. The pulse drops from childhood rates to average 60–70 beats per minute. Females have a slightly lower systolic blood pressure and a slightly higher pulse and body temperature than males (French, Perry, Leon, & Fulkerson, 1994; Katchadourian, 1977). Red blood cell mass and hemoglobin concentrations increase and the white blood cell count is decreased in both genders dur-ing adolescence. Platelet count and sedimen-tation rates are increased in females, whereas hematocrit levels and blood volume are increased in males (Katchadourian, 1977).

The lungs increase in length and diameter during adolescence, and the respiratory rate averages 16–20 breaths per minute. Males have greater vital capacity, volume, and rate because of their greater shoulder width and chest size. Their lung capacity, however, matures later than in females, probably due to their general later maturation. The slow-ness of respiratory system growth relative to the growth of other body systems may be another cause of the inadequate oxygenation and fatigue sometimes experienced by ado-lescents (Murray & Zentner, 2001).

Neurological System

Brain growth continues during adolescence. The cells that support and nourish the neu-rons proliferate, even though the number of neurons does not increase. Continued growth of the myelin sheath allows faster neural processing (Graber & Peterson, 1991), and is reflected in the adolescent's increasing ability to think abstractly and hypothesize.

Gastrointestinal System

Rapid maturation of the gastrointestinal sys-tem occurs during adolescence, and by the 21st birthday, all 32 teeth have erupted. Gastric acidity and capacity increase (up to 1,500 mL) to accommodate and facilitate digestion of the increased food intake that occurs in response to rapid growth. Adult size, function, and location of the liver is attained, as are adult elimination patterns (Katchadourian, 1977).

A summary of physiological milestones appears in Table 8-1.

PSYCHOSEXUAL DEVELOPMENT

For Freud, the physical changes of puberty reawaken the sexual and aggressive energies felt toward parents during early childhood, but that were repressed during latency or late childhood. To effectively cope, adoles-cents need to redirect these newly reemerg-ing energies from parental relationships to nonfamilial relationships (friendships, love interests) and career endeavors. For this to occur, a separation or detachment from par-ents is necessary, sometimes resulting in con-flict between adolescents and their parents. As adolescents struggle with the inner ten-sion brought on by pubertal change, Freud believed anxiety, heightened distress over how to act out their inner conflict, and a likely demonstration of psychologically regressive or immature behavior occurred.

TABLE 8-1 PHYSIOLOGICAL MILESTONES IN ADOLESCENCE

Stage	Boys	Girls	Both
Early (11–14)	Testes, scrotum, penis growing	Breast development occurs	Appetite increases
	Pubic hair curly, abundant	Menarche	PWV achieved
	Facial hair fine, downy	Ovulation	Immature cardiovascular pumping mechanism
	Axillary hair present	Pubic hair curly, thick, triangular distribution	Muscle mass increases
	PHV 9.4 cm/yr	PHV 8.3 cm/yr	Gangly, awkward
	Gynecomastia	Heavier than males	Fine motor coordination increases
			Permanent teeth present
Middle (15–17)	Adult genitalia	Skeletal growth ends	Increased fine motor coordination
	Mature sperm production	Sexual maturation achieved	Physical endurance increases
	Facial/body hair present	% of body fat decreases	Sweat glands function
	Muscle mass and strength greater than females	Appetite decreases	Increased capacity of cardiovascular system
	Increased appetite	Height gain 6–10.4 cm/yr	Acne
	Gynecomastia decreases		
	Voice changes		
Late (18–21)	Skeletal growth ends		Cardiovascular/respiratory/gastrointestinal/hematopoietic/sexual maturity achieved
			Stable appetite
			Motor activity increases
			Endurance increases
			Dentition complete

Thus, Freud argued, many psychological issues adolescents face are attributable to physiological changes. Most researchers now contend the implications of these physiological changes are much more complex than Freud or the psychosexual perspective originally indicated, and in fact, are more a result of how the individual and others respond to the adolescent's physiological changes than to the changes themselves.

PSYCHOSOCIAL DEVELOPMENT

Two major tasks for adolescents are answering the question "Who am I?" and attempting to understand the unique place they have in their world.

Adolescents' understanding of who they are is based on a global sense of their own identity, the value they place on that identity, and a sense of what they are able to do. How adolescents define themselves depends on several distinct physiological, psychological, and social changes, including (1) their own pubertal development and the biologic changes of their agemates; (2) the shift to formal operational thought, the resulting changes in their interpersonal behavior, and the moral explanations for that behavior; (3) the increasing level of responsibility they assume at home, at school, and in the workplace; (4) the need to begin thinking about their career; and (5) the need to begin considering their religious beliefs and political ideology.

An important part of adolescents' self-understanding is the value they place on their definition of who they are, which involves self-competency and self-worth. Self-competency is adolescents' sense of how well they can function within a particular realm, as for example in scholastic activities, sports, with friends, or in other activities defined as important by adolescents or those around them. In contrast, self-worth indicates the extent to which adolescents perceive themselves as individuals of worth, either as defined by themselves or those

around them. While these two definitions are related, it is possible for young people to feel they are not very competent in many areas, but still believe they have worth; or they may recognize their competence in many areas, but have little sense of personal worth.

According to Erikson (1968), the major crisis of adolescence is establishing an identity based on three primary factors: (1) individual identifications (parents, peers, teachers, folk heroes) as well as group ones ("my group of friends," "our generation," other blacks, other Americans) established during childhood; (2) their ability to master each developmental task (i.e., trust versus mistrust, autonomy versus shame and doubt, etc.) presented to them by society; and (3) the establishment of their own ideology, based on the social, political, and religious attitudes and values they adopt (Conger & Petersen, 1984).

Marcia (1980) recognized that there are different paths young people take to establish their sense of identity, resulting in one of four identity statuses: identity achievement, foreclosure, identity diffusion, and moratorium. Identity achievement indicates individuals experienced a crisis period and achieved a sense of commitment to their resulting decisions. These individuals are generally well-adjusted, stable, and mature. Foreclosed individuals demonstrate a strong sense of commitment, but have not experienced the crisis or exploratory period necessary for arriving at their sense of commitment. These individuals have typically "borrowed" or been given their ideology or career aspirations by their parents or other authority figures, and appear very mature in their belief systems. On further inspection, however, they generally have difficulty explaining why they believe as they do. Identity diffusion refers to individuals who have not experienced an identity crisis or made a commitment to any ideologic or occupational direction. These individuals are immature and tend to follow popular fads or trends. Finally, moratorium status indicates individuals are experiencing an occupational and/or ideological crisis that has not yet been resolved and delays socially expected actions.

An important determinant of adolescents' identity status appears to be the parenting they receive, especially the extent to which parents promote a strong sense of connectedness among family members while providing their adolescents appropriate opportunities for developing a sense of individuality, presenting their own point of view and verbally defining who they are (Grotevant, 1998).

Gender identity refers to the way we think about ourselves as either male or female, and is a culmination of biological makeup, personal, and social expectations and recommendations about how males and females should think and behave.

Erikson (1968) considered gender to be an important part of establishing young people's individual identity. In fact, one explanation for adolescents' more intolerant attitudes about certain cross-sex behaviors is that this more rigid perspective may help adolescents as they attempt to make sense of who they are (Shaffer, 2000). Gilligan, Lyons, and Hanmer (1990) contend that males and females experience different developmental paths and suggest that gender is particularly important in early adolescent girls' sense of identity formation—girls have a greater relationship orientation regarding their interactions with others. During the onset of adolescence, girls become aware that their innate relational orientation is not valued by the male-dominated culture, where a rules-based orientation is dominant. As a result, many girls silence their unique perspective or "different voice," becoming less willing to assert themselves and their opinions. Others (Archer, 1992; Waterman, 1992) have found that males and females are becoming increasingly similar in their patterns of identity formation.

Erikson (1968) contends that once young people have achieved a sense of who they are, they are better able to commit themselves intimately to another person. According to Erikson (1968), the youth who is not sure of his identity "shies away from interpersonal intimacy or throws himself into acts of intimacy which are 'promiscuous'" (p. 135). Such an individual may be involved

Family Teaching

Psychosocial Development

- Provide positive role models.
- Encourage efforts to establish a sense of hope about the world around them and a purpose and determination about themselves.
- Create a secure environment where adolescents can grow.
- Assist adolescents in finding and developing unique strengths.
- Allow adolescents to participate in family decision making while providing guidance and structure regarding the decisions they make about themselves.
- Create a learning and social environment where young people are encouraged to think and solve problems for themselves.
- Provide opportunities to begin exploring various career options.

in intimate relationships, but is likely to settle for highly stereotyped interpersonal relations, resulting in a lack of fulfillment and "a deep sense of isolation."

COGNITIVE DEVELOPMENT

During adolescence (Piaget's stage of formal operations), the most distinct feature of young people's thinking is that they can now consider what is possible rather than just what is real. Thinking is no longer constrained by the concrete, physical world of their existence; rather, they are now capable of considering abstract possibilities. No longer are potential solutions based only on previous experiences; young people are able to consider all possible solutions to a problem, both real and abstract, and they can assess options and determine the best solution. Young people can now consider their own thoughts as real objects to be studied and analyzed—they can think about their own thoughts (Piaget, 1972).

One outcome of adolescents' ability to consider abstract possibilities is that they begin to recognize the distinction between how things are and how things could be (the difference between the "real" and the "ideal"). Out of this ability comes a new sense of idealism and a new set of standards whereby they begin comparing themselves to the world around them.

Another significant cognitive change is language development. Adolescents generally become more sophisticated in their ability to understand words and their related abstract concepts. Because of this increased sophistication, adolescents experience a whole new world regarding the meaning of words, including metaphors and satire. During adolescence, young people also begin to find great joy in the double meaning of puns, satire, and parodies.

Lev Vygotsky, a Soviet cognitive theorist who did not base his work on Piaget's, considered the differences among adolescents' cognitive abilities to be a function of identifiable features of their cognitive environment (Santrock, 2001), and emphasized the way society promotes cognitive growth. For example, Vygotsky believed cognitive development was the result of social relationships with important others (e.g., parents, teachers and peers), rich in cognitively challenging interactions. One of Vygotsky's most important concepts is the zone of proximal development (ZPD)—tasks that are too difficult for individuals to master alone but that can be mastered with the guidance and assistance of adults or more skilled adolescents (Santrock, 2001). The lower limit of this zone is the level of problem solving reached by the adolescent working independently; the upper limit is the level of additional responsibility the adolescent can accept with the assistance of an able instructor. According to Vygotsky, the greatest growth occurs when adolescents are stretched to perform at the upper limit of their ZPD. Cognitive development, therefore, is a function of the social

Family Teaching

Cognitive Development

- Provide opportunities to explore the reasons for different religious and political values, attitudes about sexuality and social responsibility, or explanations about injustices they see.

- Clearly explain values and the reasoning behind them.

- Demonstrate greater willingness to listen to and understand adolescents' evolving opinions.

relationships adolescents experience and the extent to which they are challenged to think at a level beyond their independent capability.

Another important aspect of adolescents' cognitive development is their broadening ability to assume another person's perspective. Based on Piaget's work and the symbolic interaction theory of George Herbert Mead, Selman (1980) proposed an individual's interactions are in large part due to their social perspective taking ability. For Selman, an adolescent interacts or communicates with others according to the social–cognitive understanding they have about who they are in relation to those around them. Maturation and social experience change this over time. During adolescence, cognitive reasoning continues to become more complex, where simultaneous, mutual (third-person) perspective taking becomes possible. This allows young people to think not about what is best for each individual in an interaction, but rather what would be best for the relationship between them. Early adolescents' initial attempts to focus on the relationship between self and others is particularly evident in their best friendships, in which there is a high expectation regarding uniformity in dress, interests, and activities in which individual differences are considered threats to friendship. According to Selman, as this mutual perspective taking ability matures, young people come to recognize that relationship needs can be fulfilled through more than one or two relationships, and individual differences can be an asset rather than a threat.

Formal operational thought enables adolescents to think about their own thoughts, and also permits them to realize other people's thoughts are separate and distinct from their own. According to Elkind (1967), this capacity to consider other people's thoughts is the crux of adolescent egocentrism, when one is unable to appropriately differentiate between oneself and the objects of one's attention. With the onset of formal operational thought, adolescents are now able to consider the thoughts of others. However, their cognitive immaturity presents difficulties in differentiating their own thoughts and others' thoughts. Although adolescents realize others' thoughts are not the same as their own, they have the mistaken notion others know what they are thinking, and assume others are as obsessed with their behavior and appearance as they are themselves, resulting in an even greater sense of self-consciousness.

As a function of this egocentrism, Elkind identified two types of social thinking particularly evident during adolescence—imaginary audience and personal fable. Imaginary audience refers to the adolescents' beliefs of always being on stage. Because adolescents confuse their ability to focus on their own thoughts with others' ability to know what they are thinking, they believe others are just as concerned about their appearance and behavior as they are. This is most evident in concerns about dress or appearance.

Connected to the adolescents' imaginary audience is their belief in their own personal fable, where adolescents have an exaggerated notion of their own uniqueness. Because adolescents frequently believe they are important to so many people (i.e., the imaginary audience), they regard themselves, and particularly their feelings, as special and unique. This personal uniqueness is

> ## Reflective Thinking
>
> ### Personal Fable
>
> Can you recall any friends you had as a teenager who clearly demonstrated a personal fable? Did you have a personal fable? What was it?

expressed in two ways—an extreme sense of isolation, believing no one has ever had to endure the feelings or difficult situations they are experiencing, or they believe they are immortal and thus immune to the bad things that happen to others, including death.

MORAL DEVELOPMENT

Kohlberg's (1976) conventional level of moral reasoning, which has been shown to emerge during adolescence (Rest, Davison, & Robbins, 1978) and to persist as the predominant stage of moral functioning throughout adulthood, focuses on the acceptance by individuals of those norms and rules defined either by their close social network or by the more formal governmental systems of their culture/society (i.e., local, state, or federal laws). This level of moral thinking is occupied by two stages or primary orientations; stage 3, or the "good-boy" morality, where the focus is on maintaining good relationships; and stage 4, or the authority-maintaining morality, where the focus is on upholding the law. Gilligan (Gilligan, 1982; Gilligan, Lyons, & Hanmer, 1990) has argued that Kohlberg's stages of moral development are biased toward the rule-oriented reasoning she contends is more evident among males, and more valued by society. As a result, Gilligan believed adolescent males would more likely reflect judgement-based reasoning of the fourth stage of moral thinking, whereas female adolescents would more likely reflect the relationship-based reasoning of the third stage. Most recent research on this issue, however, has failed to support Gilligan's contentions, generally finding no gender differences, or moderate differences favoring females, when using measures of Kohlberg's stages.

SPIRITUAL DEVELOPMENT

Religious beliefs become more abstract and principled during adolescence, and it is not uncommon for this age group to examine parental religious standards and decide if they will be incorporated into their own lives. Religious and scientific views are often compared as teens decide what is true. More emphasis is placed on internal aspects of religious commitment (what a person believes) rather than on attending church as adolescents become more oriented toward spiritual and ideologic matters and less oriented towards practice, rituals, and strictly observing religious customs (Elkind, 1978). Generally, the importance of participating in organized religion declines during the adolescent years, and the younger the adolescent, the more important religion is to them. Late adolescents tend to reexamine and reevaluate the beliefs and values of childhood, and become more personalized and less bound to the traditional religious practices exposed to when younger (Steinberg, 1989).

HEALTH SCREENING

The Department of Adolescent Health, American Medical Association has developed Guidelines for Adolescent Preventive Services (GAPS) in response to recent changes in adolescent morbidity and mortality (AMA, 1997). These comprehensive recommendations provide a framework for organizing and delivering preventative health services to this age group, and emphasize annual screening visits addressing not only developmental and psychological aspects of health, but also traditional physiological conditions. GAPS recommends that adolescents be screened for eating disorders, sexual activity, alcohol and other drug use including tobacco, abuse, school performance, depression, risk for suicide, diet and physical activity, and injury prevention. The guidelines also recommend that adolescents be tested for TB, cholesterol, and HIV, GC, chlyamydia, syphilis, and HPV if sexually active. Physical assessment of adolescents should be comprehensive, and include height, weight, vision and hearing screening, BP, BMI index, urinalysis, and hematocrit/hemoglobin. Anticipatory guidance for adolescents at these screening visits should include injury and violence prevention and nutritional counseling.

HEALTH PROMOTION

General Nursing Interactions

Any adolescent health promotion effort needs to incorporate the adolescents' perspective of what health means and consider their priorities and concerns relative to health and health care services, as well as the level of their cognitive development. Often, developmental tasks and crises in the physiological, psychosexual, psychosocial, or cognitive domains have an impact on adolescent concerns related to health since the concerns usually have something to do with their own point of view or context.

Many adolescents are reluctant to seek health care because of financial concerns, geographical access, characteristics of the health care provider, or the perceived notion of unavailability of confidential services. Therefore, it is critical that providers be respectful, demonstrate openness, competence, honesty, warmth, compassion, and understanding, and have the ability to communicate effectively with adolescents and their families.

Several guidelines are also important for nurses to remember when interacting with adolescents. First, the environment should be caring—positive relationships are encouraged, individual differences are valued, and strengths and weaknesses acknowledged. Second, treat adolescents with dignity and make it a priority to know them as individuals. Third, assessment with the purpose of improving health, describing health promoting behaviors, and understanding is crucial. Fourth, relationships with families are important to develop and maintain. This means frequent communication between nurses, adolescents, and families and encouraging family participation in many health and other issues.

Effective nurses also need to know and understand age and maturational level, physiological changes have an impact on development, and the specific psychosocial needs and developmental changes expected during adolescence. Interactions should always be individualized, and communications need to convey honesty, general concern, and acceptance. Confidentiality and trust can be important issues for adolescents, which nurses must acknowledge. The physiological, psychosexual, psychosocial, and cognitive changes that normally occur during this period and the many issues and concerns adolescents face today need discussion and explanation. Any program developed for adolescents and/or their caregivers should present information objectively and accurately, and adolescents themselves should be allowed and encouraged to identify and discuss issues and problems they consider important and to provide input into planning.

To work effectively with adolescents, nurses should demonstrate poise, tolerance, warmth, and empathy. They should encourage independence and be aware of hidden adolescent fears or concerns that may be subtly expressed. Nurses also need to be aware of their own biases, which may have an impact on interactions or care delivered. Adolescents should be allowed and encouraged to be responsible for as much of their own personal health care as possible, and helped as needed. Finally, adolescents should be assisted in making appropriate decisions that have an impact on their lives. If they do not know how to make wise decisions and careful choices, nurses should teach them principles of effective decision making and problem solving.

Nursing care should be provided in settings, sometimes away from caregivers, where the self-conscious adolescent feels welcome and comfortable. Allowing sufficient time and privacy for all interactions is essential, so sensitive topics related to physiological growth, sexuality, personal goals, and behaviors (drug abuse, gang membership, promiscuity) can be discussed in an unhurried and nonjudgemental atmosphere. It is not uncommon for successful interactions to resemble conversations between persons with common interests. The interviewer applies developmental principles, so concrete-thinking early adolescents understand answers to their specific questions and older adolescents understand answers to their open-ended and more abstract questions. Confidentiality issues should be discussed early in interactions, since adolescents may confide information to nurses that they prefer their caregivers not know about. It is important to make clear early on, however, that some issues may need to be shared with caregivers, especially when they are younger adolescents still living at home.

Even though adolescence is generally a time of wellness, these young people will seek health care for skin conditions, minor illnesses, school/sports physicals, management of chronic illness, high-risk behaviors, and conditions related to sexuality.

Immunizations

Until recently, immunization or vaccination programs have not focused on improving coverage for adolescents. Since adolescents continue to be adversely affected by preventable diseases such as measles, rubella, hepatitis B, and varicella, it is important to improve the delivery of immunization services to this age group by implementing the recommended childhood immunization schedule (see Appendix F).

Nutrition

Adolescence is a time of rapid growth in muscle mass, weight, and height. These physical changes mean increased nutritional needs, especially calories, proteins, and minerals (calcium, zinc, and iron). Calcium is needed to meet skeletal growth requirements, prevent fractures, and help prevent osteoporosis later in life (Committee on Nutrition, 1999). Zinc is necessary for final body growth and sexual maturation. Iron intake should be increased to meet normally expanding blood volume needs, the increase in lean body mass, and to replace iron lost through menstruation. Iron requirements increase to as much as 2.2 mg/day and are associated with the size and timing of the growth spurt, sexual maturation, and menses (Beard, 2000). Males will need more calories than females, especially if they are involved in athletics. Typically, female requirements are around 2,000 calories per day; males will need from 2,500 to 3,000 calories per day. Protein needs also increase. Recommended allowances for females range from 44–46 grams per day and for males, from 45–59 g/day (Committee on Dietary Allowances, 1989).

Adolescents always seem hungry but often do not eat appropriate, well-balanced meals. Instead, they prefer snack foods that are easy to prepare, faddish, and often full of empty calories. Adolescent food habits are influenced by concerns of their body image, peer pressure, emotional problems, their busy schedules, or unsupervised meal preparation/purchase. It is also not unusual for teenagers to skip meals (breakfast most commonly), eat fast foods, or snack frequently. Therefore, nurses can help caregivers and adolescents improve their nutrition by explaining the importance of a good diet and encouraging adolescents to be involved in meal planning. Caregivers also need to realize that the adolescents' need for freedom, independence, and peer acceptance may be reflected in their eating habits. If nutritious foods and snacks are available (milk, cheese, yogurt, fruits, vegetables, juices), adolescents are regularly allowed to be responsible for preparing family meals, and food preferences (hamburgers, pizza, burritos) are integrated into meal plans, conflicts about nutritional concerns may decrease. Adolescents and their caregivers also need to be aware of the recommended dietary allowances, and know which foods are high in calcium (milk and milk products), iron (green vegetables, meats), and zinc (milk, meat, fish, eggs). Adolescents should also receive information about nutritious snacks and fast foods available in restaurants (salads, pasta, grilled meats, vegetables, fruits).

All health screening visits for adolescents need to include height and weight measurements as well as questions about eating habits, including dieting, changes in weight, meal patterns, and consumption of empty-calorie, high-fat, high-salt foods. Nutritional evaluations should also include information about family cultural preferences related to food, whether psychological or psychosocial problems affect eating, and whether nutritional requirements are understood or being met.

Elimination

The elimination patterns for adolescents are similar to adults. They should void an average of 700 to 1400 mL per day and have a stool every day or so. Constipation in adolescents may be due to a physiologic disorder, eating disorder (anorexia nervosa), or improper nutritional patterns.

Hygiene

Adolescents are able to be responsible for their own hygiene. In fact, because they tend to be quite conscientious about their appearance and hygiene, they often wash their hair every day and may bathe or shower more than once a day. Skin care is especially important during this age because of the increased activity of the sebaceous glands, which contributes to acne. Increased sweat gland activity requires careful cleansing as well as the use of deodorant and body powders. For females, menstrual hygiene is especially important and may require extra attention. It is important to remind parents and other adults as well as the adolescent that these physical changes that may require more attention to hygiene are normal.

Dental Health

During adolescence dental visits occur twice a year, good oral hygiene habits have been established, the majority of orthodontic work has begun, and most permanent teeth have erupted. Third molars, however, may erupt in later adolescence (Grover, 1996) or may become impacted, requiring surgical removal. Although the incidence of dental caries decreases during this time, fluoride supplements (or the need for fluoridated water) should continue until age 16 (Committee on Nutrition, 1995).

During adolescence, malocclusion, gingivitis, and dental trauma may occur. Malocclusion occurs due to dental crowding or mandibular/facial bone growth changes. Usually, braces are needed to redirect facial/mandibular growth and correct tooth positioning. Gingivitis, the inflammation and consequent breakdown of the gingival epithelium, may be seen during adolescence because of ineffective cleaning, high sugar/simple carbohydrate diets, or increased hormonal activity. The gums may bleed easily and appear swollen and pale. Treatment involves brushing the teeth at least twice a day using a soft-bristled brush and fluoride toothpaste, flossing daily, eating a well-balanced diet, and regular dental visits (American Dental Association, 1998).

Rest and Sleep

Adolescents need approximately 8 hours of sleep per night. Because of their busy schedules (social activities, obligations at school, employment commitments) and rapid physical growth, adolescents often do not receive enough sleep. Many appear fatigued, their schoolwork may suffer, and parents may complain that their teens rarely have time to help around the house. Nurses need to educate both parents and adolescents on the importance of adequate rest and sleep and

encourage teens to have realistic activity schedules that do not overextend their time. An adolescent's excessive anxiety and fatigue may also result in sleep disturbances, which can continue into adulthood since adult sleep cycles and habits are formed during adolescence.

Activity and Play

Many adolescents are not as physically active as they should be, even though they are very busy. Others exercise regularly and develop physically fit bodies. Often, fitness behaviors adopted during adolescence are predictors of fitness habits later in life (Green, 1994). Adolescents need daily exercise to provide an outlet for tension and anxiety and to maintain muscle tone and development. Regular exercise will also promote healthy sleep patterns and enhance emotional development. Physical activity and fitness may also reduce cardiovascular disease risk factors such as hyperlipidemia, hypertension, and obesity.

The Physical Activity Guidelines for Adolescents (1994) suggest that adolescents should be involved in moderate to vigorous physical activity three or more times a week for at least 30 minutes per session, and be active daily, or nearly every day. *Healthy People 2010* (U.S. Department of Health and Human Services, 2000) goals for adolescents validate these recommendations by encouraging adolescents to increase vigorous activity to at least 20 minutes or more a day for 3 days a week in at least 75% of children and adolescents. However, strength training in adolescence can occasionally lead to significant musculoskeletal injury, such as ruptured intervertebral disks, epiphyseal fractures, and low back bony disruptions (AAP Committee on Sports Medicine, 1990). Injuries can be lessened or prevented if the program followed is based on the physical maturity of the individual. The AAP Committee on Sports Medicine (1990) recommends that if adolescent athletes have reached Tanner stage 5 development, they will have experienced their period of maximal height velocity and be less vulnerable to injury.

Family Teaching

Activity

- Initiate exercise programs that are enjoyable, realistic, and consider physical limitations and capabilities. 30 to 60 minutes per day three to four times per week will enhance fitness and set the stage for a lifetime of health. However, sports involving physical contact are not recommended until after PHV.

- Seek out physical education courses at times and places conducive to adolescent participation

- Evaluate physical development regarding PHV before allowing participation in contact sports.

Family Teaching

Health Promotion

- Adopt a flexible approach to meals.
- Provide healthy snacks.
- Set realistic sleeping schedules that provide an average of 8 hours of sleep per night.
- Participate in sports according to size rather than according to chronologic age.
- Encourage schools to offer nutritious options that appeal to adolescents.
- Search for a variety of activities (tennis, basketball, baseball, softball, hockey, skateboarding, etc.).

Adolescents should be cautioned about involvement in contact sports and encouraged to participate in sports according to their size rather than according to their chronologic age. Weight-lifting is especially dangerous if the body is not physiologically ready. Sports injuries to late maturing boys are more likely to occur if they participate in contact sports with early maturing, muscular agemates. It is better to direct adolescents into activities in which they will succeed rather than those at which they will experience physical and psychological failure. Tennis, swimming, and horsemanship may be some suggestions for alternative, more appropriate activities for adolescents who develop more slowly.

Even though being involved in sports is advantageous for adolescents and participation is increasing, injuries account for substantial cost and morbidity (Cheng, Fields, Brenner, Wright, Lomax, & Scheidt, 2000). Most injuries involve falls or being struck by or against objects. Injury rates are higher for males than females, and even noncontact sports (soccer, basketball, baseball, bicycling) may result in head injuries and collisions with other persons (Cheng, et al., 2000).

Nurses can help adolescents increase their physical activity as appropriate to meet the physical activity guidelines for adolescents and avoid injury by considering the adolescent's physical development and capabilities. Therefore, it is important to inquire about an adolescent's activity program, including frequency, vigor, and preferences, before making any recommendations, as well as to determine Tanner staging. Adolescents can also be encouraged to develop interests in sports, recreation, active play, or exercise at home, school, or in the community.

Safety and Injury Prevention

Unintentional injury is the leading cause of death in adolescents. Nearly half the deaths occurring to individuals between ages 16 and 19 are caused by motor vehicle accidents, and these are more common with teenage drivers who use marijuana, alcohol, or other drugs (Clemen-Stone, McGuire, & Eigsti, 2002; Escobedo, Chorba, & Waxweiler, 1995). Automobiles, motorcycles, motor scooters, mopeds, snowmobiles, minibikes, and all-terrain vehicles cause many adolescent skeletal, head, and spinal cord injuries and abrasions and burns. Approximately 14% of teens report they rarely or never wear seat belts; of those who ride motorcycles, 37.2% rarely or never wear helmets; 84.7% rarely or never wear helmets when riding their bicycles (CDC, 2002). Adolescents are also more at risk for sports-related injuries and accidents. Therefore, accident prevention and safety promotion programs are extremely important for the adolescent. Nurses can initiate such programs or become involved in them through clinics, schools, or community agencies serving adolescents. In addition, nurses need to educate adolescents and their caregivers about safety issues and accident prevention (seat belts, helmets while riding bicycles, motorcycles, skateboards, and the use of protective equipment while participating in baseball, football, and soccer), and remind them they are not immortal or immune from being injured (personal fable) if they take unnecessary chances.

ANTICIPATORY GUIDANCE

Body Image

Body image encompasses positive or negative feelings, and the self-perception of physical attractiveness. Implicit in the definition is the assumption that one's body image varies with maturation, and changes across time, situations, and experiences one has with others. Constant changes in appearance—including increases in weight and height, appearance of body hair, oversized hands and feet, developing sex organs, and facial blemishes—present the adolescent with new challenges, both real and imagined, that affect their body image.

This is particularly significant because the adjustment required by rapid physiological changes affect self-esteem; few adolescents are satisfied with their physical appearance (Guinn, Semper, Jorgensen, & Skaggs, 1997). Adolescent females tend to be more dissatisfied with their appearance and more likely to be concerned about particular parts of their

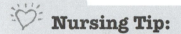

Nursing Tip:

Concerns about body image
Nurses need to be aware of the importance physical appearance has to adolescents, and offer reassurance and encouragement to late maturing adolescents that they will catch up with their counterparts. Suggestions for becoming involved in activities they may enjoy or do well in can help maintain self-esteem and perhaps make up for slower physiologic development or unhappiness with body type, height, or weight. Early maturing adolescents can be directed to activities in which they will succeed and encouraged to be understanding of their later maturing peers who are not as capable. Parents need to understand the importance of body image to adolescents and refrain from commenting negatively about weight and general appearance. If comments are necessary, they should be couched with tact, understanding, and nurturance.

bodies than their male counterparts (Berger, 1994; Blyth, Simmons, & Zakin, 1985; Rozin & Gross, 1987). Often, they perceive themselves as weighing more than they actually do (Feldman, Feldman, & Goodman, 1988). This distortion of body image is not only a potentially significant emotional problem for adolescents, but also may motivate the adolescent female to engage in potentially dangerous and life-threatening weight-reducing behaviors such as anorexia, bulimia, vigorous aerobic exercise, or special diets (Whitaker, Davies, Shaffer, Abrams, Walsh, & Kalikow, 1989).

While developing a sense of body image, most adolescents look to the cultural ideal valued by their society. In Western culture, this traditionally has been the shapely, thin woman and the muscular, tall man. However, few adolescents can successfully measure up to these standards. More than vanity, the adolescent's preoccupation with appearance is a recognition of the role physical attractiveness plays in gaining the attention and admiration of the opposite sex. The fact that physique is valued by both genders is understandable. There is a strong relationship between how adolescents feel about themselves and how they feel about their bodies. Looking "awful" or believing others view them as looking "awful" is the same as being "awful."

Many factors influence body image, including present and past experiences, level of cognitive development, and identity formation. Other factors are one's degree of attractiveness, size and physique appropriate to gender (including weight and body type), name/nickname, cultural ideals and values, degree of identification with same-sexed parent, peer and sibling relationships, level of aspiration, and ability to reach societal or individual ideals (Berger, 1994; Duke-Duncan, 1991; Murray & Zentner, 2001; Sprinthall & Collins, 1995; Wright & Whitehead, 1987). The rate and timing of maturation can also be an important factor in an adolescent's self-image. The young people who have the most difficult time adjusting to their physical development and body image are those whose body is on a different schedule from their peers. For example, late maturing adolescents may feel a sense of failure about their body if they are not as fully developed as their friends, which affects self-esteem and causes them to feel uncomfortable and insecure. Since, on average, early maturing males and females are shorter than their later maturing counterparts, they too may have difficulties with body image as their later maturing peers catch up and overtake them in height.

Social experiences are different for early and late maturing males and females. For boys, early maturation (appearance of secondary sexual characteristics during early adolescence) is associated with favorable social adjustment, whereas for females the picture is more complex. Some findings suggest that early maturation is associated with high social status and prestige in the peer group, whereas other findings indicate greater vulnerability to social pressures, leading to problems in social adjustment (Magnussen, Stattin, & Allen, 1988).

Early maturing females on the other hand, may be socially disadvantaged because they are out of step with their peer group. They may become lonely and experience pressure to become involved in sexual relationships beyond the level of their maturity and coping ability (Simmons & Blyth, 1987). This can result in damaged self-esteem or unwanted sexual activities. Early maturing females are also less satisfied with their weight and less positive about their bodies than late maturers (Koff & Rierdan, 1991). Often, they violate norms more frequently than their late maturing peers (Magnussen, Stattin, & Allen, 1988; Silbereisen & Kracke, 1993). They are also at heightened risk for engaging in delinquent behavior (Caspi & Moffitt, 1991; Simmons & Blyth, 1987) and are more vulnerable to eating disorders, depression, and deviant peer pressures (Brooks-Gunn & Paikoff, 1993; Ge, Conger, & Elder, 1996; Stattin & Magnussen, 1990) as compared with their late maturing or on-time peers.

About 20% of late maturing adolescents feel a sense of failure about their body because their development lags behind that of their friends. This also influences self-esteem and causes them to feel shy, uncomfortable, and insecure. Later maturing males tend to be less relaxed, poised, and popular with peers; feel more restless and talkative and feel socially inadequate and inferior. Later maturing females on the other hand, are higher on scales of activity, sociability, leadership, prestige, popularity, and expressivity during their early adolescence (Sprinthall & Collins, 1995). They also are twice as likely as early maturing girls to continue their education beyond the compulsory number of years of high school (Steinberg, 2001).

Nutritional Issues

Obesity is one of the most serious health problems facing today's adolescents. At least 11% of U.S. children and adolescents are obese, and as many as 22% are overweight (Strauss & Knight, 1999). In some ethnic groups these numbers may even be higher (Hill & Trowbridge, 1998). The rate is increasing (Birch & Fisher, 1998), and adolescents of obese parents are at greater risk of being obese than adolescents whose parents are thin.

Adolescents today are more sedentary as compared with a generation ago. One reason for this decline in physical activity may be that mandatory physical education classes are decreasing in schools, and television, computer games and use, and video games are popular with young people (Berkey, Rockett, Field, Gillman, Frazier, Camargo, & Colditz, 2000).

Second, today's diets (high in fat, low in fruits and vegetables and complex carbohydrates) promote obesity. High-fat foods tend to be palatable, less satiating, higher in total energy, and of smaller volume, leading to overconsumption (Berkey et al., 2000; Birch & Fisher, 1998; Troiano & Flegal, 1998). In addition, fruits, vegetables, and complex carbohydrates may not be popular with children and adolescents.

Finally, factors related to the home environment—parental obesity (more often maternal than paternal), low family income, lower levels of cognitive stimulation in the home, and parental occupation—promote obesity in adolescents. Parental obesity is an important risk factor because of parent modeling and genetics. Low family income may be related to obesity because of less healthy eating patterns, decreased activity, and an environment that provides high-fat foods and few fruits and vegetables (Kennedy & Powell, 1997). Lower levels of cognitive development may be related to obesity.

Adolescents in stimulating and interactive home environments may engage in fewer sedentary activities and more regular physical activity. Parental occupation is a factor if a parent's education is not used in the occupation or if the occupation is nonprofessional. All these factors are important independently of other socioeconomic factors, including race and caregiver marital status or education (Strauss & Knight, 1999).

Obesity in adolescence may also be connected to not being able or wanting to master the psychosocial and psychosexual tasks of adolescence. Overeating compensates as a regression tactic for self-satisfaction or as a coping mechanism for stress. The resulting obesity becomes yet another obstacle to overcome in achieving developmental milestones. Obesity can ward off the pressures associated with puberty and societal expectations and, as long as an adolescent is obese, can repress emotional maturation. For some, obesity can be the reason for their disappointments and eating a method of coping that keeps them connected to their family. This dependence on food/family also interferes with the developmental tasks of separation and individuation. In addition, obesity can interfere with sexuality issues; excess weight protects the adolescent from unwanted sexual advances or attention. Obesity may also represent a way to bring embarrassment and shame to others (caregiver, family), a way of becoming larger than a person not liked (peer), or aggression directed at the self. It is not unusual for obese adolescents to dislike their own physical appearance, express admiration for thin people, and judge others in terms of their own weight. Psychological counseling as well as nutritional and activity counseling may help adolescents develop more mature methods of coping if their obesity is connected to psychosocial or psychosexual issues.

The obese adolescent's sense of identity can also be affected by derogatory comments made by others, leading to guilt, shame, and consequent overeating, which results in more weight gain, more derogatory comments, and even more poor self-esteem. Box 8-1 provides suggestions on ways to help overweight/obese adolescents lose weight.

Box 8-1 Helping adolescents with their weight

Instruct obese adolescents to:

1. Avoid purchasing empty-calorie foods; remove empty-calorie snack foods from home.
2. Ask self before eating, "Am I hungry?"
3. Make dining pleasurable.
4. Eat only at mealtimes and at the table; avoid empty-calorie snacks, reduce dietary intake by at least 500 calories daily to lose 1 lb a week.
5. Serve individual portions on smaller plates; avoid second helpings.
6. Eat slowly by cutting food into small mouthfuls and putting eating utensils down between bites.
7. Keep a food diary; examine for empty calories and to see if you are eating traditional food groups.
8. Participate in regular exercise (walking, bicycle riding, swimming, etc.).
9. Maintain attractive appearance and proper posture.
10. Avoid using food as a reward.
11. Praise and feel proud of small weight losses.

Mechanical methods of weight loss frequently advertised in popular magazines are another option that can be used alone or in combination with diet and exercise programs. These methods include steam baths, sauna suits, spot reducers, and special exercise outfits. However, they offer only short-term weight loss. Use of appetite-suppressant drugs, a final treatment option, are typically reserved for adolescents who are severely obese. This option should be managed by a physician or nurse practitioner. On a final note, it is uncommon for weight-reduction plans to be successful with adolescents, even though many are used. A more realistic alternative goal for those who have difficulty losing weight and keeping if off may be just to not gain any additional weight.

Two other issues related to nutrition in adolescence are anorexia nervosa and bulimia nervosa. Although related, they may have different causes and long-term complications. Both, more commonly seen in females (Green, 1994), are characterized by having a distorted self-image and are psychological illnesses with accompanying physical symptoms. People with anorexia severely limit their food intake; those with bulimia have repeated episodes of binge eating followed by the use of laxatives or vomiting. The diagnosis of either should be considered when the adolescent appears underweight, has not achieved normal reproductive milestones for gender, follows a poor diet, or has not achieved anticipated height (Rees, 1996; Sifuentes, 2000). It is important to refer these clients to professionals who specialize in treating eating disorders.

Attachment and Autonomy

As young people approach adulthood, they want more autonomy and need to have a sense of self-direction and independence. Caregivers, however, are often unsure of how to provide their children with opportunities for establishing autonomy. They may even feel threatened by their child's desire for more independence, therefore responding by exerting ever greater control.

The interesting dilemma for adolescents is that although they are attempting to establish a sense of autonomy and, as a result often act as if they would rather die than be seen with their parents, the unsureness of this period makes the safety found in the caregiver–child relationship no less important. The task for caregivers is to recognize the normalcy of their adolescents' needs to push away and begin to explore the world around them, while at the same time recognizing their need to know there is a secure base to return to if their world becomes too unfamiliar or frightening. Indeed, adolescents' attachment to caregivers is important and has been linked to characteristics such as self-esteem and emotional adjustment (Armsden & Greenberg, 1987; Paterson, Pryor, & Field, 1994; Raja, McGee, & Stanton, 1992).

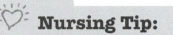

Nursing Tip:

Caregiver–adolescent conflict
Adolescents' attempts for greater autonomy can often result in an escalation in the amount of conflict they have with their caregivers. Discuss with caregivers why adolescents may disagree with rules and expectations. Suggest that caregivers "choose their battles" with adolescents. That is, keeping a bedroom neat and clean may not need to be as important as who their adolescent chooses as peers or what time they need to be home at night. Sometimes allowing adolescents to "win" may be all it takes for them to realize they are "in control" over some parts of their life.

Caregiver–Adolescent Conflict

As a result of their desire for greater autonomy, and their increased level of reasoning and the associated questioning, adolescents are likely to experience conflict in their relationships with their caregivers. Most arguments are the "normal, everyday, mundane family matters such as school work, social life and friends, home chores, disobedience, disagreements with siblings, and personal hygiene" (Montemayor, 1983, p. 91). Rarely do they argue about the hot topics that are typically identified with adolescence, such as sex, drugs, religion, or politics. This is surprising considering the differences in adult and youth attitudes about these topics. Caregivers may indirectly attempt to influence their children's behavior regarding these "hotter" issues through rules and interactions over the more mundane matters families are willing to discuss. For example, caregivers may be uncomfortable discussing their attitudes and beliefs about adolescent sexuality, but will evidence those beliefs through the rules they establish about acceptable clothing, curfews, and dating. Montemayor also found most caregiver–adolescent interactions were peaceful and free of stress. More recently, Barber (1994) found that Caucasian, African-American, and Hispanic caregivers and adolescents all disagree about similar issues (e.g., chores and dress). While there were similar proportions of each group reporting chronic (i.e., daily) conflict, substantially lower levels of conflict were reported by both minority groups as compared to Caucasian families. Barber speculated that this may be a function of Caucasians' greater use of an authoritative parenting style, which encourages adolescents to have a greater say in issues relevant to themselves.

Sibling Relations

Siblings provide a unique relationship for adolescents because they are generally close in age and are likely to spend a great deal of time with one another. Interestingly, their relationship is one in which there is no choice about membership. Thus, while conflict in friendships may be avoided, sibling relationships have more warmth and conflict since they do not operate under the same threat of termination (Brody, Stoneman, & McCoy, 1994; Furman & Buhrmester, 1992).

Siblings can have an impact on one another for both good or ill. For example, older adolescents' involvement in illicit drugs and alcohol (Brook, Whiteman, Gordon, & Brenden, 1986; Clayton & Lacy, 1982; Rowe & Gulley, 1992), as well as deviant and sexual behavior (Rowe & Britt, 1991; Rogers & Rowe, 1990), are predictive of their younger siblings' involvement in similar behavior. In contrast, siblings also provide a buffering effect against challenging experiences such as parental divorce (Kempton, Armistead, Wierson, & Forehand, 1991) or poor peer relationships (East & Rook, 1992).

As youths approach adolescence, several changes occur in their relationships with their siblings. Furman and Buhrmester (1992) found that progression through adolescence was associated with a reduction in perceived sibling support and a corresponding increase in perceived sibling conflict, which apexed between the ages of 12 and 13 years old, followed by an increase in support and a decrease in conflict when youths reached the age of 15 or 16 years old.

For adolescents who are "only" children—about 20% of all adolescents in the United States—there appears to be little research indicating they are at a loss because of the absence of a brother or sister. Only children have been found to have a fairly high sense of self-esteem and achievement motivation as compared with those with siblings (Falbo, 1992). This may be a result of their increased level of interaction with parents and other adults.

Schools

Schools and academic achievement are important in shaping the developing adolescents' sense of autonomy and identity. This is because almost 90% of adolescents attend public secondary school (grades 9 to 12), and spend an average of 180 days per year in school. In fact, during most of the year, typical adolescents spend more than one-third of their waking hours every week in school or school-related activities. In addition, adolescents remain in school for more years now than they did in the past (Sprinthall &

Collins, 1995; Steinberg, 2001). This is due to not having to drop out to support their families. Academic achievement during adolescence is important because it often reflects not only how well the individual accomplishes long- and short-term goals, but also the feelings of success one has in one's own as well as society's eyes. To be effective, schools and curricula for adolescents should be based on principles of learning and development and provide a climate that encourages exploring future directions and goals.

Schools can have a positive or negative effect on adolescents. Often, a student's experience varies according to parent and family context, peer group, size of the school, extracurricular activities, and academic track. Berndt and Keefe (1995) also found an adolescent's adjustment to school was influenced not only by the behavior of their friends, but also by the characteristics of the friendship. Students whose friends described themselves as disruptive in the fall of the academic year described themselves as increasing their disruptive behavior during the year. Students whose friendships had positive features increased their involvement in activities during the year; students whose friendships had more negative features were less involved in activities and became more disruptive as the year progressed.

For some adolescents, school is a stabilizing, friendly force in their lives. It can encourage cognitive development, establish a climate for social interaction, and provide an environment that encourages task completion. School also allows adolescents to have contact with peers and teachers, test new ideas, and validate their thoughts. Activities and opportunities at school can provide safe, acceptable outlets for their energy and foster development. Groups such as the honor society, musical and dance groups, student council, athletic teams, school yearbook and newspaper staff, debate teams, special interest clubs, pep squads, cheerleading, and ethnic-identity groups give adolescents a chance to participate in activities with young people who have similar interests, provide experiences in organizations working toward common goals, and allow development of cohesiveness and group loyalty. Schools also can help break barriers related to ethnicity, social class, race, and gender.

School is more likely to have a positive effect on adolescents if they have close friends before, during, and after the transition to secondary school. Academically talented and economically advantaged students also tend to have a more positive experience as compared with their less-affluent or less capable counterparts. These adolescents are more likely to hold positions of leadership, experience classes that are challenging and enjoyable, and have teachers who pay more attention to them (Steinberg, 2001).

For other adolescents, however, school can be a source of stress, where threats to safety and self-esteem and constant change occur (Freiberg, 1992). Some adolescents may experience depression, decreases in perceptions of their athletic and academic abilities or actual academic and athletic performance, or dissatisfaction with school (Sprinthall & Collins, 1995). Moving from an elementary school, where they were the oldest and tallest to a middle school or high school where they are now the youngest and shortest may also cause stress. This "top-dog" phenomenon, where they move from the top position in elementary school to the lowest position in middle school can be difficult and may result in less commitment and satisfaction with school as well as liking their teachers less than they did in earlier years. There are also shifts from the personal to the impersonal; from smaller to larger classes and buildings; from the same class with the same peers and teachers to different classes, different peers, and different teachers; from simple to complex classroom organization; and from slower paced to faster paced curricula.

In addition, adolescents are dealing with physiological, psychosocial, and cognitive changes that affect their adjustment; junior and senior high schools often have a more open, frightening, combative, and academically taxing environment than elementary school. Teachers provide fewer opportunities for decision making and choices, student–teacher relationships tend to be less positive

Reflective Thinking

School Experiences

What do you remember about the high school you attended? Was the experience primarily negative or positive? Why? What suggestions would you give an adolescent concerned about school experiences?

and personal than in elementary school (Sprinthall & Collins, 1995), and control and discipline are emphasized. Learning activities may often emphasize individual achievement and competition rather than learning for learning's sake. As a result, students may be alienated from the subject matter since these experiences and approaches are not well matched to their developmental needs of greater autonomy and independence.

It is difficult to generalize about the role school plays in adolescent development, however, since different adolescents have different experiences within the same school. Many schools do not promote psychosocial development and have higher dropout rates because of their focus on obedience and conformity and their lack of encouragement for self-reliance, creativity, and independence. However, there are also many good schools that emphasize these qualities and intellectual activities, have classrooms where students actively participate in their own learning, employ committed and autonomous teachers who continually evaluate their programs, and invite parent involvement. They also encourage adolescents to learn about themselves, their relationships with others, the academic material, and society so the students are better able to experience the challenges of adulthood.

Nurses can work closely with parents and school officials to provide accurate, objective information related to health-promotion activities and issues adolescents are concerned about and see as important. School-based health centers (SBHCs) afford unique opportunities for nurses to provide accurate information and nonjudgmental counseling about adolescent issues. Located in or adjacent to schools, these centers provide physical examinations; health education programs; screenings; counseling related to substance abuse, mental health, and sexuality; dental care; and treatment of minor injuries (Anglin, Naylor, & Kaplan, 1996). Often set up to serve poor young people, who are less likely to receive health care than more affluent students, these local centers are in a position to address important adolescent health issues, such as confidentiality, underused services, and preventable diseases (Steinberg, 2001). Adolescents who use SBHCs are more likely to use them for mental health, medical, and substance abuse counseling (Anglin, Naylor, & Kaplan, 1996).

Part-Time Employment

Adolescents' direct experience with the workplace through part-time employment and their preparation for entering the adult workplace through their exploration of potential career opportunities are important. Greenberger and Steinberg (1986) have identified three important issues to consider: the amount of time adolescents work, the type of work in which they are likely to be involved, and the implication of the work experience on adolescents' lives.

First, nearly two-thirds of all 16-year-olds in the United States will have some kind of part-time work while attending school. Although there is a general conception that adolescents today are lazier than they were a few generations ago, it is interesting to note that adolescents today are twice as likely to have some kind of part-time employment as compared with adolescents in 1960, when only one-third of all adolescents worked part-time while attending school.

Secondly, approximately half of all adolescent work opportunities fall into one of two areas; fast food and retail sales. Greenberger and Steinberg (1986) expressed concern over the number of useful skills adolescents are likely to develop as a function of their work experience. In the past young people were likely to receive training to prepare them

for the jobs they would take on as adults; however, most of the work available to adolescents today is dull and repetitive. Because adolescents were found to spend only about 5 minutes per hour using skills they were likely to have learned in school, little opportunity is offered for gaining skills with long-term benefits. A second possible benefit of adolescents' part-time work experience is their potential exposure to the adult workplace and the opportunity to better prepare for full-time entry into the adult world. Again, Greenberger and Steinberg (1986) found that most adolescents worked in age-segregated workplaces, where teens are generally supervised by other teens, and have little opportunity for adult contact or to learn how to interact more effectively in the adult world. The authors concluded the workplace was just as likely as schools to segregate adolescents from adults and the adult world.

A final important issue addressed by Greenberger and Steinberg and others (Mortimer, Finch, Ryu, Shanahan, & Call, 1996; Steinberg & Dornbusch, 1991) has to do with the potential risks and benefits to adolescents' development that may result from part-time work experiences. While a number of benefits do appear to be related to adolescents working (e.g., learning about the business world, learning how to manage money, a greater sense of control over one's own life, and the opportunity to develop a sense of pride in one's abilities and accomplishments), these benefits are most evident among adolescents who work a limited number of hours per week and when adolescents see their work experiences as stimulating and good preparation for later life (Mortimer, et al., 1996). However, when adolescents work more hours per week or are employed in jobs that seem to provide little personal growth, there appear to be a number of potentially negative outcomes.

Peers

Friends have long been considered to be of central importance to adolescents. Erikson (1968) believed the peer group provides a sanctuary of group identity while a young person is passing between the dependency of childhood and the independence of adulthood. Piaget considered peer relationships crucial to understanding rules and moral behavior and argued that while young children's interactions with adults and siblings tended to emphasize the divine structure of rules, the informal and unsupervised play among peers during childhood and adolescence fosters the kind of spontaneous, flexible rule making and rule enforcing that is necessary in developing a mature moral orientation (Hoffman, 1980).

Because of the developmental importance of peers during early to middle adolescence, friendships experienced during this period are unlike those encountered at any other stage of life (Douvan & Adelson, 1966; Elkind, 1984; Selman, 1980). Friendships during this period demonstrate higher levels of mutuality, interaction, and interdependency.

Peer relationships generally exist at one of three levels; the friendship dyad, the clique, and the crowd. The friendship dyad, or coming together of two friends, is the most fundamental peer relation and the one most likely to be based on similar interests and emotional support in comparison to friendships that exist largely as part of a larger association of peers. Cliques, three to nine "buddies" or "mates" who exhibit a strong sense of cohesion, have been described as constituting an alternative family structure for its members as they acclimate to the world outside the home (Dunphy, 1963). The crowd is an association of two to four cliques in which relations are less intimate than in the smaller groups (Dunphy, 1963). Formation of the crowd is usually based on a common distinguishing characteristic, evidenced by the labels often associated with different adolescent crowds (e.g., "preppies," "brains," "jocks," "normals," "druggies") (Brown, Mounts, Lamborn, & Steinberg, 1993).

As youths develop, the structure of their peer relationships changes as it passes through five stages of development (Dunphy, 1963). Beginning with the isolated, unisexual cliques established during childhood, early adolescents begin to explore, as unisexual cliques, interactions with cliques of

the opposite sex. During this early period, interaction with the opposite sex is considered daring and only approached in the security of a group setting. Unisexual cliques eventually begin to merge to form heterosexual crowds, where dating begins. In late adolescence, crowds no longer serve a purpose and are replaced by loosely associated groups of heterosexual couples.

Another important aspect of adolescents' peer relationships is the *quality* of the friendships. Quality friendships are characterized by high levels of mutual caring, respect, and trust, in a context of balanced give and take (Youniss & Smollar, 1985). Adolescents who experience these types of close friendships generally report more intimate self-disclosure, more prosocial behavior, and more emotional support or encouragement from their friends, while also reporting less conflictual, domineering, or rivalrous behavior (Berndt & Savin-Williams, 1989; Furman & Robbins, 1985).

For most adolescents, ethnicity or culture appear to be very important in determining who they select as friends. For example, in one study of an ethnically integrated school (DuBois & Hirsch, 1990) while most students reported having an other-ethnic school friend, only about a quarter of the students reported having contact with those friends outside of school. For many ethnic minority youths, especially immigrants, peer relations formed from their own ethnic group can provide an adaptive support against the sense of isolation that can often exist among their peers of the majority population (Santrock, 2001).

Peer Influence

A major concern for many parents is whether their adolescents are being adversely influenced by their friends. The extent to which adolescents influence friends or are influenced by them varies according to their ability to establish and maintain supportive peer relationships as well as the type of group they belong to. Teevan (1972) contends compliance with peers is often based on the expectation that "such conformity will be rewarded with eventual acceptance into the group" (p. 283). Whether responding to actual peer pressure or merely to perceived expectations, young people who are less secure in their relations with friends are more likely to engage in behavior they would otherwise avoid. The importance of peer influence may be evaluated according to how closely associated the individual is to their friendship group or clique. Most adolescents would be expected to fit into the *core* of a particular peer circle, where there is a strong sense of commitment and collegiality. However, many adolescents instead fit into the *peripheral* region of one or more groups, where there is a sense of tentative belonging and a desire to become a part of the core group. Finally, others float unattached, *outside* any particular peer group. Adolescents who exist at the periphery of their identified peer group would be most vulnerable to peer influence as a result of their insecure position in the group. Out of a desire to become a core member of the peer group they identify with, peripheral group members would be most likely to allow peer expectations, or at least perceived peer expectations, to dictate their behaviors. In addition to group placements, the type of group one belongs to is also an important predictor of participation in antisocial or self-destructive behavior. Adolescents identified as being in the "druggies" or "toughs" peer groups are much more likely to report participating in groups encouraging antisocial or self-destructive behaviors as compared with those identified as being "populars," "brains," or "normals" (Stone & Brown, 1998).

Reflective Thinking

Friendship

Were the friendships you had during early adolescence different from the friendships you have now? How were they different? What advice would you give an adolescent worried about their friends?

Parents and Peers

A major parental concern is that family values will be displaced by peer values. Although there is some justification for this concern, several factors influence whom adolescents are likely to select as peers (Conger & Petersen, 1984). First, there is usually considerable overlap between parental and peer values because of common backgrounds; many adolescents select friends whose values are congruent with their parents'. Second, parents often are unsure of appropriate expectations for certain areas of adolescents' lives, and are thus willing to defer to the expectations of their adolescents' friends. This is especially apparent in current fashions, music, and leisure activities. Third, parents and peers have an impact on different aspects of adolescents' lives; peers are more likely to be influential in matters of short-term importance (i.e., tastes in music and entertainment, fashions in clothing and language, dating and friendship behavior), whereas parents are more likely to be influential in matters of greater and longer-term permanence (i.e., moral and social values, educational aspirations, and occupational choice) (Kandel & Lesser, 1972). Fourth, when adolescents do turn to peers for support, frequently it is not a displacement of parental influence but rather an attempt to fill a void left by their parents' lack of support and involvement. Finally, adolescents' orientations toward parents as compared with peers varies as a function of individual differences within adolescents and their social contexts (Conger & Petersen, 1984). As a result, the degree of conflict between parental and peer influence is less than assumed.

Caregivers can also have an impact on the quality of adolescents' friendships directly, according to four mechanisms: (1) their expectations about the positive and negative implications of peer relations; (2) their monitoring of adolescents' peer activity; (3) their direct interactions with adolescents' friends; and (4) their perceptions of their own roles in their adolescent's friendships (McCoy, 1992). In another study McCoy, Corey, and Owen (1999) found that while many adolescents do seem to determine whether their parents are involved in their friendships, the involvement level of many more parents seemed to be determined by the parents' own desire or availability to be involved. Finally, parents' involvement in adolescents' peer relations can be both positive and negative (Ladd & Golter, 1988; Parke et al., 1989) and depends on whether parents act as facilitators, spectators, or controllers of their children's peer relations.

Dating

Since World War II, we have seen a dramatic shift in the purpose and events that define adolescent dating. Although some adolescents still view early dating experiences as a means of sorting and selecting an appropriate mate, for most, dating has taken on much more of a recreational role. In addition, dating is seen as providing other functions, including a source of status and achievement; a unique socializing experience in which to learn about intimacy, sexuality, and a sense of identity; and an opportunity to develop new and deeper forms of companionship (Paul & White, 1990).

Males more frequently listed "sexual activity" as a reason for dating while females were more likely to list "intimacy." When 15-year-old males and females were asked what they liked about their girlfriend or boyfriend, boys were more likely to mention physical attractiveness, whereas girls were more likely to mention support and intimacy (Feiring, 1996).

The extent to which adolescents' dating experiences have an impact on individual development remains largely unknown. Although this area has received limited exploration, there are some ways in which dating has been found to be important. First, because boys are not encouraged to develop the capacity to be emotionally expressive in their same-sex peer relationships, opposite sex relationships may provide boys with an opportunity to explore intimacy development in a context that is much more socially acceptable (Steinberg, 2001). Second, becoming seriously involved in a steady dating relationship before age 15 can have a

somewhat stunting effect on adolescents' psychosocial development, particularly for girls (Neemann, Hubbard, & Masten, 1995). Girls who begin early to date seriously have been found to be less mature, less imaginative, less oriented toward achievement, less happy with who they are, and more superficial. In contrast, adolescent girls who have not dated at all by the time they reach late adolescence have been identified as having a more retarded social development, excessive dependency on their parents, and greater feelings of insecurity (McDonald & McKinney, 1994; Neemann, Hubbard, & Masten, 1995).

If adolescents postpone dating, and dating behavior remains light to moderate, it can provide a positive opportunity for social development. What has been difficult to determine is whether adolescents' dating experiences are themselves an important positive factor for social development or whether more socially advanced adolescents are simply more likely to date.

Sexual Activity

Today, 45.6% of high school students have engaged in sexual intercourse, and 6.6% experience intercourse before they turn 13 years of age (CDC, 2002). In fact, 56% of female and 73% of male adolescents report having had sexual intercourse before turning 18. First intercourse occurs at an average age of 17 years for females and at an average age of 16 for males. One-fourth of adolescents report having had their first intercourse experience by 15. Nineteen percent of sexually active high school students report having had four or more partners (American Academy of Pediatrics Committee on Adolescence, 2000a).

Adolescents' reasons for becoming sexually active include but are not limited to feeling grown-up; to enhance self-esteem; to experiment; to be accepted by friends; to have someone to care about, love, and be close to; for pleasure; to gain control over one's life; to seek revenge; and to prove they are "normal" (American Academy of Pediatrics Committee on Adolescence, 2000a; Murray & Zentner, 2001).

Predictors of early sexual activity include lack of attentive or nurturing parents, early pubertal development, poverty, history of sexual abuse, cultural and family patterns of early sexual experience, poor school performance, lack of school or career goals, and dropping out of school. Factors associated with delay in initiating intercourse include regular attendance at worship services, stable home environment, and higher family income (AAP Committee on Adolescence, 2000a).

Sexually active young people participate in behaviors that put them at risk for sexually transmitted diseases and pregnancy because they frequently have multiple partners or do not use condoms or other forms of contraception. Sexually transmitted diseases (STDs), defined as any disease spread from person to person during sexual contact, are highly communicable, currently considered a public health epidemic, and affect an increasing number of persons (Murray & Zentner, 2001). Reasons for the increased incidence of sexually transmitted diseases include lack of understanding about transmission; breakdown of the family unit; increased use of contraceptives; changing sexual patterns, attitudes, and mores; the feeling "it can't happen to me"; and increased societal mobility. Common STDs include chlamydia

papilloma infections, genital herpes, gonorrhea, trichomonas, and acquired immunodeficiency syndrome (AIDS).

Most teen pregnancies occur in those 18–19 years old—51% end in a live birth, 35% are aborted, and 14% are miscarriages or still births (AAP Committee on Adolescence, 2000a). Although birth rates to women under 20 have declined since the 1970s, the United States continues to have one of the highest teenage pregnancy rates among developed countries (Hewell & Andrews, 1996; Ventura, Peters, Martin, & Mauer, 1997). African-American teen pregnancy rates are higher than rates in Caucasians, and continue to increase (Murray & Zentner, 2001). Most teenage mothers are unmarried. The resulting unplanned pregnancy affects not only the mother and child, but also the child's father and the respective families because adolescents are often not socially, emotionally, educationally, economically, or physically ready for pregnancy and parenthood.

Several factors related to individual, family/friend, and society influence the incidence of adolescent pregnancy. Individual factors include self-destructive or self-hate feelings and behaviors, egocentrism, low self-esteem, loneliness, recent loss, early maturation, independence from family, lack of responsibility, plea for attention, personal fable, self-punishment, and need to prove one's womanhood. Family/friend factors include having a close relative who has experienced an adolescent pregnancy, conflictual mother–daughter or father–daughter relationships, sexually permissive peer group, inadequate communication, history of sexual abuse or incest, few girlfriends, an older boyfriend, lack of religious affiliation, substance abuse by family/friends, and fulfilling caregiver prophecy when parents suggest their daughter will become pregnant if she does not change her behavior. Societal factors include implied acceptance of intercourse outside marriage, a variety of adult behavioral values, media pressure, inadequate access to contraception, and the availability of public assistance/welfare for single young mothers (AAP Committee on

Adolescence, 2000a; Clemen-Stone, Eigsti, & McGuire, 1998; Dworetzky,1995).

There are risks associated with adolescent pregnancies—medical and psychological. Medical risks include low birth weight and neonatal death. The mortality rate for the teenaged pregnant woman is twice as high as for adult pregnant women. Other problems include poor maternal weight gain, pregnancy-induced hypertension, STDs, anemia, and prematurity. Psychological complications include persistent poverty, separation from the child's father, repeat pregnancy, divorce, school interruption, and limited vocational opportunities (AAP Committee on Adolescence, 2000a).

Improved methods of contraception and the increased number of sex education courses in the schools reach only a small percentage of adolescents. Not all those students who are sexually active attend such courses or have them readily available, and those adolescents who do participate in the courses may not integrate this information into their behavior because they do not see pregnancy as a concern for themselves or their partners. Therefore, during routine interactions and/or health assessments, nurses should determine an adolescent's understanding about intercourse, contraception, and reproduction before screening or providing necessary information and support. This includes assessing their understanding and accurate interpretation of risks of being sexually active and then discussing sexual responsibility, including abstinence, how STDs are transmitted, and possible consequences of infection and pregnancy. Adolescents who are sexually active should also receive information about the potential outcomes of their behavior, including ways to reduce their risk of becoming pregnant or infected with STDs or AIDS by limiting the number of sexual partners, using appropriate birth control methods, and consistently using condoms. When adolescents with STDs are identified, they should receive appropriate counseling and medical care. When pregnant adolescents are identified, comprehensive prenatal care is essential to reduce maternal and neonatal complications.

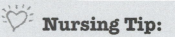

Reflective Thinking

Adolescent Pregnancy

Imagine yourself as a pregnant adolescent. What would you feel? How would your future have been affected? Do you know someone who was pregnant as an adolescent? How did she feel?

Nursing Tip:

Sexual activity
Assess adolescent's knowledge, feelings, and concerns about sexual preference and activity. Provide accurate information using correct terminology. Refer to appropriate agencies, resources, or caregivers. Ensure that adolescents understand that what they are experiencing is a normal part of moving into adulthood.

Pregnant adolescents should also receive information about available options. Teens who keep their infants need help becoming effective, secure, and comfortable parents. Information about normal infant growth, development, and care should be provided in an accepting, nurturing environment.

Homosexuality

Adolescence is also an important time for developing one's sexual orientation. In fact, in a sample of over 34,000 Minnesota junior and high school students, 10.7% were "unsure" of their sexual orientation, 88.2% described themselves as predominantly heterosexual, and 1.1% described themselves as bisexual or predominantly homosexual. As the age of the subjects increased, uncertainty about their sexual orientation diminished (Remafedi, Resnick, Blum, & Harris, 1992).

Most gay adolescents felt different from other boys as children. The average age they realized they were gay was 12.5 years and the average age of their first crush was 12.7 years. Almost half say they initially tried to deny their identity as a gay person and many were confused when they first became aware of their preferences.

In contrast, development of a same-sex orientation for young females is likely to occur much later and more abruptly (Diamond, 1998). Although development of a same-sex identity for many adolescent females will be similar to the developmental trajectory of adolescent males, most females' progression toward a same-sex orientation is likely to be more subject to nonsexual influences (emotions, personal experience, ideological or political beliefs), less associated with childhood indicators (early and pervasive sense of feeling different and gender-atypical behavior or ideation during childhood), and less stable as compared with adolescent males' development of a same-sex orientation (Diamond, 1998).

Nurses need to recognize that even though many young people explore their own sexual orientation or homosexual attractions, few who engage in homosexual behavior during adolescence continue the practice into adulthood (Santrock, 2001). Thus, nurses and caregivers need to help young people recognize that homosexual experimentation is not the same as establishing a homosexual orientation, acknowledge same and bisexual relationships and attractions, and phrase questions about sexuality and sexual activity carefully.

Violence

The second leading cause of death for individuals ages 15–19 and the third leading cause of death for adolescents ages 10–14 is homicide, most due to handgun use (American Academy of Pediatrics Committee on Injury and Poison Prevention, 2000; Webster, Gainer, & Champion, 1995). Six percent of high school students reported that they had carried a gun during the past year; 17.4% reported that they had carried a

Critical Thinking

Violence in the Home

How do you help a child who lives in a home that puts them at risk for violence? How can you help their parents?

Nursing Tip:

Violence
When working with youths who are victims of violence, ask about the victim's relationship to the perpetrator, circumstances surrounding the event, use of alcohol/drugs, predisposing risk factors (violence in the family, unemployment, truancy), and intentions regarding seeking revenge. (Danielson, 1998).

weapon at least once during the past 30 days (CDC, 2002). The homicide rate for black teens is eight times higher than that for whites of the same age (Danielson, 1998). The World Health Organization reports that the homicide rate for males aged 15 to 24 in the United States is 10 times higher than in Canada, 15 times higher than in Australia, and 28 times higher than in Germany or France (World Health Statistics Annual, 1995). During 2001, comparing school-grounds with violent neighborhoods, there was an increasing likelihood of violence having an impact on adolescents. Almost 7% of students felt too unsafe to go to school, and 6.4% said they had carried a gun, knife, or club onto school property at least once in the month preceding the survey. Almost 9% claimed they had been injured or threatened with a weapon on school property during the year before being surveyed (CDC, 2002). Delinquency rates have increased faster among girls than among boys, and adolescent-related violence in rural areas is rising (Danielson, 1998). Even though most gang-related problems occur in large cities, gang conflict is also seen in smaller cities. Gangs in schools almost doubled between 1989 and 1995, with a simultaneous 25% increase in the number of students victimized by violent crime.

The cause of violent crime committed by young people today has been traced to individual, family, community, and social circumstances. Violent delinquency tends to be more common in working-class than in middle-class teens, and a relationship exists between money-making crimes, unemployment, and poverty. It is not uncommon for violent youth to associate with delinquent peer groups and experience violence at home where there is access to illicit drugs, alcohol, and guns. Violent behaviors in adolescence are also associated with depression, drug abuse, lower church attendance, and hopelessness (DuRant, Treiber, Goodman, & Woods, 1996).

Suicide

The number of adolescents committing suicide has increased dramatically over the last few decades. Now, suicide is the third leading cause of death during adolescence (15-19 years) and the fourth leading killer of younger adolescents (American Academy of Pediatrics Committee on Adolescence, 2000). Over 19% of high schoolers nationally have considered suicide; 8.8% have attempted suicide, and 2.6% required medical attention after a suicide attempt (CDC, 2002b). Sixty-three percent of adolescent suicides in 1997 were committed with a firearm; 91% of suicide attempts involving a firearm are fatal, whereas only 23% of adolescents using a drug overdosage die (American Academy of Pediatrics Committee on Adolescence, 2000b).

Frequently, suicide is reported as an accidental death. Even though suicide affects adolescents from all races and socioeconomic groups, some groups have higher rates than others: African American females have the lowest rate; Native American males have the highest rates. Gay and bisexual adolescents have rates of attempting suicide three times higher than other adolescents

⚡ **Nursing Alert:**

At-Risk for Suicide

- *Experiencing loss (death, divorce, move)*
- *Unable to meet scholastic expectations*
- *Depression*
- *Changes in habits*
- *Drop in performance*
- *Loneliness*
- *Truancy*
- *Accident proneness*
- *Mood swings*
- *Increasing alcohol or drug use*
- *Hopelessness*
- *Giving away possessions*
- *Withdrawing*
- *Writing/talking about death/suicide*

Source: Potts, N., and Mandleco, B. (2002). Pediatric nursing: Caring for children and their families. *Clifton Park, NY: Delmar Learning.*

(American Academy of Pediatrics Committee on Adolescence, 2000b). Females are three times as likely to attempt suicide, whereas males are three times as likely to succeed in their attempts.

Stresses related to psychosocial, psychosexual, or physiological issues have been identified as causes for the increasing number of adolescent suicides in the United States (Murray & Zentner, 2001). Often, those adolescents attempting suicide come from families with inconsistent behavioral reinforcement, nonproductive communication patterns, and high levels of conflict/abuse. These youngsters may also feel inadequate or unacceptable, have underlying emotional disturbances, or fail to achieve desired goals. It is not uncommon for seemingly insignificant frustrations and disappointments to precipitate such impulsive acts, which may be committed to increase family and/or friends's attention.

Several warning signs of adolescents who might be at risk for committing suicide have been identified (Conrad, 1991; Fritz & Barbie, 1993). They include but are not limited to experiencing loss due to death or divorce; moving to a different neighborhood, city or state; the appearance of health problems they did not have before; being unable to meet scholastic expectations of teachers, parents, or self; being depressed; changes in eating and sleeping patterns or daily habits; drop in school performance; being lonely or a loner with few friends; truancy; accident proneness; mood swings; increasing alcohol or drug use; feeling rejected, guilty, or hopeless; giving away possessions; withdrawing from people and activities; and writing or talking about death or suicide. Other risk factors are previous suicide attempts, family history of psychiatric disorders, living out of the home, history of physical or sexual abuse, physical ailments, and a recent relationship breakup (American Academy of Pediatrics Committee on Adolescence, 2000b).

Suicide prevention programs for teens should be directed at school staff (counselors, school health nurses, teachers), community agency personnel (clergy, police, health care providers, merchants), and students themselves by providing information relative to warning signs, facts, and programs which can enhance self-esteem and social competence. Methods of screening at-risk youth, programs offering peer support, crisis centers, and hotlines as well as restricting the access to handguns, drugs, and other common means of suicide have also been successful. Interventions after a suicide are designed to help prevent or contain suicide clusters and help adolescents cope effectively with feelings of loss they experience with the suicide of a peer.

Nurses working with adolescents need to recognize the seriousness of any of these signs or symptoms, convey concern to the adolescents about those signs, help them feel things will change, listen to and ask about their problems, and refer adolescents with these signs and symptoms to a mental health professional experienced in working with adolescents. Nurse's should not be afraid to ask adolescents directly if they have or are considering suicide, and in fact, the adoles-

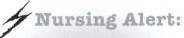

Nursing Alert:

Suicide

Take any suicide gesture seriously; convey concern, love, and acceptance; and refer and follow-up to mental health professionals experienced in working with adolescents.

cent may be relieved to finally be able to talk about it. It is not uncommon for adolescents unsuccessfully attempting suicide to be merely crying out or asking for help rather than actually wanting to check out or end their life. However, those merely asking for help must be differentiated from those who actually want to end their life because some adolescents attempting suicide later actually succeed. Therefore, followup care after gestures is extremely important and crisis intervention for suicide attempts is essential since it can often help the adolescent identify and work through problems, learn alternative ways of coping with stress, and help family and friends be supportive and caring.

Drug Abuse

Drug abuse (illicit and prescription) is defined as the use of any drug in excess because of the feeling it arouses (Murray & Zentner, 2001). Illicit drug use is reported by 15.9% of adolescents 12–17 years of age. More than 42% of American high school students have tried marijuana; 23.9% use the drug monthly. Over 9% of high school students have tried cocaine at least once; 3% have tried heroin and 14.7% have inhaled or sniffed intoxicating substances. Almost 10% had used methamphetamines. Twenty-two percent of teens report having smoked a whole cigarette by the age of 13 (CDC, 2002). Even though there has been a decrease in smoking over the last several years, teenagers still do smoke, and often, cigarette smoking begins in adolescence and continues into adulthood (Coleman & Hendry, 1999). Teens who do smoke tend to come from single parent families, may have low self-confidence and self-esteem, have poor educational aspirations, are more anxious, spend their leisure time working part time or "hanging out," and have family members and friends who also smoke (Holland & Fitzsimons, 1991; Jacobson & Wilkenson, 1994; Lloyd & Lucas, 1997).

Twenty-eight and one half percent of adolescents have been offered, sold, or given an illegal drug at school (CDC, 2002). Often adolescents abuse drugs because of curiosity, availability, rebellion, peer pressure, exhilaration, unhappiness at home, the need to overcome feelings of loneliness/insecurity, to be more accepted, to imitate family and friends, to escape, and as an attempt to be mature/sophisticated (Dworetzky, 1995; Kafka & London, 1991; Turner & Helms, 1995).

Nurses, family members, teachers, and community leaders suspecting drug abuse may observe irrational behavior, preoccupation with the occult, decreased quality of schoolwork, irresponsibleness, changes in personality, friends, activities, or appearance, difficulty communicating, rebelliousness, mental or physiological deterioration, unexplainable loss of money or the appearance of new possessions (clothes, CDs, stereo equipment, etc.), and actual drug paraphernalia or drugs, including marijuana.

Alcohol Abuse

Alcoholism and alcohol abuse in adolescence are increasing. Over 78% of high school students nationally have tried alcohol; 47.1% reported drinking alcohol at least once over the preceding month of being surveyed; 29.9% report consuming 5 or more drinks at least once over the past month (CDC, 2002). Forty-one percent of adolescents report using alcohol and 10% to 20% of adolescents are problem drinkers. It is not uncommon for drinking patterns to begin in the eighth grade (Escobedo, Chorba, & Waxweiler, 1995). Often, adolescent behavior relative to alcohol consumption is associated with parenatal

behavior, especially if they are alcoholic or have a drinking problem, peer pressure, or because it makes them feel more mature and is a common social custom. Many adolescents who do drink use it as a mind altering device since it allows participation in risk taking activities they might otherwise avoid.

There are numerous hazards of alcohol ingestion. Some may be seen in adolescents, including hepatitis, pancreatitis, gastritis, neuritis, cirrhosis, ulcers of the gastrointestinal tract, impotence, esophageal varices and cancer, cerebellar degeneration, delirium tremens, or birth defects (Murray & Zentner, 2001).

Parents and nurses working with adolescents who abuse alcohol or other mind altering drugs and their family members need to avoid lectures and judgements. It would be much better to educate adolescents about the detrimental effects of alcohol by describing people who have experienced the effects of excessive alcohol intake. Clarifying values and behaviors relative to leading a healthy lifestyle are also important topics for discussion.

Television/Media

Media in America contribute to more adverse health outcomes than to prosocial or positive outcomes. This is especially true with regard to violence, guns, sex, and drugs. For example, cross-sectional, naturalistic, and longitudinal studies as well as several meta-analyses suggest that there is a relationship between media violence, real-life aggression, and acceptance of aggressive attitudes. Those exposed to violence on television and the media tend to be more likely to commit violent acts. In addition, guns are glamorized in the media; 26% of violent acts committed on the media use guns. Research also suggests that adolescents exposed to greater amounts of alcohol or tobacco advertising are more likely to use or intend to use those products as compared with those adolescents who are not exposed to those products. One-third of teens who smoke could link their smoking to tobacco promotional activities. Alcohol advertising in the media stimulates favorable predispositions, greater problem drinking, and higher consumption by young people (Strasburger & Donnerstein, 1999.) Box 8-2 lists the effects of television and other media on adolescents.

Caregivers need to control or monitor the media programming their teens watch, and remove television sets from teens' bedrooms. Specifically, this means to limit all media use to no more than 1 to 2 hours per day, view television with their adolescents, and monitor their child or adolescent's use of the media (Strasburger & Donnerstein, 1999).

Box 8-2 Effect of television and other media on adolescents

1. 2–3 hours/day mean less physical activity, reading, and interaction with friends.

2. 10,000 acts of violence viewed/year; 26% involve use of guns.

3. 15,000 sexual references, innuendoes, jokes per year; <170 deal with abstinence, birth control, pregnancy, STDs.

4. 70% of content from prime-time dramatic programs contains references to alcohol, tobacco, illicit drugs; over 50% of movies contain references to tobacco/smoking; for every "just say no" public service announcement, 25–50 beer and wine advertisements will be viewed.

REFERENCES

American Academy of Pediatrics Committee on Adolescence (2000a). Adolescent pregnancy—Current trends and issues: 1998. *Pediatrics, 103*(2), 516–520.

American Academy of Pediatrics. Committee on Adolescence. (2000b). Suicide and suicide attempts in adolescents. *Pediatrics, 104*(4), April, 871-874.

American Academy of Pediatrics Committee on Injury and Poison Prevention (2000, April). *Pediatrics, 105*(5), 888–895.

American Academy of Pediatrics Committee on Sports Medicine (1990, November). Strength training, weight and power lifting, and body building by children and adolescents. *Pediatrics, 86*(5) 801–803.

American Dental Association. (1998). Cleaning your teeth and gums (oral hygiene) [On-line]. Available: www.ada.org/public/ faq/cleaning. html#daily

American Medical Association (1997). Guidelines for adolescent preventable services (GAPS): Recommendations for physicians and other health professionals. Available: www.ama-assn.org

Anglin, T., Naylor, K., & Kaplan, D. (1996). Comprehensive school-based health care: high school students' use of medical, mental health, and substance abuse services. *Pediatrics, 97*(3), 318–330.

Archer, S. L. (1992). A feminist's approach to identity research. In G. R. Adams, T. P. Gullotta, & R. Montemayor (Eds.), *Adolescent identity formation.* Newbury Park, CA: Sage.

Armsden, G., & Greenberg, M. T. (1987). The inventory of parent and peer attachment: Individual differences and their relationship to psychological well-being in adolescence. *Journal of Youth and Adolescence, 16,* 427–454.

Barber, B. (1994). Cultural, family, and personal contexts of parent-adolescent conflict. *Journal of Marriage and the Family, 56,* 375–386.

Beard, J. (2000). Iron requirements in adolescent females. *Journal of Nutrition, 130,* 440S–442S.

Berger, K. (1994). *The developing person through the life span* (3rd ed.). New York: Worth.

Berkey, C. S., Rockett, H. R. H., Field, A. E., Gillman, M. W., Frazier, A. L., Camargo, C. A., Jr., & Colditz, G. A. (2000). Activity, dietary intake, and weight changes in a longitudinal study of preadolescent and adolescent boys and girls. *Pediatrics. 105*(4), 56.

Berndt, T., & Keefe, K. (1995). Friends' influence on adolescents' adjustment to school. *Child Development, 66,* 1312–1329.

Berndt, T. J., & Savin-Williams, R. C. (1989). Peer relations and friendships. In P. Tolan & B. Cohler (Eds.), *Handbook of clinical research and practice with adolescents* (pp. 203–219). New York: Wiley.

Birch, L. L., & Fisher, J. O. (1998). Development of eating behaviors among children and adolescents. *Pediatrics, 101*(3), 539–549.

Blyth, D. A., Simmons, G. G., Zakin, D. F. (1985). Satisfaction with body image for adolescents. *Journal of Youth and Adolescence, 14,* 207–225.

Brody, G. H., Stoneman, Z., & McCoy, J. K. (1994). Contributions of family relationships and child temperaments to longitudinal variations in sibling relationship quality and sibling relationship styles. *Journal of Family Psychology, 8,* 274–286.

Brook J. S., Whiteman M., Gordon A. S., & Brenden C. (1986). Older brother's influence on younger sibling's drug use. *Journal of Psychology, 114,* 83–90.

Brooks-Gunn, J. (1988). Antecedents and consequences of variations in girls' maturational timing. *Journal of Adolescent Health Care, 9,* 365–373.

Brooks-Gunn, J., & Paikoff, R. (1993). Sex is a gamble, kissing is a game: Adolescent sexuality and health promotion. In S. G. Millstein, A. C. Petersen, & E. O. Nightengale (Eds.). *Promoting the health of adolescents.* New York: Oxford University Press.

Brown, B., Mounts, N., Lamborn, S., & Steinberg, L. (1993). Parenting practices and peer group affiliations in adolescence. *Child Development, 64,* 467–482.

Caspi, A., & Moffitt, T. (1991). Individual differences are accentuated during periods of social change: The sample case of girls at puberty. *Journal of Personality and Social Psychology, 61,* 157–168.

Centers for Disease Controls and Prevention. (2002). *Youth risk behavior surveillance survey—U.S.— 2001.* MMWR, June 28, 2002/51 (SS04); 1-64.

Cheng, T., Fields, C., Brenner, R., Wright, J., Lomax, T., Scheidt, P., & DC Child/Adolescent Injury Research Network (2000). Sports injuries: An important cause of morbidity in urban youth. *Pediatrics, 105*(3), e32.

Clayton R. R., & Lacy W. B. (1982). Interpersonal influences on male drug use and drug use intentions. International *Journal of the Addictions, 17*(4), 655–666.

Clemen-Stone, S., McGuire, S., & Eigsti, D. (2002). *Comprehensive community health nursing* (6th ed.). St. Louis: Mosby-Year Book.

Committee on Dietary Allowances, Food and Nutrition Board, National Research Council. (1989). *Recommended dietary allowances* (10th ed.). Washington, DC: National Academy Press.

Committee on Nutrition. (1995). Fluoride supplementation for children: Interim policy recommendations. *Pediatrics, 95,* 777.

Committee on Nutrition. (1999). Calcium requirements of infants, children, and adolescents. *American Academy of Pediatrics, 104*(5), 1152–1157.

Conger, J. J., & Petersen, A. C. (1984). *Adolescence and youth.* New York: Harper & Row.

Conrad, N. (1991). Where do they turn? Social support systems of suicidal high school adolescents. *Journal of Psychosocial Nursing, 29*(3), 14-20.

Danielson, R. (1998). Adolescent violence in America. *Clinician Reviews, 8*(5), 167–184.

Diamond, L. M. (1998). Development of sexual orientation among adolescent and young adult women. *Developmental Psychology, 34,* 1085–1095.

Douvan, E., & Adelson, J. (1966). *The adolescent experience.* New York: Wiley.

DuBois, D. L., & Hirsch, B. J. (1990). School and neighborhood friendship patterns of blacks and whites in early adolescence. *Child Development, 61,* 524–536.

Duke-Duncan, P. (1991). Body Image. In R.M. Lerner, A.C. Petersen, & J. Brooks-Gunn (Eds.). *Encyclopedia of adolescence* (pp. 90–94). New York: Garland.

Dunphy, D. C. (1963). The social structure of urban adolescent peer groups. *Sociometry, 26,* 230- 246.

DuRant, R., Treiber, F., Goodman, E., & Woods, E. (1996). Intentions to use violence among young adolescents. *Pediatrics, 98*(6), 1104–1108.

Dworetzky, J. (1995). *Human development: A lifespan approach* (6th ed.). St. Paul: West.

East, P. L., & Rook, K. S. (1992). Compensatory patterns of support among children's peer relationships: A test using school friends, non-school friends, and siblings. *Developmental Psychology, 28,* 163–172.

Elkind, D. (1967). Egocentrism in adolescence. *Child Development, 38,* 1025–1034.

Elkind, D. (1978). Understanding the young adolescent. *Adolescence, 13,* 128-134.

Elkind, D. (1984). *All grown up and no place to go: Teenagers in crisis.* Reading, MA: Addison-Wesley.

Erikson, E. H. (1968). *Identity: Youth and crisis.* New York: Norton.

Escobedo, L., Chorba, J., & Waxweiler, R. (1995). Patterns of alcohol use and the risk of drinking and driving among U.S. high school students. *American Journal of Public Health, 85,* 976–978.

Eveleth, P.B., & Tanner, J.M. (1990). *Worldwide variation in human growth* (2nd ed.). Cambridge, UK: Cambridge University Press.

Falbo, T. (1992). Social norms and the one-child family: Clinical and policy implications. In F. Boer & J. Dunn (Eds.), *Children's sibling relationships* (pp. 71–82). Hillsdale, NJ: Erlbaum.

Feiring, C. (1996). Concepts of romance in 15-year-old adolescents. *Journal of Research on Adolescence, 6,* 181–200.

Feldman, W. R., Feldman, E., & Goodman, J. (1988). Culture versus biology: Children's attitudes toward thinness and fatness. *Pediatrics, 81,* 190–194.

Freiberg, K. (1992). *Human development: A life-span approach.* Boston: Jones and Bartlett.

French, S., Perry, C., Leon, G., & Fulkerson, J. (1994). Weight concerns, dieting behavior, and smoking initiation among adolescents: A prospective study. *American Journal of Public Health, 84,* 1818–1820.

Fritz, T., & Barbie, M. (1993). What are the warning signs for suicidal adolescents? *Journal of Psychosocial Nursing, 32*(2), 37-40.

Furman, W., & Buhrmester, D. (1992). Age and sex differences in perceptions of networks of personal relationships. *Child Development, 63,* 103–115.

Furman, W., & Robbins, P. (1985). What's the point? Issues in the selection of treatment objectives. In B. Schneider, K. Rubin, & J. Leddingham (Eds.), *Children's relations: Issues in assessment and intervention* (pp. 41–54). New York: Springer-Verlag.

Gallahue, D., & Ozmun, J. (1995). *Understanding motor development* (3rd ed.). Madison, WI: Brown & Benchmark.

Ge, X., Conger, R., & Elder, G. (1996). Coming of age too early: Pubertal influences on girl's vulnerability to psychological distress. *Child Development, 67,* 3386–3400.

Gilligan, C. (1982). *In a different voice.* Cambridge, MA: Harvard University Press.

Gilligan, C., Lyons, N., and Hanmer, T. (Eds.). (1990). *Making connections: The relational worlds of adolescent girls at Emma Willard School.* Cambridge, MA: Harvard University Press.

Graber, J., & Peterson, A. (1991). Cognitive changes at adolescence: Biological perspectives. In K. Gibson & A. Peterson (Eds.). *Brain, maturation and cognitive development.* New York: Aldine de Gruyter.

Graber, J., Brooks-Gunn, J., & Warren, M. (1995). The antecedents of menarchial age: Heredity, family environment, and stressful life events. *Child Development, 66,* 346–359.

Green, E. W. (Ed.). (1994). *Bright futures: Guidelines for health supervision of infants, children, and adolescents.* Arlington, VA: National Center for Education in Maternal and Child Health.

Greenberger, E., & Steinberg, L. (1986). *When teenagers work.* New York: Basic Books.

Grotevant, H. D. (1998). Adolescent development in family contexts. In W. Damon (Ed) & N. Eisenberg (Vol. Ed.), *Handbook of child psychology* (5th ed.) Vol. xx, *Social, emotional, and personality development.* New York: Wiley.

Grover, G. (1996) Dental care. In C. Berkowitz, (Ed.). *Pediatrics: A primary care approach* (pp. 45–49). Philadelphia: Saunders.

Guinn, B., Semper, T., Jorgensen, L., & Skaggs. (1997, March). Body image perception in female Mexican-American adolescents. *Journal of School Health, 67*(3), 112–116.

Hewell, S., & Andrews, J. (1996). Contraceptive use among female adolescents. *Clinical Nursing Research, 5*(3), 356–363.

Hill, J. O., & Trowbridge, F. L. (1998). Childhood obesity: future directions and research priorities. *Pediatrics, 101*(3), 570–574.

Hoffman M. L. (1980). Moral development in adolescence. In J. Adelson (Ed.), *Handbook of adolescent psychology* (pp. 295–343). New York: Wiley.

Kafka, R., & London, P. (1991, Fall). Communication in relationships and adolescent substance use: The influence of parents and friends. *Adolescence, 26*(103), 587–597.

Kandel, D. B., & Lesser, G. S. (1972). Parental and peer influences on educational plans of adolescents. *American Sociological Review, 34,* 213–223.

Katchadourian, H. (1977). *The biology of adolescence.* San Francisco: Freeman.

Kempton, T., Armistead, L., Wierson, M., & Forehand, R. (1991). Presence of a sibling as a buffer following parental divorce: An examination of young adolescents. *Journal of Clinical Child Psychology, 20,* 434–438.

Kennedy, E., & Powell, R. (1997). Changing eating patterns of American children: a view from 1996. *Journal of the American College of Nutrition, 16,* 524–529.

Koff, E., & Rierdan, J. (1991). Menarche and body image. In R.M. Lerner, A. C. Petersen, & J. Brooks-Gunn (Eds.), *Encyclopedia of adolescence* (pp. 631–636). New York: Garland.

Kohlberg, L. (1976). Moral stages and moralization: The cognitive-development approach. In T. Lickona (Ed.), *Moral development and behavior.* New York: Holt, Rinehart and Winston.

Ladd, G. W., & Golter, B. S. (1988). Parents' management of preschooler's peer relations: Is it related to children's social competence? *Developmental Psychology, 24,* 109–117.

Magnussen, D., Stattin, H., & Allen, V. (1988). Differential maturation among girls and its relations to social adjustment: A longitudinal perspective. In E. M. Hetherington, & R. Parke, (Eds.), *Contemporary readings in child psychology* (3rd ed.; pp. 97–116). New York: McGraw-Hill.

Malina, R., & Bouchard, C. (1991). *Growth maturation and physical activity.* Champaign, IL: Human Kinetics.

Mandleco, B. (2002). Care of infants, children and adolescents. In J. Hitchcock, P. Schubert, & S. Thomas (Eds.), *Community health nursing* (2nd Ed.). Clifton Park, NY: Delmar, 521–562.

Marcia, J. E. (1980). Identity in adolescence. In J. Adelson (Ed.), *Handbook of Adolescent Psychology* (pp. 159–187). New York: Wiley.

Marshall, W.A., & Tanner, J.M. (1969). Variations in the pattern of pubertal changes in girls. *Archives of Disease in Childhood, 44,* 291–303.

Marshall, W.A., & Tanner, J.M. (1970). Variations in the pattern of pubertal changes in boys. *Archives of Disease in Childhood, 45,* 13–23.

McCoy, J. K. (1992). *The importance of individual and family characteristics in predicting adolescent friendship quality.* Unpublished doctoral dissertation, University of Georgia, Athens, GA.

McCoy, J. K., Corey, A. M., & Owen, C. L. (1999, April). *Early adolescents' relationship patterns with parents and peers and parents' involvement in their children's friendships.* Paper presented at the Biennial Conference of the Society for Research in Child Development, Albuquerque, NM.

McDonald, D., & McKinney, J. (1994). Steady dating and self-esteem in high school students. *Journal of Adolescence, 17,* 557–564.

Mortimer, J., Finch, M., Ryu, S., Shanahan, M., & Call, K. (1996). The effects of work intensity on adolescent mental health, achievement, and behavioral adjustment: New evidence from a prospective study. *Child Development, 67,* 1243–1261.

Moffitt, T., Caspi, A., Belsky, J., & Silva, P. (1992). Childhood experience and the onset of menarche: A test of a sociobiological model. *Child Development, 63,* 47–58.

Montemayor, R. (1983). Parents and adolescents in conflict: All families some of the time and some families most of the time. *Journal of Early Adolescence, 3,* 83–103.

Murray, R., & Zentner, J. (2001). *Health assessment and promotion strategies throughout the lifespan.* (7th ed.). Stamford, CT: Appleton & Lange.

Neemann, J., Hubbard, J., & Masten, A. (1995). The changing importance of romantic relationship involvement to competence from late childhood to late adolescence. *Development and Psychopathology, 7,* 727–750.

Parke, R. D., MacDonald, K. B., Burks, V. M., Carson, J., Bhavnagri, N., Barth, J. M., & Beitel. A. (1989). Family and peer systems: In search of the linkages. In K. Kreppner & R. M. Lerner (Eds.), *Family systems and life-span development.* Hillsdale, NJ: Erlbaum.

Paterson, J., Pryor, J., & Field, J. (1994). Adolescent attachment to parents and friends in relation to aspects of self-esteem. *Journal of Youth and Adolescence, 24,* 365–376.

Paul, E. L., & White, K. M. (1990). The development of intimate relationships in late adolescence. *Adolescence, 25,* 375–400.

Physical Activity Guidelines for Adolescents. (1994). *Pediatric Exercise Science, 6,* 299–463.

Piaget, J. (1972). Intellectual evolution from adolescence to adulthood. *Human Development, 15,* 1–12.

Potts, N. & Mandleco, B. (Eds). (2002). *Caring for children and their families.* Clifton Park, NY: Delmar Learning.

Raja, S. N., McGee, R., & Stanton, W. R. (1992). Perceived attachments to parents and peers and psychological well-being in adolescence. *Journal of Youth and Adolescence, 21,* 471–485.

Rees, J. (1996). Eating disorders in adolescence: A model for broadening our perspective. *Journal of the American Dietetic Association, 96*(1), 22–24.

Remafedi, G., Resnick, M., Blum, R., & Harris, L. (1992). Demography of sexual orientation in adolescents. *Pediatrics, 89*(4), 714–721.

Rest, J., Davison, M., & Robbins, S. (1978). Age trends in judging moral issues: A review of cross-sectional, longitudinal, and sequential studies of the Defining Issues Test. *Child Development, 49,* 263–279.

Rogers, J. L., & Rowe, D. C. (1990). Influence of siblings on adolescent sexual behavior. *Developmental Psychology, 24*(5), 722–728.

Rowe, D. C., & Britt, C. L. (1991). Developmental explanation of delinquent behavior: Common vs. transmitted effects. *Journal of Quantitative Criminology, 7,* 315–322.

Rowe, D. C., & Gulley, B. L. (1992). Sibling effects on substance use and delinquency. *Criminology, 30,* 217–233.

Rozin, J. C., & Gross, J. (1987). Prevalence of weight reducing and weight gaining in adolescent boys and girls. *Health Psychology, 6,* 131–147.

Santrock, J. W. (2001). *Adolescence* (8th ed.). Dubuque, IA: Brown & Benchmark.

Selman, R. L. (1980). *The growth of interpersonal understanding.* New York: Academic.

Shaffer, D. R. (2000). *Social and personality development,* (4th ed.). Pacific Grove, CA: Brooks/Cole.

Sharabany, R., Gershoni, R., & Hofman, J. E. (1981). Girlfriend, boyfriend: Age and sex differences in intimate friendship. *Developmental Psychology, 17,* 800–808.

Sifuentes, M. (2000). Eating disorders. In C. Berkowitz, (Ed.). *Pediatrics: A primary care approach* (2nd ed., pp. 429–433). Philadelphia: Saunders.

Silbereisen, R., & Kracke, B. (1993). Variation in maturational timing and adjustment in adolescence. In S. Jackson & H. Rodriguez-Tome (Eds.), *Adolescence and its social worlds* (pp. 67–94). Hillsdale, NJ: Erlbaum.

Simmons, R., & Blyth, D. (1987). *Moving into adolescence: The impact of pubertal change and school context.* New York: Aldine de Gruyter.

Sprinthall, N. A., & Collins, W. A. (1995). *Adolescent psychology: A developmental view.* New York: McGraw-Hill.

Stattin, H., & Magnussen, D. (1990). *Pubertal maturation in female development: Paths through life* (Vol. 2). Hillsdale, NJ: Erlbaum.

Stein, K., Roeser, R., & Markus, H. (1998). Self-schemas and possible selves as predictors and outcomes of risky behaviors in adolescents. *Nursing Research, 47*(2), 96–106.

Steinberg, L. (1989). *Adolescence* (2nd ed.). New York: McGraw-Hill.

Steinberg, L. (2001). *Adolescence* (5th ed.). New York: McGraw-Hill.

Steinberg, L., & Dornbusch, S. (1991). Negative correlates of part-time work in adolescence: Replication and elaboration. *Developmental Psychology, 17.* 304–313.

Stone, M. R., & Brown, B. B. (1998). In the eye of the beholder: Adolescents' perceptions of peer crowd stereotypes. In R. E. Muuss & H. D. Porton (Eds.) *Adolescent behavior and society: A book of readings* (pp. 158–169). Boston: McGraw-Hill College.

Strasburger, V., & Donnerstein, E. (1999, January). Children, adolescents, and the media: Issues and solutions. *Pediatrics, 103*(1), 129–139.

Strauss, R. S., & Knight, J. (1999). Influence of the home environment on the development of obesity in children. *Pediatrics, 106*(6), 85.

Tanner, J. M., (1990). *Fetus into man: Physical growth from conception to maturity* (2nd ed.). Cambridge, MA: Harvard University Press.

Teevan, J. J., Jr. (1972). Reference groups and premarital sexual behavior. *Journal of Marriage and the Family, 34,* 283–291.

Troiano, R. P., & Flegal, K. M. (1998). Overweight children and adolescents: Description, epidemiology, and demographics. *Pediatrics, 101*(3), 497–504.

Turner, J., & Helms, D. (1995). *Lifespan development* (5th ed.). New York: Holt, Rinehart & Winston.

U.S. Department of Health and Human Services. (1997). Guidelines for school and community programs to promote lifelong physical activity among young people. *MMWR 46*, 1–36.

U.S. Department of Health and Human Services. (2000). *Healthy People 2010: National health promotion and disease prevention objectives.* Washington DC: Author.

Ventura, S. J., Peters, K. D., Martin, J. A., & Maurer, J. D. (1997). Births and deaths: United States 1996. *Monthly Vital Statistics Report, 46*(1), Supplement 2.

Warren, M., Brooks-Gunn, J., Fox, R., Lancelot, C., Newman, D., & Hamilton, W. (1991). Lack of bone accretion and amenorrhea in young dancers: Evidence for a relative osteopenia in weight bearing bones. *Journal of Clinical Endocrinology and Metabolism, 72*, 847–853.

Waterman, A. S. (1992). Identity as an aspect of optimal psychological functioning. *Adolescent identity formation.* Newbury Park, CA: Sage.

Webster, D., Gainer, P., & Champion, H. (1995). Weapon carrying among inner-city junior high students: Defensive behavior vs. aggressive deliquency. *American Journal of Public Health, 85*, 1604–1608.

Whitaker, A., Davies, S., Shaffer, D., Abrams, S., Walsh, B., & Kalikow, K. (1989). The struggle to be thin: A survey on anorexic and bulimic symptoms in a non-referred adolescent population. *Psychological Medicine, 19*, 143–163.

Wright, E., & Whitehead, T. (1987). Perceptions of body size and obesity: A selected review of the literature. *Journal of Community Health, 12*, 117–129.

World Health Statistics Annual, 1994 (1995). Geneva, Switzerland: World Health Organization.

Youniss, J., & Smollar, J. (1985). *Adolescent relations with mothers, fathers, and friends.* Chicago: University of Chicago Press.

SUGGESTED READINGS

Adler, E., & Clark, R. (1991). Adolescence: A literary passage. *Adolescence, 26*(104), 757–768.

Amato, P. R. (1993). Children's adjustment to divorce: Theories, hypotheses, and empirical support.. *Journal of Marriage and the Family, 55*, 23–38.

American Academy of Pediatrics Committee on Infectious Diseases (1997, March). Immunization of adolescents: Recommendations of the Advisory Committee on Immunization Practices, the American Academy of Pediatrics, the American Academy of Family Physicians, and the American Medical Association (RE9711). *Pediatrics, 99*(3), 479–488,

Anderson, R., Crespo, C., Bartlett, S., Cheskin, L, & Pratt, M. (1998, March). Relationship of physical activity and television with body weight and level of fatness among children. *Journal of the American Medical Association, 279*(12): 938–942.

Behrman, R., & Kleigman, B. (2002). *Nelson's essentials of pediatrics* (4th ed.). Philadelphia: Saunders.

Berndt, T. J., & Perry, T. B. (1986). Children's perceptions of friendships as supportive relationships. *Developmental Psychology, 22*, 640–648.

Bradford, M. (1996). Health concerns and prevalence of abuse and sexual activity in adolescents at a runaway shelter. *Applied Nursing Research, 8*(4), 187–190.

Connelly, C. (1998). Hopefulness, self-esteem, and perceived social support among pregnant and nonpregnant adolescents. *Western Journal of Nursing Research, 20*(2), 195–209.

Dietz, W. H. (1998). Health consequences of obesity in youth: Childhood predictors of adult disease. *Pediatrics, 101*(3), 518–525.

Dryfoos, J. (1998). *Safe passage: Making it through adolescence in a risky society.* New York: Oxford University Press.

Estes, M. E. (2002). *Health assessment & physical examination* (2nd ed.). Clifton Park, NY: Delmar.

Gordon-Larsen, P., McMurray, R., & Popkin, B. (2000, June). Determinants of adolescent physical activity and inactivity patterns. *Pediatrics, 105*(6), e83 ff.

Herman-Giddens, M., Slora, E., Wasserman, R., Bourdony, C., Bhapkar, M., Koch, G., & Hasemeier, C. (1997). Secondary sexual characteristics and menses in young girls seen in office practice: A study from the pediatric research in office settings network. *Pediatrics, 99*(4), 505–512.

Hetherington, E. M., Bridges, M., & Insabella, G. M. (1998). What matters? What does not? Five perspectives on the association between marital transitions and children's adjustment. *American Psychologist, 53*(2), 167–184.

Lee, S., & Gruggs, L. (1995). Pregnant teenagers' reasons for seeking or delaying prenatal care. *Clinical Nursing Research, 4*(1), 38–49.

Mahon, N., Yarcheski, A., & Yarcheski, T. (1993). Health consequences of loneliness in adolescents. *Research in Nursing and Health, 12,* 23-31.

McCoy, J. K., Brody, G. H., & Stoneman, Z. (1994). A longitudinal analysis of sibling relationships as mediators of the link between family processes and youths'

best friendships. *Family Relations, 43,* 400–408.

Parker, J. G., Rubin, K. H., Price, J. M., & DeRosier, M. (1995). Peer relationships, child development, and adjustment: A developmental psychopathology perspective. In D. Cicchetti & D. J. Cohen (Eds.), *Developmental psychopathology, Vol 2. Risk, disorder, and adaptation* (pp. 96–161). New York: Wiley.

Rosenbaum, M., & Leibel, R. L. (1998). The physiology of body weight regulation: relevance to the etiology of obesity in children. *Pediatrics, 101,* 525–539.

Troiano, R. P., Flegal, K. M., Kuczmarski, R. J., Campbell, S. M., & Johnson, C. L. (1995). Overweight prevalence and trends for children and adolescents: The National Health and Nutrition Examination Surveys, 1963 to 1991. *Archives of Pediatric Adolescent Medicine, 149,* 1085–1091.

Wagner, W. (1996). Optimal development in adolescence: What is it and how can it be encouraged? *The Counseling Psychologist, 24*(3), 360–399.

Williams, J. O., Achterberg, C., & Sylvester, G. P. (1995). Targeting marketing of food products to ethnic minority youths. In C. L. Willams & S. Y. Kim (Eds.), Prevention and treatment of childhood obesity. *Annals of the New York Academy of Sciences, 699,* 107–114.

Yarcheski, A., Mahon, N., & Yarcheski, T. (1997). Alternate models of positive health practices in adolescents. *Nursing Research, 46*(3), 85–92.

Yarcheski, A., Mahon, N., & Yarcheski, T. (1998). A study of introspectiveness in adolescents and young adults. *Western Journal of Nursing Research, 20*(3), 312–324.

APPENDIX **A**

Normal Vital Signs and Growth Parameters

NORMAL TEMPERATURES IN CHILDREN

Age	Temperature (in degrees)	
	Fahrenheit	Celsius
3 mo	99.4	37.5
6 mo	99.5	37.5
1 yr	99.7	37.7
3 yr	99.0	37.2
5 yr	98.6	37.0
7 yr	98.3	36.8
9 yr	98.1	36.7
11 yr	98.0	36.7
13 yr	97.8	36.6
	$F = (C \times 9/5) + 32$	
	$C = (F - 32) \times 5/9$	

NORMAL HEART RATES IN CHILDREN

Age	Awake at rest (bpm)	Asleep (bpm)	Exercise/Fever (bpm)
Newborn	100–180	80–160	up to 220
1 wk to 3 mo	100–220	80–200	up to 220
3 mo to 2 yr	80–150	70–120	up to 200
2 to 10 yr	70–110	60–90	up to 200
10 yr to adult	55–90	50–90	up to 200

bpm, beats per minute.

Adapted from Potts, N. L., & Mandleco, B. L. (2002). *Pediatric nursing: Caring for children and their families*. Clifton Park, NY: Delmar Learning.

GRADING OF PULSES

Grade	Description
0	Not palpable
+1	Difficult to palpate; thready; weak; can be easily obliterated with pressure
+2	Difficult to palpate; may be obliterated with pressure
+3	Easy to palpate; not easily obliterated
+4	Strong; bounding; not obliterated with pressure

NORMAL RESPIRATORY RATES FOR CHILDREN

Age	Rate (breaths per minute)
Newborn	35
1–11 mo	30
2 yr	25
4 yr	23
6 yr	21
8 yr	20
10–12 yr	19
14 yr	18
16 yr	17
18 yr	16–18

Adapted from Potts, N. L., & Mandleco, B. L. (2002). *Pediatric nursing: Caring for children and their families*. Clifton Park, NY: Delmar Learning.

ASSESSMENT OF NORMAL BREATH SOUNDS

Classification	Description
Vesicular	Heard over entire lung surface, except upper intrascapular area and below manubrium
Bronchovesicular	Heard over manubrium and in upper intrascapular areas where trachea and bronchi bifurcate; inspirations are louder and higher in pitch than in vesicular breathing
Bronchial	Heard only near suprasternal notch over trachea; inspiratory phase is short and expiratory phase is long

NORMAL BLOOD PRESSURE RATES IN CHILDREN
(BASED ON 50TH PERCENTILE)

Note: Blood pressure is frequently not monitored in children unless their condition warrants it.

	Females		Males	
Age	Systolic	Diastolic	Systolic	Diastolic
1 day	65	55	73	55
3 days	72	55	74	55
7 days	78	54	76	54
1 mo	84	52	86	52
2 mo	87	51	91	50
3 mo	90	51	91	50
4 mo	90	52	91	50
5 mo	91	52	91	52
6 mo	91	53	90	53
7 mo	91	53	90	54
8 mo	91	53	90	55
9 mo	91	54	90	55
10 mo	91	54	90	56
11 mo	91	54	90	56
1 yr	91	54	90	56
2 yr	90	56	91	56
3 yr	91	56	92	55
4 yr	92	56	93	56
5 yr	94	56	95	56
6 yr	96	57	96	57
7 yr	97	58	97	58
8 yr	99	59	99	60
9 yr	100	61	101	61
10 yr	102	62	102	62
11 yr	105	64	105	63
12 yr	107	66	107	64
13 yr	109	64	109	63
14 yr	110	67	112	64
15 yr	111	67	114	65
16 yr	112	67	117	67
17 yr	112	66	119	69
18 yr	112	66	121	70

Adapted from Potts, N. L., & Mandleco, B. L. (2002). *Pediatric nursing: Caring for children and their families.* Clifton Park, NY: Delmar Learning.

NORMAL GROWTH PARAMETERS RELATED TO WEIGHT, HEIGHT, AND HEAD CIRCUMFERENCE

Age	Weight	Height	Head Circumference
1–6 mo	Gains 5–8 oz per wk	Grows 1 inch per mo	
7–12 mo	Gains 4–5 oz per wk	Grows ½ inch per mo	
12–18 mo	Gains 2–6 lb in next 6 mo	Grows to 33 inches by 18 mo	Head circumference equals chest circumference at 12 mo
	Average weight is 20–24 lb		
	Birth weight is tripled by 12 mo		
18 mo–3 yr	Average weight is 28–30 lb	Grows to 33–37 inches	
	Birth weight is quadrupled by 2 yr	Approximately 50% of adult height by 2 yr	
3–6 yr	Average weight is 44 lb	Grows to 44 inches	
		Birth length doubles by 4 yr	
		Height and weight are even at 5 yr	
7–11 yr	Gains 5–7 lb per year	Growth appears in spurts	
		Increases 3 inches per year to 52 inches at 7–10 yr	

Physical Growth Charts

Birth to 36 months: Girls
Length-for-age and Weight-for-age percentiles

NAME _____

RECORD # _____

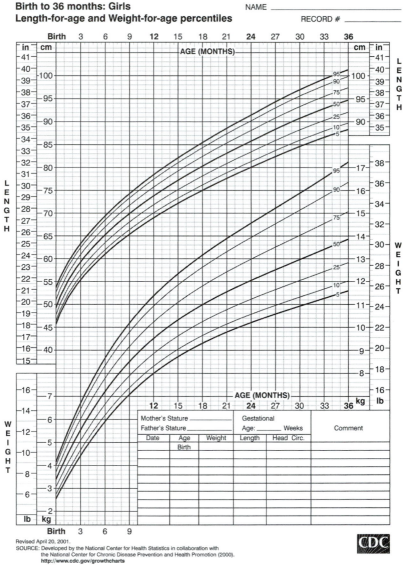

Revised April 20, 2001.
SOURCE: Developed by the National Center for Health Statistics in collaboration with
the National Center for Chronic Disease Prevention and Health Promotion (2000).
http://www.cdc.gov/growthcharts

CDC

A. Girls: Birth to 36 Months (Length and Weight)

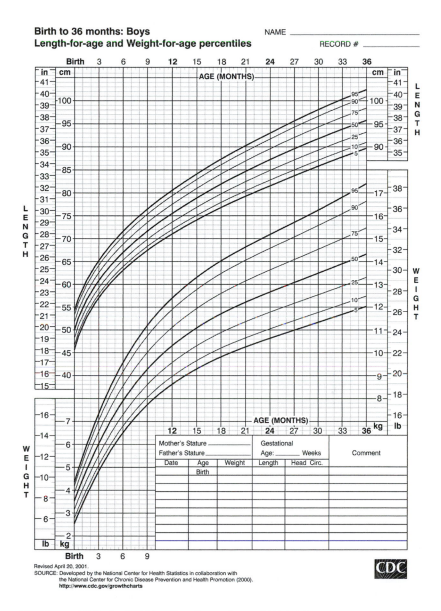

Birth to 36 months: Boys
Length-for-age and Weight-for-age percentiles

NAME _____

RECORD # _____

Revised April 20, 2001.
SOURCE: Developed by the National Center for Health Statistics in collaboration with
the National Center for Chronic Disease Prevention and Health Promotion (2000).
http://www.cdc.gov/growthcharts

CDC

B. Boys: Birth to 36 Months (Length and Weight)

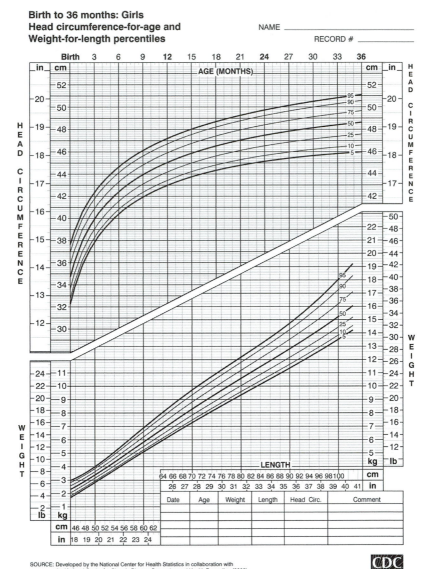

**Birth to 36 months: Girls
Head circumference-for-age and
Weight-for-length percentiles**

NAME _____

RECORD # _____

C. Girls: Birth to 36 Months (Head Circumference)

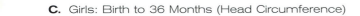

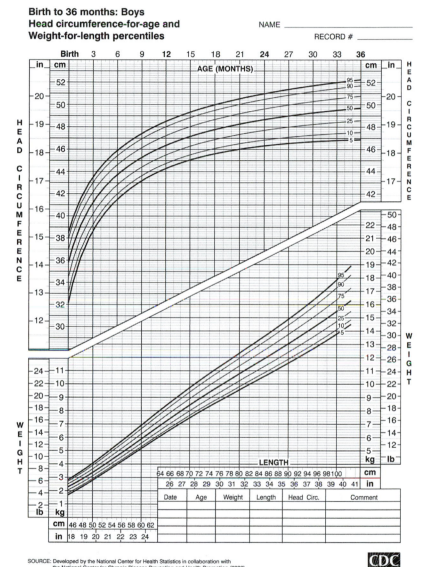

Birth to 36 months: Boys
Head circumference-for-age and
Weight-for-length percentiles

NAME _____

RECORD # _____

SOURCE: Developed by the National Center for Health Statistics in collaboration with
the National Center for Chronic Disease Prevention and Health Promotion (2000).
http://www.cdc.gov/growthcharts

D. Boys: Birth to 36 Months (Head Circumference)

2 to 20 years: Girls
Stature-for-age and Weight-for-age percentiles

NAME _____

RECORD # _____

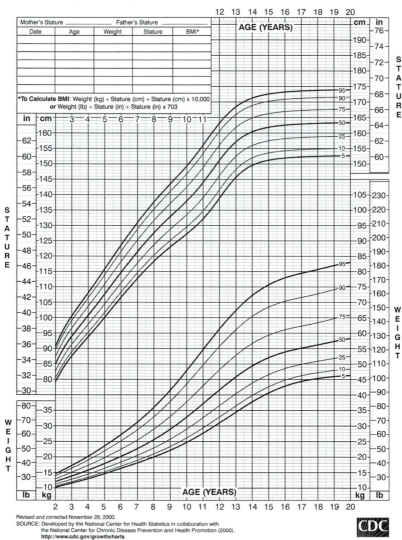

Revised and corrected November 28, 2000.
SOURCE: Developed by the National Center for Health Statistics in collaboration with
the National Center for Chronic Disease Prevention and Health Promotion (2000).
http://www.cdc.gov/growthcharts

E. Girls: 2-20 Years (Stature and Weight)

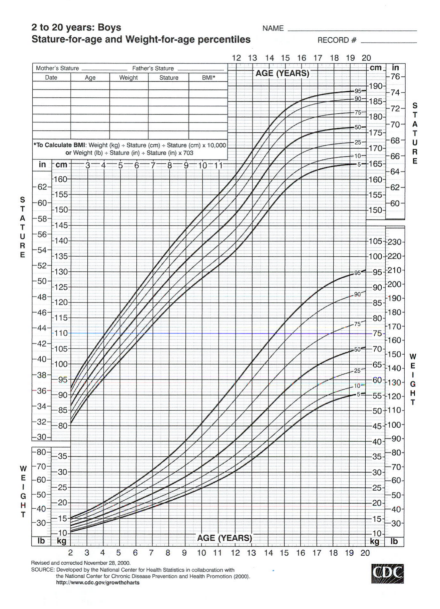

2 to 20 years: Boys
Stature-for-age and Weight-for-age percentiles

NAME _____

RECORD # _____

F. Boys: 2-20 Years (Stature and Weight)

Common Laboratory Tests and Normal Values

Acetaminophen (serum or plasma)
Therapeutic concentration
                     10–30 µg/ml
Toxic concentration   >200 µg/ml

Albumin (plasma)
Newborn   2.5–3.4 g/dl
< 5 yr   3.4–5.0 g/dl
5–19 yr   4.0–5.6 g/dl

Alkaline phosphatase (ALP) (serum)
infant   150–400 U/L
2–10 yr   100–300 U/L
11–18 yr male   50–375 U/L
11–18 yr female   30–300 U/L

Ammonia nitrogen (serum or plasma)
Newborn   90–150 mg/dl
Child   40–80 mg/dl

Amylase (serum)
1–19 yr   35–127 U/L

Antistreptolysin O titer (ASO titer)
(serum)
2–4 yr   <166 Todd units
School-aged   170–330 Todd units

Bicarbonate (HCO$_3$) (serum)
Infant (venous)   20–24 mEq/L
>2 years (venous) 22–29 mEq/L
>2 years (arterial) 21–28 mEq/L

Bilirubin (total) (serum)
Premature Infant
  Cord blood   <2 mg/dl
  0–1 day   <8 mg/dl
  1–2 days   <12 mg/dl
  2–5 days   <16 mg/dl
  >5 days   <20 mg/dl

Full-term Infant
  Cord   <2.8 mg/dl
  0–1day   <2–6 mg/dl
  1–2 days   <6–8 mg/dl
  2–5 days   <4–6 mg/dl
  >5 days   <10 mg/dl

Bilirubin (conjugated) (serum)
0.0–0.2 mEq/L

Blood volume (whole blood)
Female   50–75 ml/Kg
Male   52–83 ml/Kg

C-reactive protein (CRP) (serum)
2–12 yr   67–1800 ng/ml

Calcium (Ca)—Total (serum)
Newborn   9.0–10.6 mg/dl
Child   8.8–10.8 mg/dl

Carbon dioxide

  Partial pressure (PCO$_2$)
  (whole blood, arterial)

  Newborn   27–40 mm Hg
  Infant   27–41 mm Hg

  Thereafter:
  Male   35–48 mm Hg
  Female   32–45 mm Hg

  Total (tCO$_2$) (serum or plasma)

  Newborn   13–22 mmol/L
  Infant   20–28 mmol/L
  Child   20–28 mmol/L
  Thereafter   23–30 mmol/L

Chloride (Cl) (serum)
Newborn   97–110 mmol/L
Thereafter   98–106 mmol/L

Chloride (sweat)

Normal	<40 mmol/L
Borderline	45–60 mmol/L
Cystic Fibrosis	>60 mmol/L

Cholesterol (total)

Newborn	53–135 mg/dl
Infant	70–175 mg/dl
Child	120–200 mg/dl
Adolescent	<200 mg/dl

Creatine kinase (CK, CPK) (serum)

Newborn	87–725 U/L

Creatine (serum)

Newborn	0.3–1.0 mg/dl
Infant	0.2–0.4 mg/dl
Child	0.3–0.7 mg/dl
Adolescent	0.5–1.0 mg/dl

Digoxin (serum or plasma)
Therapeutic concentration
  Congestive heart failure (CHF)

	0.8–1.5 ng/ml
Arrhythmias	1.5–2.0 ng/ml
Toxic concentration	>2.5 ng/mt

Erythrocyte (RBC) count (whole blood)

Newborn	4.8–7.1 million/mm^3
3–6 mo	3.1–4.5 million/mm^3
0.5–2 yr	3.7–5.3 million/mm^3
2–6 yr	3.9–5.3 million/mm^3
6–12 yr	4.0–5.2 million/mm^3
12–18 yr: Male	4.5–5.3 million/mm^3
Female	4.1–5.1 million/mm^3

Erythrocyte sedimentation rate (ESR)
(whole blood)
Westergren (modified)

Child	0–10 mm/hr
Wintrobe	
Child	0–13 mm/hr

Fibroginogen (plasma)

Newborn	125–300 mg/dl
Thereafter	200–400 mg/dl

Glucose (serum)

Newborn	50–90 mg/dl
Child	60–100 mg/dl
Thereafter	70–105 mg/dl

Growth hormone (hGH, somatotropin)
(plasma, fasting)

Newborn	5–40 ng/ml
Child	0–10 ng/ml

Hematocrit (HCT, Hct) (whole blood)

Newborn	44–72%
2 mo	28–42%
6–12 yr	35–45%
12–18 yr: Male	37–49%
Female	36–46%

Hemoglobin (Hb) (whole blood)

Newborn	14–27 g/dl
2 mo	9–14 g/dl
6–12 yr	11.5–15.5 g/dl
12–18 yr: Male	13–16 g/dl
Female	12–16 g/dl

Iron (serum)

Newborn	100–250 µg/dl
Infant	40–100 µg/dl
Child	50–120 µg/dl
Thereafter: Male	50–160 µg/dl
Female	40–150 µg/dl

Lead (whole blood)

Child	<10 µg/dl

Leukocyte (WBC) Count (whole blood)

Newborn	9–30 × 1000 cells/mm^3
1–3 yr	6.0–17.5 × 1000 cells/mm^3
4–7 yr	5.5–15.5 × 1000 cells/mm^3
8–13 yr	4.5–13.5 × 1000 cells/mm^3
Adult	4.5–11.0 × 1000 cells/mm^3

Leukocyte differential count
(whole blood)

Myelocytes	0%
Neutrophils—"bands"	3–5%
Neutrophils—"segs"	54–62%
Lymphocytes	25–33%
Monocytes	3–7%
Eosinophils	1–3%
Basophils	0–0.75%

Osmolality (serum)

Child, adult	275–295 mOsmol/kg H_2O

Oxygen, partial pressure (PO$_2$)
(whole blood, arterial)

Birth	8–24 mm Hg
1 d	54–95 mm Hg
Thereafter (decreased with age)	83–108 mm Hg

Oxygen saturation (SaO$_2$) (whole blood, arterial)

Newborn	85–90%
Thereafter	95–99%

Partial thromboplastin time (PTT)
(whole blood) (Na citrate)

Nonactivated	60–85 seconds (Platelin)
Activated	25–35 seconds (differs with methods)

Phenylalanine (serum)

Premature	2.0–7.5 mg/dl
Newborn	1.2–3.4 mg/dl
Thereafter	0.8–1.8 mg/dl

Plasma volume (plasma)

Male	25–43 ml/kg
Female	28–45 ml/kg

Platelet count
(thrombocyte count) (whole blood)

Newborn (After 1 wk. same as adult)	$84–478 \times 10^3$ mm^3 (µl)
Adult	$150–400 \times 10^3$ mm^3 (µl)

Potassium (serum)

<2 yr	3.0–6.0 mmol/L
2–12 yr	3.5–7.0 mmol/L
>12 yr	3.5–5.0 mmol/L

Protein (serum, total)

Premature	4.3–7.5 g/dl
Newborn	4.6–7.4 g/dl
1–7 yr	6.1–7.9 g/dl
8–12 yr	6.4–8.1 g/dl
13–19 yr	6.6–8.2 g/dl

Prothrombin time (PT)
One-stage (Quick) (whole blood)

In general	11–15 seconds (varies with type of thromboplastin)
Newborn	Prolonged by 2–3 sec

Sodium (serum or plasma)

Newborn	136–146 mmol/L
Infant	139–146 mmol/L
Child	138–145 mmol/L
Thereafter	136–146 mmol/L

Specific gravity (urine)

Newborn	1.016–1.030
Infants	1.002–1.006
Thereafter	1.016–1.030

Thyroxine (T$_4$, T$_4$ total, T$_4$ RIA) (serum)

Newborn	9–18 µg/dl
Infant	7–15 µg/dl
1–5 yr	7.3–15 µg/dl
5–10 yr	6.4–13.3 µg/dl
Thereafter	5–12 µg/dl

Thyrotropin (thyroid stimulating hormone [TSH])

Newborn	3–18 µIU/L by day 3 of life
Thereafter	2–10 mU/L

Triglycerides (TG) (serum)
(after ≥12 hr fast)

	M	F
0–5 yr	30–86 mg/dl	32–99 mg/dl
6–11 yr	31–108 mg/dl	35–114 mg/dl
12–15 yr	36–138 mg/dl	41–138 mg/dl
16–19 yr	40–163 mg/dl	40–128 mg/dl

Triiodothyronine (T$_3$, T$_3$ total, T$_3$ RIA)
(serum)

Newborn	72–260 ng/dl
1–5 yr	100–260 ng/dl
5–10 yr	90–240 ng/dl
10–15 yr	80–210 ng/dl
Thereafter	115–190 ng/dl

Urea nitrogen (serum or plasma)

Newborn	3–12 mg/dl
Infant/child	5–18 mg/dl
Thereafter	7–18 mg/dl

Urine volume (urine, 24 hr)

Newborn		50–300 ml/d
Infant		350–550 ml/d
Child		500–1000 ml/d
Adolescent		700–1400 ml/d
Thereafter:	Male	800–1800 ml/d
	Female	600–1600 ml/d
		(varies with intake and other factors)

Note: Normal lab values differ depending on lab used. Verify your facility's normal values.

Modified from *Delmar's Guide to Laboratory and Diagnostic Tests* by R. Daniels. (2001). Clifton Park, NY: Delmar; *Nelson's Textbook of Pediatrics* (17th ed.), by R. Behrman, R. Kliegman, and H. Jenson. (2000). Philadelphia, PA: W. B. Saunders; *A Manual of Laboratory and Diagnostic Tests* (6th ed.) by F. Fischbach. (1999). Philadelphia, PA: Lippincott.

Denver II

DIRECTIONS FOR ADMINISTRATION

1. Try to get child to smile by smiling, talking or waving. Do not touch him/her.
2. Child must stare at hand several seconds.
3. Parent may help guide toothbrush and put toothpaste on brush.
4. Child does not have to be able to tie shoes or button/zip in the back.
5. Move yarn slowly in an arc from one side to the other, about 8" above child's face.
6. Pass if child grasps rattle when it is touched to the backs or tips of fingers.
7. Pass if child tries to see where yarn went. Yarn should be dropped quickly from sight from tester's hand without arm movement.
8. Child must transfer cube from hand to hand without help of body, mouth, or table.
9. Pass if child picks up raisin with any part of thumb and finger.
10. Line can vary only 30 degrees or less from tester's line.
11. Make a fist with thumb pointing upward and wiggle only the thumb. Pass if child imitates and does not move any fingers other than the thumb.

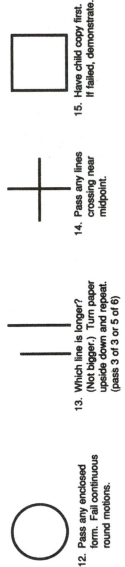

12. Pass any enclosed form. Fail continuous round motions.

13. Which line is longer? (Not bigger.) Turn paper upside down and repeat. (pass 3 of 3 or 5 of 6)

14. Pass any lines crossing near midpoint.

15. Have child copy first. If failed, demonstrate.

When giving items 12, 14, and 15, do not name the forms. Do not demonstrate 12 and 14.

16. When scoring, each pair (2 arms, 2 legs, etc.) counts as one part.
17. Place one cube in cup and shake gently near child's ear, but out of sight. Repeat for other ear.

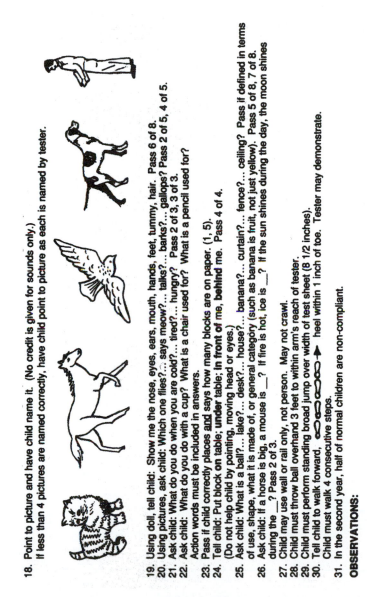

18. Point to picture and have child name it. (No credit is given for sounds only.)
    If less than 4 pictures are named correctly, have child point to picture as each is named by tester.

19. Using doll, tell child: Show me the nose, eyes, ears, mouth, hands, feet, tummy, hair.   Pass 6 of 8.
20. Using pictures, ask child: Which one flies?... says meow?... talks?... barks?... gallops? Pass 2 of 5, 4 of 5.
21. Ask child: What do you do when you are cold?... tired?... hungry?   Pass 2 of 3, 3 of 3.
22. Ask child: What do you do with a cup? What is a chair used for? What is a pencil used for?
    Action words must be included in answers.
23. Pass if child correctly places and says how many blocks are on paper. (1, 5).
24. Tell child: Put block on table, under table; in front of me, behind me.   Pass 4 of 4.
    (Do not help child by pointing, moving head or eyes.)
25. Ask child: What is a ball?... lake?... desk?... house?... banana?... curtain?... fence?... ceiling?   Pass if defined in terms
    of use, shape, what it is made of, or general category (such as banana is fruit, not just yellow).   Pass 5 of 8, 7 of 8.
26. Ask child: If a horse is big, a mouse is ___? If fire is hot, ice is ___? If the sun shines during the day, the moon shines
    during the ___? Pass 2 of 3.
27. Child may use wall or rail only, not person.   May not crawl.
28. Child must throw ball overhand 3 feet to within arm's reach of tester.
29. Child must perform standing broad jump over width of test sheet (8 1/2 inches).
30. Tell child to walk forward, ⌒⌒⌒⌒➤ heel within 1 inch of toe. Tester may demonstrate.
    Child must walk 4 consecutive steps.
31. In the second year, half of normal children are non-compliant.

OBSERVATIONS:

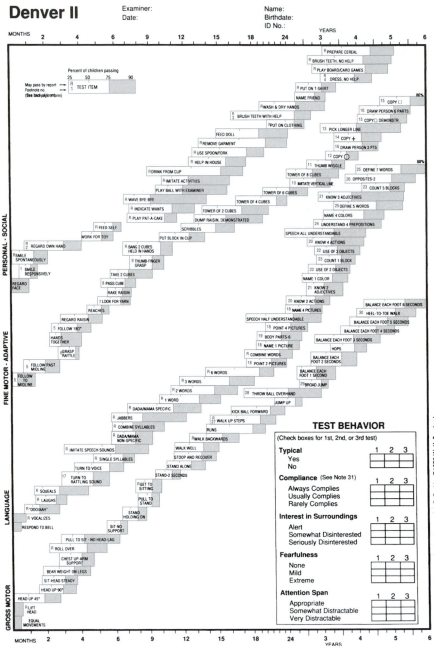

Reprinted with permission of Denver Developmental Materials, Denver, CO.

APPENDIX E

The Friedman Family Assessment Model (Short Form)

Before using the following guidelines in completing family assessments, two words of caution: First, not all areas included will be germane for every family. The guidelines are comprehensive and allow depth when probing is necessary. The student should not feel that every subarea needs be covered when the broad area of inquiry poses no problems to the family or concern to the health care professional. Second, by virtue of the interdependence of the family system, one will find unavoidable redundancy. For the sake of efficiency, the assessor should try not to repeat data, but to refer the reader back to sections where this information has already been described.

Identifying Data

1. Family Name
2. Address and Phone
3. Family Composition
   See Table A-1.
4. Type of Family Form
5. Cultural (Ethnic) Background
6. Religious Identification
7. Social Class Status
8. Family's Recreational or Leisure Time Activities

Developmental Stage and History of Family

9. Family's Present Developmental Stage
10. Extent of Family Developmental Tasks Fulfillment
11. Nuclear Family History
12. History of Family of Origin of Both Parents

Environmental Data

13. Characteristics of Home
14. Characteristics of Neighborhood and Larger Community
15. Family's Geographic Mobility
16. Family's Associations and Transactions with Community
17. Family's Social Support System or Network
    Ecomap
    Family genogram

Family Structure

18. Communication Patterns
    Extent of Functional and Dysfunctional Communication (types of recurring patterns)
    Extent of Emotional (Affective) Messages and How Expressed
    Characteristics of Communication Within Family Subsystems

(continues)

TABLE A-1 FAMILY COMPOSITION FORM

Name (Last, First)	Gender	Relationship	Date/Place of Birth	Occupation	Education
1. (Father)					
2. (Mother)					
3. (Oldest child)					
4.					
5.					
6.					
7.					
8.					

Extent of Congruent and Incongruent Messages

Types of Dysfunctional Communication

Processes Seen in Family

Areas of Open and Closed Communication

Familial and Contextual Variables Affecting Communication

19. Power Structure
Power Outcomes

Decision-Making Process

Power Bases

Variables Affecting Family Power

Overall Family System and Subsystem Power (family power continuum placement)

20. Role Structure
Formal Role Structure

Informal Role Structure

Analysis of Role Models (optional)

Variables Affecting Role Structure

21. Family Values
Compare the family with American or family's reference group values and/or identify important family values and their importance (priority) in family.

Congruence between the Family's Values and Values of the Family's Reference Group or Wider Community

Congruence Between the Family's Values and Family Members' Values

Variables Influencing Family Values

Values Consciously or Unconsciously Held

Presence of Value Conflicts in Family

Effect of the Above Values and Value Conflicts on Health Status of Family

Family Functions

22. Affective Function
Family Need–Response Patterns

Mutual Nurturance, Closeness, and Identification
Family attachment diagram

Separateness and Connectedness

(continues)

23. **Socialization Function**
    Family Child-Rearing Practices

    Adaptability of Child-Rearing Practices for Family Form and Family's Situation

    Who Is (Are) Socializing Agent(s) for Child(ren)?

    Value of Children in Family

    Cultural Beliefs That Influence Family's Child-Rearing Patterns

    Social Class Influence on Child-Rearing Patterns

    Estimation about Whether Family Is at Risk for Child-Rearing Problems and If So, Indication of High-Risk Factors

    Adequacy of Home Environment for Children's Needs to Play

24. **Health Care Function**
    Family's Health Beliefs, Values, and Behaviors

    Family's Definitions of Health–Illness and Their Level of Knowledge

    Family's Perceived Health Status and Illness Susceptibility

    Family's Dietary Practices

    Adequacy of family diet (recommended three-day food history record)

    Function of mealtimes and attitudes toward food and mealtimes

    Shopping (and its planning) practices

    Person(s) responsible for planning, shopping, and preparation of meals

    Sleep and Rest Habits

    Physical Activity and Recreation Practices (not covered earlier)

    Family's Drug Habits

    Family's Role in Self-Care Practices

    Medically Based Preventive Measures (physicals, eye and hearing tests, and immunizations)

    Dental Health Practices

    Family Health History (both general and specific diseases— environmentally and genetically related)

    Health Care Services Received

    Feelings and Perceptions Regarding Health Services

    Emergency Health Services

    Source of Payments for Health and Other Services

    Logistics of Receiving Care

Family Stress and Coping

25. **Short- and Long-Term Familial Stressors and Strengths**

26. **Extent of Family's Ability to Respond, Based on Objective Appraisal of Stress-Producing Situations**

27. **Coping Strategies Utilized (present/past)**
    Differences in Family Members' Ways of Coping

    Family's Inner Coping Strategies

    Family's External Coping Strategies

28. **Dysfunctional Adaptive Strategies Utilized (present/past; extent of usage)**

Courtesy of Friedman, Bowden, & Jones. *Family nursing: Research, theory, & practice* (5th ed.). Upper Saddle River, NJ: Pearson Education, Inc.

Recommended Childhood Immunization Schedule

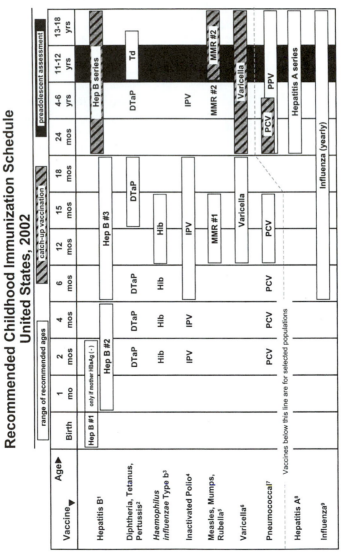

**Recommended Childhood Immunization Schedule
United States, 2002**

Vaccine ▼	Age ▶	Birth	1 mo	2 mos	4 mos	6 mos	12 mos	15 mos	18 mos	24 mos	4-6 yrs	11-12 yrs	13-18 yrs
Hepatitis B[1]		Hep B #1	only if mother HBsAg (-)									Hep B series	
				Hep B #2		Hep B #3							
Diphtheria, Tetanus, Pertussis[2]				DTaP	DTaP	DTaP		DTaP			DTaP	Td	
Haemophilus influenzae Type b[3]				Hib	Hib	Hib	Hib						
Inactivated Polio[4]				IPV	IPV		IPV				IPV		
Measles, Mumps, Rubella[5]							MMR #1				MMR #2		MMR #2
Varicella[6]							Varicella				Varicella		
Pneumococcal[7]				PCV	PCV	PCV	PCV			PCV		PPV	
Hepatitis A[8]											Hepatitis A series		
Influenza[9]									Influenza (yearly)				

range of recommended ages

catch-up vaccination

preadolescent assessment

Vaccines below this line are for selected populations

This schedule indicates the recommended ages for routine administration of currently licensed childhood vaccines, as of December 1, 2001, for children through age 18 years. Any dose not given at the recommended age should be given at any subsequent visit when indicated and feasible. ▨ Indicates age groups that warrant special effort to administer those vaccines not previously given. Additional vaccines may be licensed and recommended during the year. Licensed combination vaccines may be used whenever any components of the combination are indicated and the vaccine's other components are not contraindicated. Providers should consult the manufacturers' package inserts for detailed recommendations.

1. Hepatitis B vaccine (Hep B). All infants should receive the first dose of hepatitis B vaccine soon after birth and before hospital discharge; the first dose may also be given by age 2 months if the infant's mother is HBsAg-negative. Only monovalent hepatitis B vaccine can be used for the birth dose. Monovalent or combination vaccine containing Hep B may be used to complete the series; four doses of vaccine may be administered if combination vaccine is used. The second dose of vaccine should be given at least 4 weeks after the first dose, except for Hib-containing vaccine which cannot be administered before age 6 weeks. The third dose should be given at least 16 weeks after the first dose and at least 8 weeks after the second dose. The last dose in the vaccination series (third or fourth dose) should not be administered before age 6 months.

Infants born to HBsAg-positive mothers should receive hepatitis B vaccine and 0.5 mL hepatitis B immune globulin (HBIG) within 12 hours of birth at separate sites. The second dose is recommended at age 1-2 months and the vaccination series should be completed (third or fourth dose) at age 6 months.

Infants born to mothers whose HBsAg status is unknown should receive the first dose of the hepatitis B vaccine series within 12 hours of birth. Maternal blood should be drawn at the time of delivery to determine the mother's HBsAg status; if the HBsAg test is positive, the infant should receive HBIG as soon as possible (no later than age 1 week).

2. Diphtheria and tetanus toxoids and acellular pertussis vaccine (DTaP). The fourth dose of DTaP may be administered as early as age 12 months, provided 6 months have elapsed since the third dose and the child is unlikely to return at age 15-18 months. **Tetanus and diphtheria toxoids (Td)** is recommended at age 11-12 years if at least 5 years have elapsed since the last dose of tetanus and diphtheria toxoid-containing vaccine. Subsequent routine Td boosters are recommended every 10 years.

3. Haemophilus influenzae type b (Hib) conjugate vaccine. Three Hib conjugate vaccines are licensed for infant use. If PRP-OMP (PedvaxHIB® or ComVax® [Merck]) is administered at ages 2 and 4 months, a dose at age 6 months is not required. DTaP/Hib combination products should not be used for primary immunization in infants at age 2, 4 or 6 months, but can be used as boosters following any Hib vaccine.

4. Inactivated poliovirus vaccine (IPV). An all-IPV schedule is recommended for routine childhood poliovirus vaccination in the United States. All children should receive four doses of IPV at age 2 months, 4 months, 6-18 months, and 4-6 years.

5. Measles, mumps, and rubella vaccine (MMR). The second dose of MMR is recommended routinely at age 4-6 years but may be administered during any visit, provided at least 4 weeks have elapsed since the first dose and that both doses are administered beginning at or after age 12 months. Those who have not previously received the second dose should complete the schedule by the visit at 11-12 years.

6. Varicella vaccine. Varicella vaccine is recommended at any visit at or after age 12 months for susceptible children (i.e. those who lack a reliable history of chickenpox). Susceptible persons aged ≥13 years should receive two doses, given at least 4 weeks apart.

7. Pneumococcal vaccine. The heptavalent **pneumococcal conjugate vaccine (PCV)** is recommended for all children aged 2-23 months and for certain children aged 24-59 months. **Pneumococcal polysaccharide vaccine (PPV)** is recommended in addition to PCV for certain high-risk groups. See *MMWR* 2000;49(RR-9);1-37.

8. Hepatitis A vaccine. Hepatitis A vaccine is recommended for use in selected states and regions, and for certain high-risk groups; consult your local public health authority. See *MMWR* 1999;48(RR-12);1-37.

9. Influenza vaccine. Influenza vaccine is recommended annually for children age ≥ 6 months with certain risk factors (including but not limited to asthma, cardiac disease, sickle cell disease, HIV, and diabetes; see *MMWR* 2001;50(RR-4);1-44), and can be administered to all others wishing to obtain immunity. Children aged ≤12 years should receive vaccine in a dosage appropriate for their age (0.25 mL if age 6-35 months or 0.5 mL if aged ≥ 3 years). Children aged ≤ 8 years who are receiving influenza vaccine for the first time should receive two doses separated by at least 4 weeks.

For additional information about vaccines, vaccine supply, and contraindications for immunization, please visit the National Immunization Program Website at www.cdc.gov/nip or call the National Immunization Hotline at 800-232-2522 (English) or 800-232-0233 (Spanish).

Approved by the Advisory Committee on Immunization Practices (www.cdc.gov/nip/acip), the American Academy of Pediatrics (www.aap.org), and the American Academy of Family Physicians (www.aafp.org).

Recommended Dietary Allowances

RECOMMENDED DIETARY ALLOWANCES[a]

Category	Age (Yr) or Condition	Weight (kg)	Weight (lb)	Height (cm)	Height (in)	Kcal per Day	Protein (g)	Fat-Soluble Vitamins Vitamin A (µg RE)[c]	Vitamin D (µg)[d]	Vitamin E (mg α-TE)[e]	Vitamin K (µc)
Infants	0.0–0.5	6	13	60	24	650	13	375	7.5	3	5
	0.5–1.0	9	20	71	28	850	14	375	10	4	10
Children	1–3	13	29	90	35	1300	16	400	10	6	15
	4–6	20	44	112	44	1800	24	500	10	7	20
	7–10	28	62	132	52	2000	28	700	10	7	30
Men	11–14	45	99	157	62	2500	45	1000	10	10	45
	15–18	66	145	176	69	3000	59	1000	10	10	65
Women	11–14	46	101	157	62	2200	46	800	10	8	45
	15–18	55	120	163	64	2200	44	800	10	8	55

a The allowances, expressed as average daily intakes over time, are intended to provide for individual variations among most normal persons as they live in the United States under usual environmental stresses. Diets should be based on a variety of common foods to provide other nutrients for which human requirements have been less well defined.
b Weights and heights of Reference Adults are actual medians for the U.S. population of the designated age.
c Retinol equivalents. 1 RE = 1 µg retinol or 6 µg β-carotene.
d As cholecalciferol. 10 µg cholecalciferol = 400 U of vitamin D.
e Tocopherol equivalents. 1 mg d-α-tocopherol = 1 α-TE.
f Ne Niacin equivalent = 1 mg of niacin or 60 mg of dietary tryptophan.

RECOMMENDED DIETARY ALLOWANCES [a] *Continued*

	Water-Soluble Vitamins							Minerals						
Vitamin C (mg)	Thiamin (mg)	Riboflavin (mg)	Niacin NE[f]	Vitamin B_6 (mg)	Folate (µg)	Vitamin B_{12} (µg)	Calcium (mg)	Phosphorus (mg)	Magnesium (mg)	Iron (mg)	Zinc (mg)	Iodine (µg)	Selenium mg (µg) 35
30	0.3	0.4	5	0.3	25	0.3	400	300	40	6	5	40	10
35	0.4	0.5	6	0.6	35	0.5	600	500	60	10	5	50	15
40	0.7	0.8	9	1.0	50	0.7	800	800	80	10	10	70	20
45	0.9	1.1	12	1.1	75	1.0	800	800	120	10	10	90	20
45	1.0	1.2	13	1.4	100	1.4	800	800	170	10	10	120	20
50	1.3	1.5	17	1.7	150	2.0	1200	1200	270	12	15	150	40
60	1.5	1.8	20	2.0	200	2.0	1200	1200	400	12	15	150	50
50	1.1	1.3	15	1.4	150	2.0	1200	1200	280	15	12	150	45
60	1.1	1.3	15	1.5	180	2.0	1200	1200	300	15	12	150	50

Sexual Maturity Ratings (SMR)

Developmental Stages

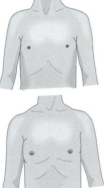

1. **Preadolescent stage**
   (before age 8).
   Nipple is small, slightly
   raised.

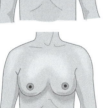

2. **Early adolescent stage.** Breast
   bud development (after age 8).
   Nipple and breast form a
   small mound. Areola enlarges.
   Height spurt begins.

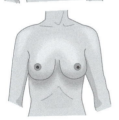
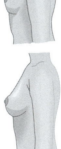

3. **Adolescent stage** (10-14 years).
   Nipple is flush with breast
   shape. Breast and areola
   enlarge. Menses begins.
   Height spurt peaks.

4. **Late adolescent stage**
   (14–17 years).
   Nipple and areola form
   a secondary mound over
   the breast. Height spurt ends.

5. **Adult stage.**
   Nipple protrudes; areola
   is flush with the breast shape.

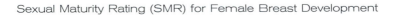

Sexual Maturity Rating (SMR) for Female Breast Development

Stage 1

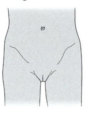

**Preadolescent
Stage**
(before age 8)
No pubic hair,
only body
hair (vellus hair)

Stage 2

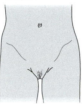

**Early Adolescent
Stage**
(ages 8 to 12)
Sparse growth
of long, slightly
dark, fine pubic
hair, slightly curly
and located along
the labia

Stage 3

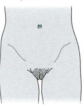

**Adolescent
Stage**
(ages 12 to 13)
Pubic hair
becomes
darker, curlier,
and spreads
over the
symphysis

Stage 4

**Late Adolescent
Stage**
(ages 13 to 15)
Texture and
curl of pubic
hair is similar
to that of an
adult but not
spread to thighs

Stage 5

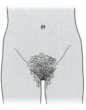

Adult Stage
Adult appearance
in quality and
quantity of pubic
hair; growth is
spread to inner
aspect of thighs
and abdomen

Sexual Maturity Rating (SMR) for Female Genitalia

Developmental Stage	Pubic Hair	Penis	Testes
1.	No pubic hair, only fine body hair (vellus hair)	Preadolescent; childhood size and proportion	Preadolescent; childhood size and proportion
2.	Sparse growth of long, slightly dark, straight hair	Slight or no growth	Growth in testes and scrotum; scrotum reddens and changes texture
3.	Becomes darker and coarser; slightly curled and spreads over symphysis	Growth, especially in length	Further growth
4.	Texture and curl of pubic hair is similar to that of an adult but not spread to thighs	Further growth in length; diameter increases; development of glans	Further growth; scrotum darkens
5.	Adult appearance in quality and quantity of pubic hair; growth is spread to medial surface of thighs	Adult size and shape	Adult size and shape

Sexual Maturity Rating (SMR) for Male Genitalia

APPENDIX I

Resources

Adolescence Directory On-Line (ADOL)
www.education.indiana.edu/cas/adol/adol.html
(An electronic guide to information on adolescent issues)

After School: School Age Resources
School-Age NOTES
PO Box 40205
Nashville, TN 37204-0205
(615) 279-0700
www.afterschoolalliance.com

AMA Archives of Pediatrics and Adolescent Medicine
www.ama-assn.org
(A vehicle for increased attention to adolescent health, the education of pediatric health care professionals, and disease prevention and health promotion.)

American Academy of Pediatrics
141 Northwest Point Blvd.
Elk Grove Village, IL 60007-1098
(847) 434-4000
www.aap.org

American Academy of Child and Adolescent Psychiatry (AACAP)
3615 Wisconsin Ave., NW
Washington, D.C. 20016-3007
(202) 966-7300
www.aacap.org

American Academy of Family Physicians
P.O. Box 11210
Shawnee Mission, KS 66207-1210
(800) 274-2237
www.aafp.org

American Association for Maternal and Child Health, Inc.
P.O. Box 965
Los Altos, CA 94022

American Pediatric Society
3400 Research Forest Drive, Suite B-7
The Woodlands, TX 77381
(281) 419-0052
www.aps-spr.org

American Psychological Association
750 First Street, NE
Washington, DC 20002-4242.
(800) 374-2721
www.apa.org

American Psychologist
www.apa.org/journals/amp.html

American School Health Association
7263 State Route 43
P.O. Box 708
Kent, Ohio 44240
(330) 678-1601
www.ashaweb.org

Association of Women's Health, Obstetric, and Neonatal Nurses (AWHONN)
2000 L Street, NW Suite 740
Washington, D.C. 20036
(800) 673-8499
www.awhonn.org

Bright Futures Project
NCEMCH
2000 15th Street, North, Suite 701
Arlington, VA 22201-2617
Phone: (703) 524-7802
www.brightfutures.org

Center for Disease Control and Prevention
1600 Clifton Rd.
Atlanta, GA 30333
(800) 311-3435
www.cdc.gov

Children's Health Information Network
1561 Clark Drive
Yardley, PA 19067
(215) 493-3068

Consumer Product Safety Commission
4330 East-West Highway
Bethesda, MD 20814-4408
(800) 638-2772
www.cpsc.gov

Denver Developmental Materials, Inc.
P.O. Box 6919
Denver, CO 80206-9019
(800) 419-4729

Developmental Psychology
www.apa.org/journals/dev.html

Healthy People 2010
www.health.gov/healthypeople/

HRSA (Health Resources and Service Administration) Information Center
1-888-Ask HRSA (275-4772)
www.ask.hrsa.gov

I am Your Child
Eastern Office
1325 6th Avenue, 30th Floor
New York, NY 10019
(212) 636-5030
Western Office
P.O. Box 15605
Beverly Hills, CA 90209
(310) 285-2385
www.iamyourchild.org
(The I am Your Child campaign stresses the importance of a child's first years and is sponsored by Rob Reiner's Families and Work Institute.)

Kidlink
www.kidlink.org

Kids Health Organization
www.kidshealth.org

KidSource OnLine
www.kidsource.com
(This is a group of parents who want to make a positive and lasting difference in the lives of parents and children. Their goal is to provide knowledge and advice to help caregivers better raise and educate children.)

La Leche League International
1400 N. Meacham Road
Schaumburg, IL 60173-4808
(800) 525-3243
www.lalecheleague.org/contact.html

Maternal and Child Health Bureau
Parklawn Building Room 18-05
5600 Fishers Lane
Rockville, Maryland 20857
www.mchb.hrsa.gov

Morbidity & Mortality Weekly Report
www.cdc.gov/mmwr/

National Association of Neonatal Nurses
4700 West Lake Avenue
Glenview, IL 60025-1485
(800) 451-3795
www.nann.org

National Association of Pediatric Nurse Associates and Practitioners
20 Brace Road Suite 200
Cherry Hill, NJ 08034-2633
(856) 857-9700
www.napnap.org

National Association of School Nurses
Eastern Office
P.O. Box 1300
Scarborough, ME 04070-1300
Western Office
1416 Park Street, Suite A
Castle Rock, CO 80109
1-866-627-6767 (1-866-NASN-SNS)
www.nasn.org

**National Center for Education
Statistics, U.S. Department of
Education**
1990 K Street, NW
Washington, DC 20006
(202) 502-7300
www.nces.ed.gov

National Center for Health Statistics
Division of Data Services
Hyattsville, MD
20782-2003
(301) 458-4636
www.cdc.gov/nchs

National Council on Family Relations
3989 Central Ave., NE, #550
Minneapolis, MN 55421
(888) 781-9331
www.ncfr.org

**National Highway Traffic Safety
Administration**
National Center for Statistics and Analysis
NRD-30
400 Seventh Street, SW
Washington, D.C. 20590
1-888-DASH-2-DOT (1-888-327-4236)
www.nhtsa.dot.gov/

**National Institute of Child Health and
Human Development**
Bldg 31, Room 2A32, MSC 2425
31 Center Drive
Bethesda, MD 20892-2425
(800) 370-2943
www.nichd.nih.gov

National Institutes of Health
Bethesda, Maryland 20892
www.nih.gov

National Institute of Nursing Research
www.nih.gov/ninr/

National Safe Kids Campaign
www.safekids.org/

National Network for Child Care
www.nncc.org

National Runaway Switchboard
3080 N. Lincoln Ave.
Chicago, IL 60657
(800) 621-4000
www.nrscrisisline.org

**National Sudden Infant Death
Syndrome Resource Center**
2070 Chain Bridge Road, Suite 450
Vienna, VA 22182
(703) 821-8955
www.sidscenter.org

Pediatrics
www.pediatrics.org

**PEDINFO: An Index of the Pediatric
Internet**
www.pedinfo.org

Planned Parenthood Federation of America, Inc.
810 Seventh Ave.
New York, NY 10019
(212) 541-7800
www.plannedparenthood.org

Pub Med National Library of Medicine
www.ncbi.nlm.nih.gov/entrez/query.fcgi

Public Health Service AIDS and STD Information Hotline
CDC NPIN
P.O. Box 6003
Rockville, MD 20849-6003
www.cdcnpin.org
(800) 342-AIDS
(800) 458-5231

SIECUS (Sexuality Information and Education Council of the U.S.)
130 West 42nd Street, Suite 350
New York, NY 10036-7802
(212) 819-9770
www.siecus.org

Society for Research in Child Development
University of Michigan
505 E. Huron, Suite 301
Ann Arbor, MI 48104-1567
(734) 998-6578
www.srcd.org

The Annual Review of Research for Neonatal Nurses
1304 Southpoint Boulevard, Suite 240
Petaluma, CA 94954-6861

The Children's Defense Fund
25 E Street NW
Washington, DC 20001
(202) 628-8787
www.childrensdefense.org

The Children's Foundation
1420 New York Ave., NW, 8th Floor
Washington, DC 20005

The Commonwealth Fund
www.cmwf.org/

The Online Safety Project
www.safekids.com
www.safeteens.com

Tough Love International
P.O. Box 1069
Doylestown, PA 18901
(215) 348-7090
www.toughlove.org/

U.S. Census Bureau
Washington DC 20233
www.census.gov/

U.S. Consumer Product Safety Commission
Eastern
201 Varick Street, Room 903
New York, NY 10014-4811
(212) 620-4120
Central
230 South Dearborn Street, Room 2944
Chicago, IL 60604-8260
(312) 353-8260
Western
1301 Clay Street, Suite 610-N
Oakland, CA 94612-5217
(510) 637-4050
www.cpsc.gov

**U.S. Department of Agriculture
Food, Nutrition & Consumer Services**
www.fns.usda.gov/fncs/

**U.S. Department of Health and
Human Services**
200 Independence Ave SW
Washington, DC 20201
www.hhs.gov

Your Amazing Baby
www.amazingbaby.com
(Information on typical infant and
toddler development.)

YouthInfo
U.S. Department of Health and
Human Services
The Administration for Children
and Families
www.acf.dhhs.gov/programs/fysb/youthinfo/
index.htm

**Youth Risk Behavior Surveillance
System**
www.cdc.gov/nccdphp/dash/yrbs/

**Zero to Three: National Center for
Infants, Toddlers and Families**
2000 M Street, NW, Suite 200
Washington, DC 20036
(202) 638-1144
www.zerotothree.org
(A national nonprofit charitable organization
whose aim is to strengthen and support
families, practitioners, and communities to
promote the health/development of babies
and toddlers and is the nation's leading
resource on the first three years of life.)

INDEX